D0579897

RADIOLOGIC INTERVENTIONS

Noncardiac Thoracic Interventions

RADIOLOGIC INTERVENTIONS

Series Editor: Helen C. Redman, M.D.

Non-Cardiac Interventions

Alan H. Matsumoto, M.D.

Embolotherapy

Douglas M. Coldwell, Ph.D., M.D.

RADIOLOGIC INTERVENTIONS

Noncardiac Thoracic Interventions

Alan H. Matsumoto

Associate Professor of Radiology
Director, Division of Angiography and
Interventional Radiology
Department of Radiology
Charlottesville, Virginia
University of Virginia Health Sciences Center

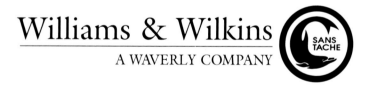

Williams & Wilkins

A WAVERLY COMPANY

BALTIMORE • PHILADELPHIA • LONDON • PARIS • BANGKOK
BUENOS AIRES • HONG KONG • MUNICH • SYDNEY • TOKYO • WROCLAW

Editor: Charles W. Mitchell
Marketing Manager: Lorraine A. Smith
Production Coordinator: Dana M. Soares
Typesetter: Digitype
Printer: Quebecor Printing Book Group

351 West Camden Street
Baltimore, Maryland 21201-2436 USA

Rose Tree Corporate Center
1400 North Providence Road
Building II, Suite 5025
Media, Pennsylvania 19063-2043 USA

Accurate indications, adverse reactions and dosage schedules for drugs are provided in this book, but it is possible that they may change. The reader is urged to review the package information data of the manufacturers of the medications mentioned.

Printed in the United States of America

First Edition,

Library of Congress Cataloging-in-Publication Data
Non-cardiac thoracic interventions / [edited by] Alan H. Matsumoto.
     p.   cm. — (Radiologic interventions)
  Includes bibliographical references and index.
  ISBN 0-683-30338-4
  1. Chest—Interventional radiology.   I. Matsumoto, Alan H.
II. Series.
  [DNLM: 1. Thoracic Arteries—radiography. 2. Vascular Diseases—
therapy. 3. Radiography, Interventional—methods. WG 595. T4 N812
1997]
RD536.N66 1997
617.5′4—DC21
DNLM/DLC
for Library of Congress   96-52547
                                  CIP

ISBN: 0-683-30338-4

The publishers have made every effort to trace the copyright holders for borrowed material. If they have inadvertently overlooked any, they will be pleased to make the necessary arrangements at the first opportunity.

To purchase additional copies of this book, call our customer service department at **(800) 638-0672** or fax orders to **(800) 447-8438.** For other book services, including chapter reprints and large quantity sales, ask for the Special Sales department.

Canadian customers should call **(800) 665-1148,** or fax **(800) 665-0103**. For all other calls originating outside of the United States, please call **(410) 528-4223** or fax us at **(410) 528-8550.**

Visit Williams & Wilkins on the Internet: http://www.wwilkins.com or contact our customer service department at **custserv@wwilkins.com.** Williams & Wilkins customer service representatives are available from 8:30 am to 6:00 pm, EST, Monday through Friday, for telephone access.

97 98 99 00
1 2 3 4 5 6 7 8 9 10

Preface

As our ability to noninvasively image internal anatomic structures grows, the potential for diagnosing and treating thoracic pathology with minimally invasive techniques will continue to expand. Because of the rapid pace of technologic advances, it is difficult for most busy interventional radiologists to "keep up" with the changes that are occurring.

The objective of this work is to provide a focused and practical interventional radiology text-book which clearly reviews the indications, contraindications, anatomic and technical considerations, devices, techniques, potential pitfalls and complications associated with procedures involving the noncardiac portions of the thorax. To this end, the contributing authors have aimed to produce a concise and comprehensive summary of information in a well illustrated manner.

The book is divided into two Sections: Section I–Vascular Interventions, and Section II–Nonvascular Interventions. Topics in Section I include basic vascular anatomy of the thorax, interventions for acute pulmonary emboli, transcatheter embolotherapy for hemoptysis, endovascular therapy for pulmonary arteriovenous malformations, management and insertion of central venous catheters, percutaneous retrieval of foreign bodies, balloon angioplasty and stenting of the brachiocephalic arteries, central venous thrombolysis and stenting, percutaneous therapy for tumors involving the thoracic vertebral bodies, and endovascular methods of managing thoracic aortic dissections and aneurysms. Topics in Section II include a review of the nonvascular thoracic anatomy, biopsies of the lung, mediastinum, pleura, breast, and musculoskeletal system, management of pleural and nonpleural fluid collections, tracheobronchial stenting, and management of esophageal strictures and foreign bodies.

The wide spectrum of topics covered herein should provide the reader with a pragmatic, state-of-the-art reference on minimally invasive, image-guided, noncardiac thoracic interventions. The hope is that this book will provide a review of interventional radiology procedures being performed in the thorax and allow practicing radiologists to refine and expand their expertise in this clinical arena.

DEDICATION

To my wife Julie, and my daughters Mallory Emiko and Monica Mary

Acknowledgments

Throughout my life, my family has provided the stability that has allowed me to pursue my career interests. My parents, George and Amy Matsumoto, have shown me the importance of a good work ethic, dedication, and honesty. This has been the foundation upon which I have based my professional endeavors. My wife Julie, despite feeling like a single parent on many occasions, has always been supportive of me as a professional, husband, and father.

I have also had the good fortune of being mentored by a number of special individuals. Drs. James H. Scatliff and Matthew A. Mauro influenced my career significantly during my residency years; and Dr. Mauro continues to be an invaluable resource to me, both as a friend and an experienced interventional radiologist. Dr. Klemens H. Barth took me under his wing during my fellowship year and provided a nurturing environment for my academic and clinical growth. He also instilled in me a fierce loyalty for, and firm belief in the sub-specialty of Interventional Radiology. In 1991, I came to the University of Virginia to work with the late Dr. Charles J. "Tunk" Tegtmeyer. Although I had not spent any time "training" with Tunk, I soon found that one cannot work with him without learning from him. He taught me the subtleties of patient care and clinical judgement, and the intangibles associated with the development of a successful Interventional Radiology Service. I miss him greatly.

I would also like to thank all of the authors for taking time from their busy schedules to contribute to this book. Lastly, I want to acknowledge Sherry Deane and Tammy Amos for their untiring assistance in preparing this book.

Foreword

Vascular radiology became a reality with the description of the Seldinger technique in 1953. Diagnostic angiography developed rapidly over the next decade accompanied by improved filming capabilities and image intensifiers, smaller, more flexible catheters that could be shaped for selective angiography; improved injectors and the development of numerous types of needles, guide wires and stopcocks. At the same time Professor Eberhardt Zeitler, in Germany and Dr. Charles Dotter were working on ways to dilate atherosclerotic arteries percutaneously. Use of caged balloons was one concept. The Dotter dilation technique that was introduced about 1964 was another. This was probably the first intravascular interventional technique that became widely used clinically. At about the same time transhepatic cholangiography was reintroduced after failure in the 1930s to be performed safely. Biliary drainage was attempted but the short straight catheters used for the diagnostic procedure generally fell out in one or two days. Dr. Stanley Baum described the diagnosis and therapy for gastrointestinal hemorrhage in the late 1960s and from then on there has been an explosion of interventional procedures introduced into clinical usage. The increased sophistication of other imaging modalities, such as ultrasound, computed tomography, and most recently, magnetic resonance imaging, has further increased the interventional possibilities over the past thirty years.

Therefore, the development of a monograph series encompassing the many faces of interventional radiology is most timely. The series encompasses the entire spectrum of procedures ranging from neuroradiological intervention to thoracic interventions to genitourinary procedures. Each monograph is designed to be a complete compendium within its sphere so, although there is some overlap among the volumes, each one can stand independently.

Readers may pick and choose from the series or may wish to obtain the entire series for reference purposes. Interventional radiology is still an expanding subspeciality and these volumes should be of use to anyone in radiology who performs interventional procedures.

The second volume in this series is on noncardiac thoracic interventions. Dr. Alan H. Matsumoto, editor and primary author and his well chosen and excellent coauthors have written a comprehensive monograph on this topic, which is divided into two sections. The first section addresses vascular interventions and the second, nonvascular interventions. Both sections start with comprehensive, well illustrated chapters on the relevant anatomy and its variations. The following chapters in each section deal with specific problems such as the acute transcatheter management of pulmonary arteriovenous malformations, percutaneous lung biopsy, management of esophageal foreign bodies, strictures and leaks and percutaneous angioplasty of the brachiocephalic arteries. The appropriate procedures are thoroughly discussed as is the rationale for their usage.

Dr. Charles Tegtmeyer is an author on three of these chapters. His untimely death in 1996 left a great void in the interventional arena. These chapters on intravascular foreign body retrieval, brachiocephalic artery angioplasty and tracheal and bronchial stenoses must be among his last projects. All of us in interventional radiology have benefited from his talents and inventiveness. This monograph is authored largely by his colleagues at the University of Virginia and its excellence is indicative of his great influence on the field.

Thoracic interventions whether vascular or nonvascular in nature are increasing in variety and numbers. While percutaneous lung biopsy has been performed for at least 30 years, techniques for this procedure have become much more sophisticated. Embolization of pulmonary arteriovenous fistulae has also been performed for many years but the currently available techniques and equipment make these procedures increasingly successful. Even more exciting are the newer procedures such as the aggressive management of intrathoracic fluid collections discussed by Drs. Nakamato and Haaga; tracheal and bronchial dilatation and stenting discussed by Drs. Matsumoto, Angle and Tegtmeyer and the exciting new procedures in the thoracic aorta and superior vena cava described by Drs. Dake, Semba and Kee. These are new arenas for the interventional radiologist and all radiologists should be aware of them and their potential.

Helen C. Redman, M.D.
Fred Bonte Professor of Radiology
Vice Chairman, Academic Affairs
The University of Texas Southwestern Medical School
Dallas, Texas

Contributors

J. Fritz Angle, M.D.
Assistant Professor
Division of Angiography and
    Interventional Radiology
Department of Radiology
University of Virginia Health Sciences
    Center
Charlottesville, Virginia

Kevin Burner, M.D.
Department of Radiology
University Hospitals of Cleveland
Case Western Reserve University School
    of Medicine
Cleveland, Ohio

William E. Campbell, Jr., M.D.
Fellow, Vascular and Interventional
    Radiology
Department of Radiology
The University of North Carolina
    School of Medicine
Chapel Hill, North Carolina

Michael D. Dake, M.D.
Assistant Professor of Radiology and
    Medicine
Chief, Cardiovascular and
    Interventional Radiology
Department of Radiology
Stanford University Medical Center
Stanford, California

Jacques E. Dion, M.D.
Professor
Department of Radiology and
    Neurosurgery
Division of Neuroradiology
University of Virginia Health Sciences
    Center
Charlottesville, Virginia

Melinda M. Dunn, M.D.
Medical College of Virginia
Department of Diagnostic Radiology
Richmond, Virginia

Robert G. Dussault, M.D.
Professor of Radiology and Orthopaedics
Department of Radiology
University of Virginia Health Sciences
    Center
Charlottesville, Virginia

Rolf W. Günther, M.D.
Professor and Chairman
Department of Radiology
University of Technology
Aachen, Germany

John R. Haaga, M.D., F.A.C.R.
Professor and Chairman
Department of Radiology
University Hospitals of Cleveland
Case Western Reserve University School
    of Medicine
Cleveland, Ohio

Phan T. Huynh, M.D.
Fellow
Medical College of Virginia
Department of Diagnostic Radiology
Richmond, Virginia

Paul F. Jaques, M.D.
Professor of Radiology and Surgery
The University of North Carolina
    School of Medicine
Chapel Hill, North Carolina

Mary E. Jensen, M.D.
Assistant Professor
Department of Radiology and
    Neurosurgery
Division of Neuroradiology
University of Virginia Health Sciences
    Center
Charlottesville, Virginia

David F. Kallmes, M.D.
Assistant Professor
Department of Radiology and
    Neurosurgery
Division of Neuroradiology
University of Virginia Health Sciences
    Center
Charlottesville, Virginia

Phoebe A. Kaplan, M.D.
Professor of Radiology and
    Orthopaedics
Department of Radiology
University of Virginia Health Sciences
    Center
Charlottesville, Virginia

Nancy Keaton, M.D.
Department of Radiology
Pitt County Memorial Hospital
East Carolina School of Medicine
Greenville, NC

Stephen T. Kee, M.B., F.R.C.R.
Visiting Assistant Professor
Department of Radiology
Stanford University Medical Center
Stanford, California

Eduard E. de Lange, M.D.
Professor of Radiology
Director, Section of Body Magnetic
    Resonance Imaging
Department of Radiology
University of Virginia Health Sciences
    Center
Charlottesville, Virginia

Peter A. Loud, M.D.
Department of Radiology
University of North Carolina School of
    Medicine
Chapel Hill, North Carolina

Alan H. Matsumoto, M.D.
Associate Professor
Director, Division of Angiography and
    Interventional Radiology
Department of Radiology
University of Virginia Health Sciences
    Center
Charlottesville, Virginia

Matthew A. Mauro, M.D., F.A.C.R.
Vice Chair, Department of Radiology
Professor of Radiology and Surgery
The University of North Carolina
    School of Medicine
Chapel Hill, North Carolina

Paul L. Molina, M.D.
Associate Professor
Department of Radiology
University of North Carolina School of
    Medicine
Department of Radiology
Chapel Hill, North Carolina

Dean A. Nakamoto, M.D.
Assistant Professor
Department of Radiology
University Hospitals of Cleveland
Case Western Reserve University School
    of Medicine
Cleveland, Ohio

Ellen Shaw de Paredes, M.D.
Professor of Radiology
Director of Breast Imaging
Department of Diagnostic Radiology
Medical College of Virginia
Richmond, Virginia

Jeffrey S. Pollak, M.D.
Associate Professor
Chief, Section of Vascular and
    Interventional Radiology
Department of Radiology
Yale University School of Medicine
New Haven, Connecticut

J. Bayne Selby, Jr., M.D.
Radiology Associates
Everett, Washington

Charles P. Semba, M.D.
Assistant Professor of Radiology and
  Medicine
Department of Radiology
Stanford University Medical Center
Stanford, California

Hubert A. Shaffer, Jr., M.D., F.A.C.R.
Professor of Radiology and Internal
  Medicine
Co-Director, Division of
  Thoracoabdominal Imaging
Department of Radiology
University of Virginia Health Sciences
  Center
Charlottesville, Virginia

William N. Snearly, M.D.
Staff, Musculoskeletal Radiology
Wilford Hall USAF Medical Center
San Antonio, Texas

Charles J. Tegtmeyer, M.D.
Professor of Radiology and Anatomy
Division of Angiography and
  Interventional Radiology
Department of Radiology
University of Virginia
  Health Sciences Center
Charlottesville, Virginia

Renan Uflacker, M.D.
Professor of Radiology
Director, Division of Vascular and
  Interventional Radiology
Medical University of South Carolina
Charleston, South Carolina

Contents

SECTION II: NONVASCULAR INTERVENTIONS

SECTION I

VASCULAR INTERVENTIONS

CHAPTER
1

Vascular Anatomy of the Thorax

David F. Kallmes, Mary E. Jensen, Jacques E. Dion

AORTIC ARCH

Normal Anatomy

The aortic arch begins at the level of the upper border of the right second costosternal articulation[1] and continues posterolaterally to pass to the left of the trachea. The arch normally contains three main branches: the brachiocephalic trunk (innominate artery), left common carotid artery, and left subclavian artery (Figure 1.1). This pattern of branching is present in 70% of individuals.[2] Normally the left common carotid artery originates in closer approximation to the brachiocephalic trunk than to the left subclavian artery.[1]

Variant Anatomy of the Aortic Arch

Minor variations in the branching pattern of the aortic arch are seen in 23% of the population.[3] A common origin of the brachiocephalic trunk and left common carotid artery occurs in 13% (Figure 1.2). Nine percent have the origin of the left common carotid artery arise directly from the brachiocephalic trunk,[3] which is often referred to as a "bovine" trunk. The remaining 1% of variations of brachiocephalic artery branching patterns include right and left brachiocephalic trunks, bicarotid trunks, common brachiocephalic trunk, right or left subclavian arteries from a bicarotid trunk, and no brachiocephalic trunk.[3] Variant anatomy of the left vertebral and right subclavian arteries are discussed below.

Right Aortic Arch

This anomaly occurs in 0.02% of the population[4] and results from persistence of the embryologic fourth branchial artery. The aortic arch passes to the right of the trachea and may descend either to the right or left of midline. Although five types of branching patterns of the brachiocephalic arteries have been described with right aortic arches, two of these constitute the vast majority.[5] The avian or mirror image branching pattern of brachiocephalic vessels from a right aortic arc is as follows: first the left bra-

3

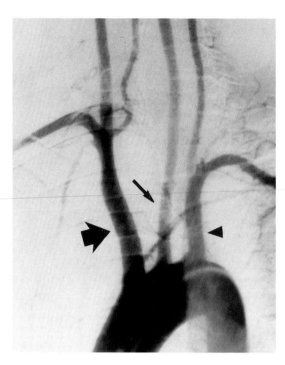

Figure 1.1 Digital subtraction aortogram (DSA) demonstrates normal configuration of the major vessels from the aortic arch. The first branch is the brachiocephalic artery (large arrow) followed by the left common carotid artery (CCA) (small arrow) and the left subclavian artery (arrowhead). Note that the origin of the left CCA is slightly closer to the brachiocephalic artery than it is to the left subclavian artery.

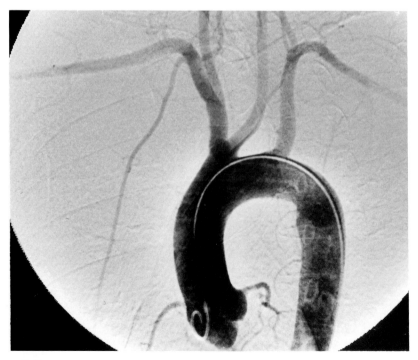

Figure 1.2 Digital subtraction aortogram in the right posterior oblique (RPO) position shows a common origin of the brachiocephalic and the left common carotid arteries, a frequent variant noted in 13% of patients.

chiocephalic trunk, then the right common carotid artery, and lastly the right subclavian artery (Figure 1.3A). This branching pattern is almost always associated with cyanotic congenital heart disease, most commonly tetralogy of Fallot.[6] The other common type of right aortic arch is associated with congenital heart disease in 10% of cases,[6] and its branching pattern is as follows: first the left common carotid, followed by the right common carotid, right subclavian, and aberrant left subclavian arteries (Figure 1.3B). The left subclavian artery usually originates from an aortic diverticulum with this type of branching pattern.

Thyroidea Ima Artery (Figure 1.4)

The thyroidea ima artery occurs in 6% of individuals[3] and ascends in the neck to supply the inferior lobe of the thyroid gland. It most often originates from the brachiocephalic trunk, but may arise directly from the aortic arch or right common carotid artery.[7] Rarely, it may originate from the internal mammary, subclavian, inferior thyroid, or suprascapular arteries.[3] It is present more commonly on the right than the left.[8] Bilateral thyroidea ima arteries have been reported.[3]

Ductus Diverticulum (Figure 1.5)

The inferior aspect of the aortic arch is usually concave. However, there may be straightening or even a mild focal convex bulge of the anteromedial aspect of the arch

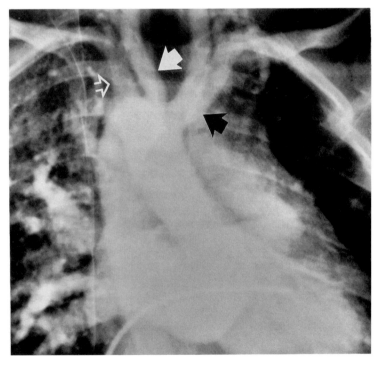

A

Figure 1.3 A. Left ventricular injection in a child with tetralogy of Fallot. Note the mirror image branching pattern with the left brachiocephalic artery (large black arrow) arising from the arch first, followed by the right common carotid artery (white arrow) and then the right subclavian artery (open white arrow). B. Following page.

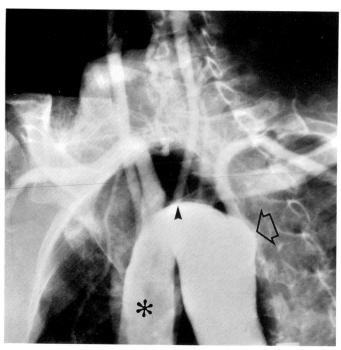

B

Figure 1.3 B. RPO injection of a right aortic arch with aberrant left subclavian artery: Evaluation of this film and other obliquities showed that the ascending aorta (asterisk) gives rise to the left common carotid artery first (arrowhead), followed by the right common carotid and the right subclavian arteries. The left subclavian artery arises last, originating from an aortic diverticulum (open black arrow). Incidentally noted is a direct origin of the vertebral artery from the arch located between the two subclavian arteries. (Courtesy of Dr. Paul Dee.)

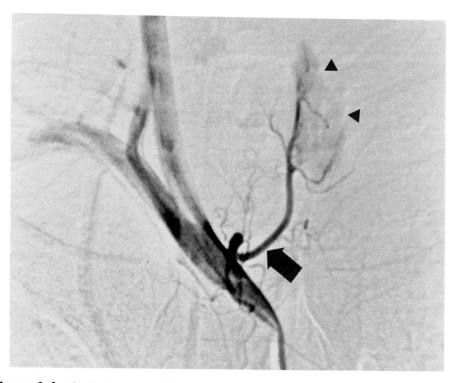

Figure 1.4 Selective injection of the brachiocephalic trunk demonstrates the thyroidea ima artery (arrow) and the blush of the inferior portion of the thyroid gland (arrowheads).

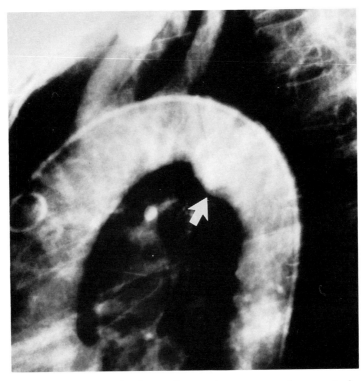

Figure 1.5 Arteriogram shows the ductus diverticulum as a smooth convexity from the anterior medial aspect of the aortic arch in the region of the true aortic isthmus (arrow).

at the level of the aortic isthmus. This bulge represents the ductus arteriosus remnant and is called a ductus diverticulum or ductus "bump". It is present in 33% of infants[9] and 9% of adults.[10] The ductus diverticulum itself has a smooth contour, and the angle between the convexity of the diverticulum and the aorta is obtuse. Washout of contrast from the ductus diverticulum is brisk. Conversely, an aortic transection, from which a ductus diverticulum must be differentiated, usually has acute angles at the junction of its convex bulge with the aorta, may have an associated intimal flap, and can be associated with a delayed washout of contrast.

Origin of Vertebral Arteries from Aortic Arch

Normally the left vertebral artery is a branch of the subclavian artery. It passes superiorly to enter the transverse foramen of C6. The left vertebral artery arises directly from the aortic arch in 6% of individuals, usually originating between the left common carotid and left subclavian arteries[4] (Figure 1.6). In this case, the artery enters the C4 or C5 transverse foramen rather than the C6 foramen. In addition, there may be a rudimentary vertebral artery present in the normal position.[4] In 0.6% of cases the vertebral artery will arise from the aortic arch distal to the left subclavian artery.[4] With this anatomic variant, the vertebral artery usually enters the C7 transverse foramen.

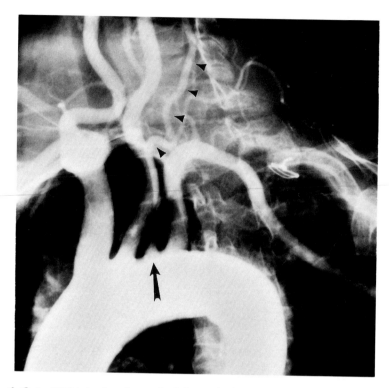

Figure 1.6 An RPO injection shows the left vertebral artery arising from the aortic arch (arrow) between the left common carotid and the left subclavian arteries. In this variant, seen in 6% of patients, the vessel enters the foramen transversarium at the level of C5 (arrowheads) instead of C6.

Cervical Aortic Arch

This rare variant probably is the result of failure of involution of the embryologic third branchial artery,[4] resulting in an aortic arch that is located more cephalad than normal. The aorta makes an abrupt turn caudally before descending posterior to the esophagus contralateral to the side of the ascending aorta. Aberrant right or left subclavian arteries as well as separate origins of the internal and external carotid arteries have been seen in association with a cervical aortic arch.[11]

Aberrant Right Subclavian Artery (Figure 1.7)

In 0.8% of individuals the right subclavian artery arises in an aberrant location as the most distal branch of the aortic arch.[8] In 29% of cases of aberrant right subclavian artery, a common origin of the right and left common carotid arteries is present.[4] Although early literature suggested that the right subclavian artery could pass either posterior or anterior to the esophagus, more recent reports suggest that in almost all cases the artery passes dorsal (posterior) to the esophagus.[12]

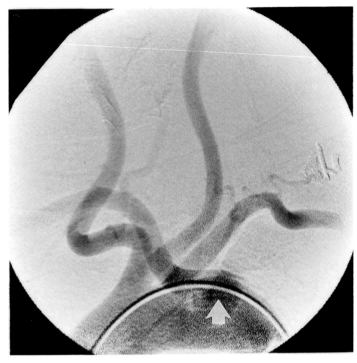

Figure 1.7 Right posterior oblique DSA demonstrates the right subclavian artery arising as the most distal branch of the aortic arch (arrow). Also noted is a common origin of the carotid arteries, frequently seen with this variant.

BRONCHIAL ARTERIES

The bronchial arteries arise from the aorta or the intercostal vessels in the midthoracic region. These vessels not only supply the major bronchi and larger bronchopulmonary lymph nodes, but also may anastomose with pulmonary, spinal and, less commonly, coronary arteries.[7] While the bronchial arteries may arise at any level between the third and seventh thoracic interspace, they arise at the T5-6 level in 80% of cases.[13] In 13%, a left bronchial artery can arise from the inferior surface of the aortic arch.[13] The bronchial arteries rarely arise from the internal mammary, subclavian, superior intercostal, thyrocervical trunk, abdominal aorta, or inferior phrenic arteries.[3,14]

Both autopsy and angiographic studies have reported on the variations in the number and branching pattern of the bronchial arteries.[13–15] Slightly more than half of individuals have a single right bronchial artery. The reported incidence of a common right intercostal–bronchial trunk ranges from 70%[7] to greater than 90%,[14] while a common left intercostal–bronchial artery is rare.[15] Right and left bronchial arteries arise as a common trunk in 43% of individuals.[14,16] The distribution of bronchial arteries is as follows: single arteries bilaterally in 30%; two left and one right in 40%; two left and two right in 20%; one left and two right in 5%; three left and one right in 4%.[7]

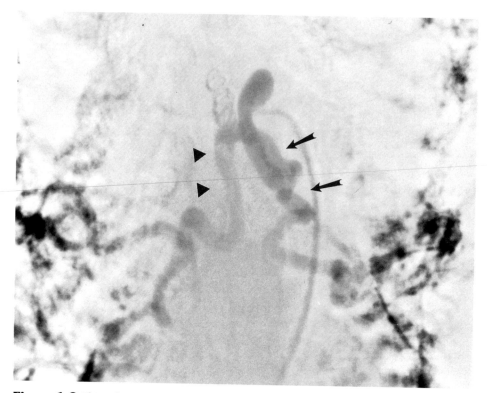

Figure 1.8 This selective injection of an enlarged common bronchial trunk demonstrates hypertrophy of the left (arrows) and right (arrowheads) bronchial arteries in a patient with chronic inflammatory lung disease.

The origin of the bronchial arteries from the aorta depends on the branching pattern of the vessels themselves. A common right and left bronchial artery trunk arises from the anterior aspect of the aorta (Figure 1.8). When the vessels originate independently, they are positioned along the anterolateral aspect of the aorta.[3,15] The right intercostobronchial trunk is usually located along the lateral or posterolateral aspect of the aorta (Figure 1.9).[15]

The radiculomedullary arteries that supply the thoracic spinal cord can arise from the bronchial arteries. This occurs more commonly on the right than on the left.[16] One author reported a 5% incidence of radiculomedullary arteries arising from the bronchial arteries.[16] Other series have noted that, while bronchial arteries can give rise to radicular arteries supplying nerve roots in more than 50% of individuals, radiculomedullary vessels supplying the spinal cord were much less common.[14]

SUBCLAVIAN ARTERY

Most frequently, the right subclavian artery is a branch of the brachiocephalic trunk, while the left subclavian artery arises as the last brachiocephalic vessel from the aortic arch. The subclavian arteries are divided into three segments: the first, or intrathoracic segment, is medial to the anterior scalene muscle;[7] the second segment is dorsal to the anterior scalene muscle; the third segment is lateral to the anterior scalene muscle.[1] The subclavian artery becomes the axillary artery as the vessel passes the lateral aspect of the first rib.

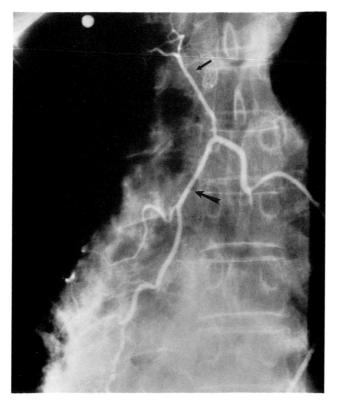

Figure 1.9 As many as 90% of patients will have the right intercostal artery (small arrow) and bronchial artery (large arrow) arise as a common trunk.

The first segment of the subclavian artery gives rise to three branches: vertebral artery, internal mammary artery, and thyrocervical trunk (Figure 1.10). Anomalous vertebral artery origins from the aortic arch have been described earlier in this chapter. Normally the vertebral artery originates just proximal to the thyrocervical trunk, but may arise more proximally. The next branch of the subclavian artery, the thyrocervical trunk, has variable branching patterns. The most common branching pattern for the thyrocervical trunk, present in 52% of individuals,[7] is as follows: suprascapular, superficial cervical, and inferior thyroid arteries. Common variants include: separate origins of all three vessels (31%);[7] presence of a common trunk for the superficial cervical and dorsal scapular arteries, called the transverse cervical artery (29%);[8] and a main thyrocervical trunk with one independent branch (16%).[7] The dorsal scapular artery usually arises as a separate vessel from the subclavian artery.[17] The inferior thyroid artery usually gives rise to the ascending cervical artery, which ascends in the anterior aspect of the neck. The ascending cervical artery may have radiculomedullary branches to the spinal artery and/or multiple anastomoses with branches of the ipsilateral vertebral artery. On rare occasions, the inferior thyroid artery arises directly from the vertebral artery before the vertebral artery enters the foramen transversarium.

The costocervical trunk arises from the first or second segment of the subclavian artery.[17,18] The two primary branches of this vessel are the deep cervical artery and the superior (supreme) intercostal artery. The deep cervical artery ascends dorsal to the transverse processes of the cervical vertebral arteries and often anastomoses with branches of the occipital artery. The supreme intercostal artery supplies the upper two intercostal arteries in 60% of individuals, but supplies only the first intercostal artery in 32%.[8]

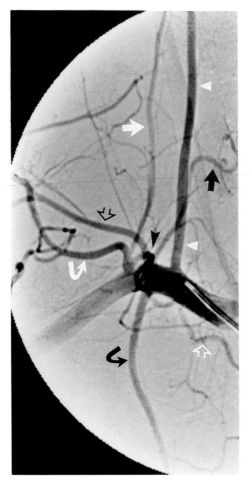

Figure 1.10 Anteroposterior injection of the right subclavian artery demonstrates the anatomy of the thyrocervical and costocervical trunks. The vertebral artery (white arrowheads) arises from the first portion of the subclavian artery, followed by the thyrocervical trunk (black arrowhead). The inferior thyroidal artery (solid black arrow) courses superiorly and medially. The transverse cervical (open black arrow) courses laterally to give rise to the dorsal scapular and superficial cervical branches. Opposite the thyrocervical trunk is the internal mammary artery (curved black arrow) traveling inferiorly. Lastly, the costocervical trunk gives rise to the deep cervical (solid white arrow) and supreme intercostal (open white arrow) arteries. In this patient, an aberrant suprascapular artery (curved white arrow) is also noted.

The internal mammary artery arises along the inferior aspect of the first segment of the subclavian artery, opposite to the origin of the thyrocervical trunk. It descends along the anterior chest wall 1 to 2 cm lateral to the sternum. After giving off several small branches, including pericardiacophrenic, mediastinal, pericardial, sternal, and anterior intercostal arteries, the internal mammary artery bifurcates into the musculophrenic and superior epigastric arteries.[1]

The axillary artery gives rise to the following vessels: the superior thoracic, which supplies the upper three intercostal spaces anteriorly; the thoracoacromial and lateral thoracic arteries, which supply the lateral chest wall; the subscapular artery; and the anterior and posterior circumflex humeral arteries.[7] There may be an additional branch, called the accessory pectoral artery.[3] Many variations of this branching pattern of the axillary artery may be seen, including absent thoracoacromial or superior thoracic arteries[8] or common trunks giving rise to two or three of the vessels listed above.[7]

VASCULAR SUPPLY TO THE SPINAL CORD

The blood supply to the spinal cord arises from multiple radicular arteries that ultimately form the midline anterior spinal artery and paired paramedian posterior spinal arteries. The radicular arteries originate from neighboring segmental arteries and pass through the intervertebral foramen medially to supply the corresponding nerve root. The larger radicular arteries that supply both the nerve root and spinal cord are called "radiculomedullary" arteries. The radiculomedullary arteries initially ascend within the spinal canal and then have a characteristic "hairpin" loop to become the midline anterior spinal artery. The radiculomedullary artery gives off small meningeal branches to the dura before dividing into ascending and descending branches to form the spinal arteries.

Although the anterior spinal artery runs the entire length of the spinal cord in the anterior median fissure, it may be discontinuous along its course. Its cephalad extent is formed by the fusion of two branches from the distal vertebral arteries. These vertebral artery branches typically are small and are responsible for vascular supply to only the upper cervical spinal cord. The longitudinally oriented anterior spinal artery receives input from multiple segmental radiculomedullary arteries. The number of radiculomedullary arteries ranges from 2 to 14.[19] The discontinuity of the anterior spinal artery increases the importance of each of its radiculomedullary branches because collateral supply to the anterior cord may be inadequate with occlusion of one radiculomedullary branch.

In the cervical spinal cord there is relatively constant input to the anterior spinal artery from the vertebral artery at the level of C3.[20] The "artery of the cervical enlargement" represents a large radiculomedullary vessel usually present at some level between C4 and C8.[21] This vessel may originate from the deep cervical artery, usually at C7 or C8,[22] or from the ascending cervical artery, usually at C4 or C5.[23] Less commonly the artery of the cervical enlargement will originate from the supreme intercostal artery[20] or directly from a subclavian artery.[24]

The upper thoracic spinal cord represents a region of relatively poor blood supply, as radiculomedullary vessels are uncommon between C8 and T6. When radiculomedullary arteries are present in this region, they usually arise from bronchial or superior intercostal arteries.

The thoracolumbar spinal cord is supplied by the artery of Adamkiewicz, otherwise known as the arteria radicularis magna[1] or the artery of the lumbar enlargement[21] (Figure 1.11). This large radiculomedullary vessel, present on the left in 80% of individuals,[22] originates as a branch of an intercostal or lumbar artery. It is present between T9 and T12 in 75% of cases, between T5 and T8 in 15%, and at L1 or L2 in 10%. If the artery of Adamkiewicz originates above T9, there is usually an additional lumbar radiculomedullary artery.[22] At the level of the conus medullaris, the anterior spinal artery forms an anastomotic loop with the terminal branches of the posterior spinal arteries.

The paired posterior spinal arteries run in the posterolateral sulci, originating from the fourth segment of each vertebral artery and receiving contributions from 10 to 23 posterior radicular arteries.[25] Below the T4 or T5 level there is usually one posterior radicular branch every other segment. Like the anterior spinal artery, these vessels traverse the entire length of the spinal cord, although they may become discontinuous.[25]

The course of segmental feeding vessels that supply the radiculomedullary vessels

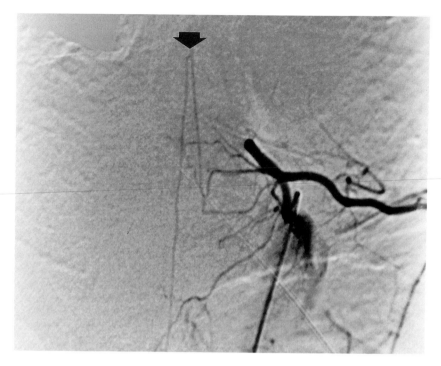

Figure 1.11 Selective injection of the left T10 intercostal artery demonstrates the radiculomedullary artery giving rise to the artery of Adamkiewicz. This vessel is the major blood supply to the anterior portion of the thoracic cord and is easily identified by the classic "hairpin" turn (arrow).

can be predicted by the ascent of the spinal cord in fetal development. In the thoracolumbar region the feeding vessel ascends at a steep angle after entering the spinal canal. In the mid and upper thoracic region the angle of ascent is shallow, and in the cervical region the course of the feeding vessels is nearly horizontal.[19]

POSTERIOR INTERCOSTAL AND SUBCOSTAL ARTERIES

Posterior intercostal arteries represent segmental dorsal branches of the descending thoracic aorta. They arise in a paramedian location along the posterior aspect of the aorta. Separate origins of right and left intercostal arteries are present in 83% of segments. In 13% of segments there is trunk formation by two adjacent vessels on a given side, often involving the third and fourth intercostal vessels.[3] A common trunk for both right and left intercostal vessels is present in 2% of segments.[3] The posterior intercostal arteries normally travel anteroinferior to the adjacent rib. Intercostal arteries may course posterior to the ribs (thoracic vertebral artery); this occurs in 5% of cases for the supreme intercostal artery and in 4% of cases for the third intercostal artery.[3]

The thoracic vertebrae derive their blood supply from branches of the proximal posterior intercostal arteries and the dorsal rami of these arteries. In the cervical region, the situation is more complex with supply from the vertebral, ascending cervical, and/or deep cervical branches. The regional arterial and venous anatomy of the vertebral bodies will be outlined in greater detail in Chapter 9.

THORACIC OUTLET SYNDROME

Nerves or vessels may be compressed at the level of the thoracic outlet by bony and/or fibrous structures, leading to upper extremity pain, numbness, or even Raynaud's phenomenon.[26] The neurovascular bundle traverses the following spaces in the region of the thoracic outlet: the interscalene triangle, formed by the anterior scalene muscle anteriorly, the middle scalene muscle posteriorly, and the first rib inferiorly; the costoclavicular space, formed by the clavicle and subclavius muscle superiorly and the first rib inferiorly; and the pectoralis minor tunnel, formed by the pectoralis minor tendon anteriorly and the coracoid process posteriorly.[27]

Cervical ribs are present in 0.5% of individuals[28] and may cause compression either at the level of the interscalene triangle or the costoclavicular space.[27] Conversely, fewer than 50% of individuals with completely formed cervical ribs will have symptoms of thoracic outlet compression.[29] Nevertheless, when the thoracic outlet syndrome is present, cervical ribs or their associated fibrous bands are the most common cause.[30] Other causes of thoracic outlet syndrome include compression from anomalous fibrous bands or muscular insertions, muscular hypertrophy,[30] anomalous vessels, malunited clavicular fractures, clavicular and other osseous lesions,[31] or an anomalous first rib that narrows the costoclavicular space.[27] Arteriographic evaluation for thoracic outlet compression should include studies with the upper extremity in a neutral position and also with the arm hyperabducted. Examinations in the neutral position alone may not demonstrate the vascular compression (Figure 1.12A, B). Similar principles apply to evaluation of the axillosubclavian venous anatomy with venography.

THORACIC VENOUS ANATOMY

The axillary vein represents the continuation of the basilic vein and enlarges in caliber as it receives the brachial and cephalic veins. The axillary vein becomes the subclavian vein as it passes medial to the lateral aspect of the first rib. The subclavian vein receives inflow from the external jugular and dorsal scapular veins before uniting with the internal jugular vein at the level of the medial border of the anterior scalene muscle to become the brachiocephalic (innominate) vein.[1]

The left brachiocephalic vein is approximately 6 cm in length and runs anteroinferiorly behind the manubrium. The right brachiocephalic vein is approximately 2.5 cm in length and courses inferiorly to a position dorsal to the lower border of the costal cartilage of the first right rib, where it joins the left brachiocephalic vein to form the superior vena cava. The tributaries that drain into the brachiocephalic veins include the vertebral, internal mammary, inferior thyroid, and superior intercostal veins.[7] The superior vena cava is approximately 7 cm in length and travels inferiorly to the right atrium (Figure 1.13).

The most common anomaly of systemic venous drainage is a persistent left superior vena cava, present in 0.3% of individuals.[32] It represents failure of portions of the left anterior and common cardinal veins to regress.[33] A right superior vena cava is present in addition to the left superior vena cava in 82% of cases.[33] The left superior vena cava empties into the coronary sinus[34] (Figure 1.14). The accessory hemiazygos vein may empty into the left superior vena cava after arching over the left mainstem bronchus.[8]

The right-sided azygos and left-sided hemiazygos veins form at the level of the L1-L2 vertebral bodies and are joined at the T12 level by the subcostal and ascending lumbar veins. At the T8 level the hemiazygos vein crosses midline to join the azygos vein. Additional tributaries of the thoracic portion of the azygos vein include the right posterior fifth to eleventh intercostal veins; the right second through fourth posterior intercostal veins via the right superior posterior intercostal vein; and the esophageal, mediastinal, and pericardial veins.

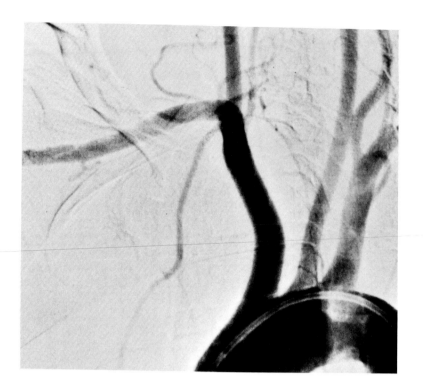

A

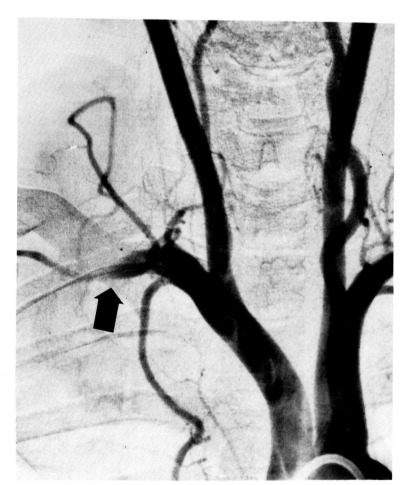

B

Figure 1.12 A. DSA with the right upper extremity in the neutral position demonstrates normal filling of the right subclavian artery. B. With the upper extremity in hyperabduction, occlusion of the right subclavian artery at the level of the junction between the first rib and the clavicle is noted (arrow).

16

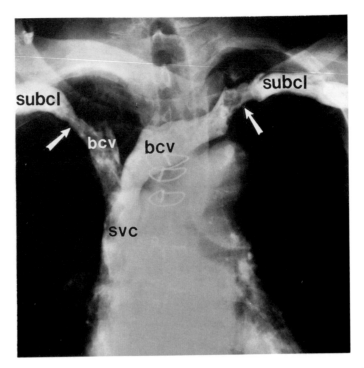

Figure 1.13 AP radiograph performed during bilateral upper extremity venography. Subclavian veins (subcl) join with internal jugular veins (wash-in of unopacified blood from internal jugular veins denoted by arrows) to form the brachiocephalic veins (bcv). These veins in turn join to form the superior vena cava (svc). Sternotomy wires are present from prior bypass surgery.

The accessory hemiazygos vein collects flow from the left fourth through eighth posterior intercostal veins before crossing the midline to join the azygos vein. The accessory hemiazygos vein may or may not communicate with the hemiazygos vein.[1] The left superior intercostal vein forms an arch on the left side of the mediastinum similar to the azygos arch on the right. This vein drains the second through fourth posterior intercostal veins before passing anterior to drain into the left brachiocephalic vein. In the majority of cases the left superior intercostal vein connects to the accessory hemiazygos vein.[33]

PULMONARY VESSELS

Pulmonary Arteries

The pulmonary trunk arises from the base of the right ventricle and runs posterosuperiorly for approximately 5 cm where it divides into the right and left pulmonary arteries. The right pulmonary artery travels horizontally and to the right before dividing into ascending (truncus anterior) and descending (interlobar) branches.[35] The truncus anterior divides into anterior, apical, and posterior segmental arteries, the latter two of which usually arise together.[7] In the majority of cases there is a small branch from the proximal aspect of the interlobar artery which supplies a portion of the posterior segment of the upper lobe.[36] The interlobar artery travels inferiorly, giving off one or two segmental branches to the middle lobe before dividing into five segmental arteries supplying each of the five lower lobe bronchopulmonary segments[35] (Figure 1.15A).

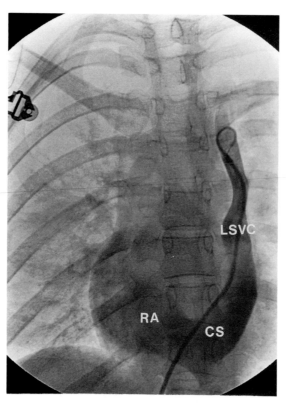

Figure 1.14 Digital subtraction venogram performed with pigtail catheter placed from a femoral approach with its tip in a left superior vena cava (LSVC). The drainage from the LSVC is via the coronary sinus (CS) into the right atrium (RA).

The left pulmonary artery is directed posterior and is shorter than the right pulmonary artery. Formation of a common upper lobe trunk is unusual on the left; rather, the five upper lobe branches (apical, posterior, anterior descending, posterior descending, and lingular)[1] arise individually and in random order.[7] The pulmonary artery then divides into the lower lobe branches. There may be formation of two major trunks: the anterolateral basal and posterior basal arteries. Alternatively, a common trunk between anterior and medial segmental arteries may be seen.[7]

Pulmonary Veins

Unlike the pulmonary arteries, the pulmonary veins do not travel with their corresponding bronchi.[35] Segmental veins from the right middle and upper lobe coalesce into the right superior pulmonary vein, which empties into the posterosuperior aspect

Figure 1.15 A. Pulmonary angiogram—AP subtraction film from a pulmonary angiogram performed with catheter positioned in the main pulmonary artery. Right pulmonary artery (RPA) is slightly longer than the left pulmonary artery (LPA). The RPA branches into the truncus anterior (TA), supplying the upper lobe segmental vessels, and the interlobular artery (ILA), supplying middle and lower lobe vessels as well as an accessory upper lobe artery (acc). Lower lobe branches include anterobasal (ab), lateral basal (lb), and posterobasal (pb) segmental arteries. The right medial

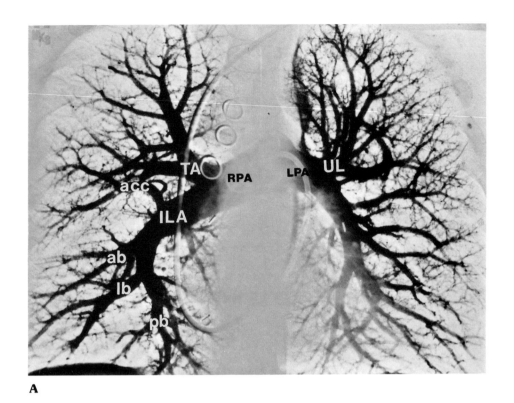

A

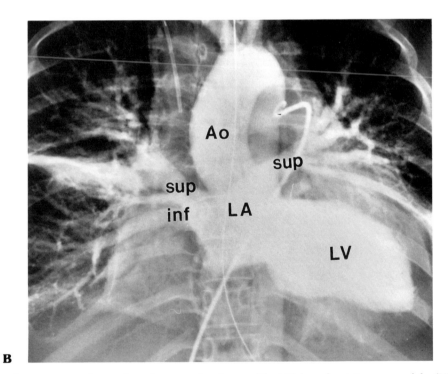

B

basal artery is superimposed on the posterobasal artery. The LPA branches into an upper lobe (UL) trunk as well as lingular and lower lobe branches. The left lower lobe segmental arteries follow similar courses to their right-sided counterparts. Note rings from prior bypass surgery. B. Pulmonary venogram–AP film during the levo-phase of a pulmonary angiogram shows the tip of catheter in the main pulmonary artery. The superior and inferior pulmonary veins (sup and inf, respectively) are opacified (the left inferior pulmonary vein is not well seen because of contrast within the left ventricle (LV). These pulmonary veins empty into the left atrium (LA). Also seen is the ascending aorta (Ao). A nasogastric tube and right subclavian venous catheter are present.

of the left atrium. The middle lobe veins may empty separately into the left atrium.[35] The right inferior pulmonary vein forms as the confluence of the lower lobe segmental veins and empties separately from the superior pulmonary vein into the left atrium (Figure 1.15B).

The left pulmonary venous drainage is similar to the right. Upper and lower lobe segmental veins coalesce to form superior and inferior pulmonary veins, which drain separately into the left atrium. The lingular veins empty into the superior pulmonary vein.

THORACIC DUCT

The thoracic duct is the common trunk of all lymph vessels of the body, except those of the right upper extremity and the right aspect of the head, neck, and trunk. The thoracic duct begins at the cephalad aspect of the cisterna chyli near the lower border of the T12 vertebral body, passes into the thorax through the diaphragmatic hiatus, and ascends within the thorax between the azygos vein and the descending aorta. At the level of T5 the duct passes upward and to the left, and continues its ascent to the left of the esophagus. At the level of C7 the duct turns laterally and arches forward to join the venous system, usually at the junction of the left subclavian and internal jugular veins[1] (Figure 1.16A and B). The thoracic duct may occasionally empty into the internal jugular or innominate veins or directly into the superior vena cava.[37] In 2% of cases the upper portion of the thoracic duct is duplicated, with each branch entering its ipsilateral subclavian vein. In 5% of cases the thoracic duct may continue cephalad in the right aspect of the thorax, without crossing to the left, and then empty into the right-sided venous system.[37]

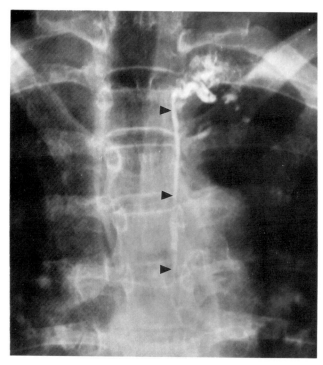

A

Figure 1.16 A. Thoracic duct (arrowheads) is shown ascending to the left of midline, coursing toward the junction of the internal jugular and subclavian veins. B. Following page.

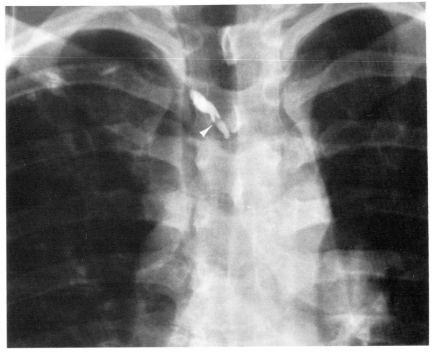

B

Figure 1.16 B. Right-sided lymphatic vessel shown draining into the junction of the right internal jugular and subclavian veins. Valve within the lymphatic channel is denoted by the arrowhead.

REFERENCES

1. Warwick R, Williams PL: Angiology. In: *Gray's Anatomy,* ed 35. Philadelphia, WB Saunders, 1973, pp 619–626.

2. Oelrich TM: The cardiovascular system. In Morris H (ed): *Human Anatomy: A Complete Systematic Treatise,* ed 12. Blakiston, New York, NY, 1966, pp 667–670.

3. Lippert H, Pabst R: *Arterial Variations in Man.* Munich, Germany, JF Bergmann, 1985, pp 3–22.

4. Haughton VM, Rosenbaum AE: The normal and anomalous aortic arch and brachiocephalic arteries. In Newton TH, Potts DG (eds): *Radiology of the Skull and Brain: Angiography.* St. Louis, CV Mosby, 1974, pp 1145–1163.

5. Shuford WH, Sybers RG: The Aortic Arch and Its Malformations. Springfield, IL, Charles C. Thomas, 1974, pp 41–92.

6. Stewart JR, Kincaid OW, Titus JL: Right aortic arch: plain film diagnosis and significance. *Am J Roentgenol* 97:377:381, 1966.

7. Kadir S: *Atlas of Normal and Variant Angiographic Anatomy.* Philadelphia, WB Saunders, 1991, pp 19–55.

8. Bergman RA, Thompson SA, Afifi AK: *Catalog of Human Variation.* Baltimore, Urban and Schwartzenberg, 1984, pp 88–103.

9. Abrams HL: The normal thoracic aorta. In Abrams HL (ed): *Abrams Textbook of Angiography,* Boston, Little, Brown, 1971, p 306.

10. Goodman PC, Jeffrey RB, Minagi H, et al: Angiographic evaluation of the ductus diverticulum. *Cardiovasc Intervent Radiol* 5:1–4, 1982.

11. Shuford WH, Sybers RG, Milledge RD, et al: The cervical aortic arch. *Am J Roentgenol* 116:519–527, 1972.

12. Proto AV, Cuthbert NW, Raider L: Aberrant right subclavian artery: further observations. *Am J Roentgenol* 148:253–257, 1987.

13. Cauldwell EN, Siekert RG, Liningar RE, et al: The bronchial arteries: an anatomic study of 150 human cadavers. *Surg Gynecol Obstet* 86:395–412, 1948.

14. Uflacker R, Kaemmaerer A, Pican P, et al: Bronchial artery embolization in the management of hemoptysis: technical aspects and long-term results. *Radiology* 157:637–644, 1985.

15. Roberts AC: Bronchial artery embolization. *J Thorac Imag* 5:60, 1990.

16. Botenga ASJ: *Selective Bronchial and Intercostal Arteriography.* Baltimore, Williams and Wilkins, 1970.

17. Huelke DF: A study of the transverse cervical and dorsal scapular arteries. *Anat Rec* 132:233–245, 1958.

18. Daseler EH, Anson BJ: Surgical anatomy of the subclavian artery and its branches. *Surg Gynecol Obstet* 108:149–174, 1959.

19. Thron AK: *Vascular Anatomy of the Spinal Cord.* New York, Springer-Verlag, 1988, pp 8–20.

20. Djindjian R: *Angiography of the Spinal Cord.* Baltimore, University Park Press, 1970, pp 6–10.

21. Lazorthes G, Gouaze A, Zadeh JO, et al: Arterial vascularization of the spinal cord. *J Neurosurg* 235:253–262,1971.

22. Turnbull IM: Blood supply of the spinal cord: normal and pathologic considerations. *Clin Neurosurg* 20:56–84, 1973.

23. Chakravorty BG: Arterial supply of the cervical spinal cord (with special reference to the radicular arteries). *Anat Record* 170:311–330, 1971.

24. Miller DL: Direct origin of the artery of the cervical enlargement from the left subclavian artery. *AJNR* 14:242–244, 1993.

25. Netter FH: *Nervous System: Anatomy and Physiology.* West Caldwell, NJ, Ciba-Geigy Corp, pp 45–46.

26. Beyer JA, Wright IS: The hyperabduction syndrome: with special reference to its relationship to Raynaud's syndrome. *Circulation* 4:161–172, 1951.

27. Kadir S: *Diagnostic Angiography.* Philadelphia, WB Saunders, 1986, pp 194–198.

28. Rainer WG, Vigor W, Newby JP: Surgical treatment of thoracic outlet compression. *Am J Surg* 116:704–707, 1968.

29. Adson AW, Coffey JR: Cervical rib: a method of anterior approach for relief of symptoms by division of the scalenus anticus. *Ann Surg* 85:839–857, 1927.

30. Teleford ED, Mottershead S: Pressure at the cervicobrachial junction. An operative study. *J Bone Joint Surg* 30B:249–265, 1948.

31. Pang O, Wessel HB: Thoracic outlet syndrome. *Neurosurgery* 22:105–120, 1988.

32. Cha EM, Khoury GH: Persistent left superior vena cava. *Radiology* 103:375–381, 1975.

33. Godwin JD, Chen JTT: Thoracic venous anatomy. *Am J Roentgenol* 147:674–684, 1986.

34. Campbell M, Deuchar DC: The left sided superior vena cava. *Br Heart J* 16:423–439, 1954.

35. Fraser RG: The normal chest. In Fraser RG, Pare JAP (eds): *Diagnosis of Diseases of the Chest,* ed 3. Philadelphia, WB Saunders, 1988, pp 85–86.

36. Jefferson KE: The normal pulmonary angiogram and some changes seen in chronic nonspecific lung disease. I. The pulmonary vessels in the normal pulmonary angiogram. *Proc R Soc Med* 58:677, 1965.

37. Kuisk H: *Technique of Lymphography and Principles of Interpretation.* St. Louis, MO, Warren H Green, Inc, 1971, pp 113–117.

C H A P T E R
2

Interventions for Acute Pulmonary Emboli

Alan H. Matsumoto, Renan Uflacker, Rolf W. Günther

Venous thromboembolic disease remains the third most common cardiovascular disease and one of the leading causes of sudden death in the United States. The true incidence of pulmonary embolism (PE) is unknown, but based on historic projections, it is estimated that more than 600,000 cases of PE occur every year in the United States.[1] Approximately 10% of patients with PE do not survive their initial event. Of those that do survive, approximately 70% fail to have the diagnosis made and experience a mortality rate of 30%. If the diagnosis of PE is made promptly and appropriate therapy initiated, the mortality rate can be reduced to less than 10%.[1-3] Despite the awareness of the incidence of PE and morbidity associated with PE, the mortality associated with PE has not significantly changed in the last 30 yr.[4] Perhaps the only exception to this statement is the orthopedic patient population, in whom effective anticoagulation prophylaxis has reduced the incidence of PE and the mortality rate associated with it.[5]

Once the diagnosis of acute PE is made, treatment should be initiated as soon as possible. The therapeutic options that are available should be tailored to each patient and clinical scenario. In this chapter, we will discuss the management of patients with acute PE using anticoagulation, catheter-directed thrombolysis, percutaneous embolectomy and embolus fragmentation techniques, and/or surgical embolectomy. The role of inferior vena cava filters will not be addressed.

ANTICOAGULATION

A patient who receives no specific treatment for acute PE has an 18% to 30% chance of suffering a subsequent lethal PE.[1,3,6] Retrospective data also suggests that anticoagulation therapy can reduce the likelihood of a recurrent fatal PE to less than 3%.[1,6,7] Patients with symptomatic deep venous thrombosis who have not had a PE and receive no treatment, have a 6% to 14% chance of sustaining a lethal PE. In this patient population, anticoagulation can reduce the incidence of lethal PE to less than 1%.[6]

In one of the few prospective studies in the literature, 35 patients with documented acute PE were randomized to receive either heparin or placebo therapy.[3] None of the 16 patients treated with heparin had recurrent PE. In the 19 patients receiving a placebo, 10 had recurrent PE of which 5 were fatal. There was one heparin-associated death secondary to a gastrointestinal hemorrhage.

Bleeding is the most frequent major complication associated with anticoagulation. The incidence of major bleeding during standard, unfractionated heparin administration varies from 1.6% to 14.2% and depends upon the amount of heparin that is being given, method of administration (continuous IV versus intermittent IV or subcutaneous), duration of administration, concomitant use of aspirin, age of the patient, and presence of underlying risk factors for bleeding.[8-10] Other complications associated with the use of heparin include thrombocytopenia, osteoporosis, skin necrosis, alopecia, and hypersensitivity reactions.[11-15]

Low-molecular-weight heparins have recently become available. They have a longer plasma half-life and a more predictable anticoagulation response than standard, unfractionated heparin. Preliminary reports have shown them to be highly effective and possibly safer than standard heparin regimens.[16,17]

The duration of anticoagulation therapy for acute PE depends upon the absence or continuing presence of a risk factor for recurrent deep venous thrombosis and PE. Patients having their first episode of acute PE are usually treated with a course of heparin and then converted to oral anticoagulants for 3 to 6 months. If there is a continuing risk factor for deep venous thrombosis and PE, anticoagulation is continued indefinitely or until the risk factor is no longer present.[18] The risk for developing a major bleeding complication associated with long-term oral anticoagulation therapy varies between 4.2% and 22.4%, and depends upon the intensity of therapy.[19,20] Concomitant use of aspirin also increases the risk for a bleeding complication.[21]

ENDOVASCULAR AND SURGICAL INTERVENTIONS

When obstruction of 70% of the pulmonary arterial circulation occurs, the right ventricle needs to be able to generate a systolic pressure in excess of 50 mm Hg and a mean pulmonary artery pressure greater than 40 mm Hg in order to maintain pulmonary perfusion. A previously normal right ventricle is incapable of generating a systolic pressure exceeding 50 mm Hg, so any incremental embolic obstruction to the vasculature beyond this point results in right ventricular failure.[22] The degree of obstruction of the pulmonary arterial circulation required to cause a change in the pulmonary hemodynamics also depends upon the amount of underlying cardiopulmonary disease prior to an embolic event. Therefore, a patient with massive PE obstructing the majority of the pulmonary circulation or a submassive PE superposed on underlying cardiopulmonary disease may present with right ventricular dysfunction or compromised hemodynamics. In this subset of patients, anticoagulation therapy alone may not be adequate, and more aggressive intervention with thrombolysis and/or pulmonary embolectomy and clot fragmentation techniques should be considered.

Thrombolysis

Although anticoagulation protocols with heparin are now more aggressive in patients with acute PE,[23] anticoagulation therapy is still directed at the source of the embolism and not at the embolism itself. The purpose of anticoagulation is to prevent propagation of thrombus, while allowing the endogenous fibrinolytic system to lyse the clot. However, up to 50% of patients with acute PE do not completely lyse clot, and chronic pulmonary hypertension from residual vascular obstruction can occur.[24,25]

In the 1970s, two randomized, prospective trials were undertaken to evaluate the efficacy of intravenous infusion of thrombolytic agents versus traditional anticoagulation therapy on the outcome of patients with acute PE.[26,27] The studies demonstrated significant improvement in perfusion lung scans and pulmonary angiograms at 12 and 24 hr in patients receiving thrombolytic therapy when compared to patients receiving heparin alone. The results of the trials also demonstrated a more rapid decrease in the mean pulmonary and right atrial pressures in patients receiving thrombolytic therapy. When these cohorts of patients were further evaluated, there were improved short- and long-term diffusion capacity in the lung and more normal pulmonary capillary blood volumes in patients receiving urokinase.[28] Patients who initially received thrombolytic agents also had significantly improved New York Heart Association classifications, lower resting and exercise pulmonary arterial pressures, and lower pulmonary vascular resistances 10 yr later.[29]

In a recent, nonrandomized, observational report of a cohort of 399 patients with acute PE, 291 (78%) of the patients were treated with anticoagulation alone and had a 19% 1-yr mortality rate. In contrast, 23 (6%) of the patients were treated with thrombolytic therapy and had a 9% 1-yr mortality rate.[7] In another study, patients who received thrombolytic therapy had a sustained improvement in pulmonary hemodynamics at rest and during exercise at 15 months follow-up.[30] Most patients treated with heparin alone were observed to have persistent pulmonary hypertension aggravated by exercise at 3–5 yr of follow-up.[31]

Despite the numerous randomized trials demonstrating faster improvement in pulmonary perfusion and hemodynamics and better lung diffusing capacities and pulmonary capillary blood volumes in patients receiving thrombolytic therapy, when symptoms and mortality rates at 6 and 12 months are analyzed, there is no statistical difference between patients who received thrombolytics versus heparin.[32] In addition, bleeding complications were more frequent in patients undergoing thrombolysis.

The problem in demonstrating a decrease in mortality with thrombolysis therapy for acute PE is the small number of patients studied. In the largest trial, only 160 patients were evaluated (78 received heparin and 82 received urokinase).[26] Since anticoagulation alone reduces the mortality associated with acute PE to less than 8%, a trial at least 10 times as large (>1,600 patients) would be necessary to demonstrate a statistically significant reduction in mortality of 25%.[33] In addition, acute PE often accompanies underlying advance illnesses that predispose the patients to thromboembolic disease. Therefore, factors unrelated to the acute PE affect mortality rates. In one prospective study, 95 (24%) of 399 patients with acute PE died within 1 yr. Of these 95 deaths, 70 (74%) were related to either cancer, sepsis, or cardiac disease.[7] In short, a study capable of demonstrating a reduction in mortality with the use of thrombolytic agents for acute PE would require a very large number of patients.

The United States Food and Drug Administration approved the use of streptokinase in 1977 and urokinase in 1978 for the treatment of acute PE. Recombinant tissue plasminogen activator (rt-PA) was approved for the treatment of acute PE in 1990. The recommendation for administration of all three thrombolytic agents is based on fixed or weight-adjusted doses given intravenously (Table 2.1). None of the FDA-approved thrombolytic regimens for acute PE employs the concomitant use of anticoagulation therapy.

TABLE 2.1 FDA-Approved Thrombolytic Regimens for PE

Streptokinase:	250,000 IU as a loading dose over 30 min followed by 100,000 IU/hr IV for 24 hr
Urokinase:	4,400 IU/kg as a loading dose over 10 min, followed by 4,400 IU/kg/hr IV for 12 to 24 hr
rt-PA:	100 mg as a continuous peripheral IV infusion administered over 2 hr

The Consensus Development Conference subsequently recommended that thrombolytic therapy be considered in any patient who has a perfusion defect equivalent to one or more lobes.[34] Additional indications for thrombolytic therapy include hemodynamic compromise regardless of the volume of thrombus, acute pulmonary hypertension, persistent hypoxemia despite anticoagulation, and evidence for right ventricular dysfunction.[33,35,36]

Contraindications for thrombolytic therapy are related to the increased risk for a bleeding complication. Unfortunately, no laboratory test will reliably predict which patient receiving a thrombolytic agent will suffer a bleeding complication.[36,37] Therefore, screening patients with a careful history and physical examination and a review of old medical records is extremely important. Absolute contraindications to thrombolytic therapy include active or recent internal bleeding, a history of a hemorrhagic stroke, intracranial or intraspinal disease, recent cranial surgery, or recent head or spinal trauma. Relative contraindications include major surgery or trauma within 14 days, recent cardiopulmonary resuscitation with active chest compressions, recent biopsy or invasive procedure in a location inaccessible to external compression, nonhemorrhagic stroke, hemorrhagic retinopathy, uncontrolled severe hypertension, or a severe coagulation defect (i.e., platelet count $< 100,000$ mm^3).

Advocates of lytic therapy suggest that treatment in this era is less risky than quoted in earlier reports since the mechanism of action of thrombolytic agents and the risk factors that predispose patients to bleeding are better understood. Indeed, a recent multicenter trial demonstrated only a 4% incidence of severe bleeding.[38] Intracranial bleeding occurs in less than 1% of patients treated with thrombolytic therapy.[36]

If major bleeding occurs, the thrombolytic therapy should be discontinued. If bleeding continues despite discontinuation of therapy, coagulation factors should be replenished. Fresh frozen plasma is a source of factors V and VIII as well as α_2-antiplasmin, fibrinogen, and several other active coagulation factors. Fresh frozen plasma may take 45 min to thaw. Cryoprecipitate can be obtained from the blood bank quicker than fresh frozen plasma. Each unit of cryoprecipitate contains about 200 to 500 mg of fibrinogen and 80 units of factor VIII in a volume of 10 to 15 cc. Therefore, 10 units of cryoprecipitate will increase the fibrinogen level by about 70 mg/dl and the factor level VIII to about 30% of normally circulating levels.[36,39] Minor oozing of blood can usually be managed with manual pressure. Occasional idiosyncratic reactions such as rigors can be managed with intravenous meperidine.[36,40]

Although complication rates associated with the use of urokinase appear to be less than with the use of streptokinase, there has been no clear demonstration of any benefit of urokinase over rt-PA.[27,41,42] When comparing the results achieved with peripheral versus intrapulmonary infusion of rt-PA, similar rates of lysis, bleeding, and induction of a systemic lytic state have been noted.[43]

Despite this, experience with peripheral arterial bypass grafts and thrombosed dialysis fistulas has demonstrated that catheter-directed thrombolysis is associated with better rates of lysis, more rapid lysis, the need for lower doses, and fewer complications.[44-48] In addition, when comparing the use of urokinase versus streptokinase with peripheral arterial occlusions, urokinase has been found to be more clinically beneficial and cost-effective.[49,50] The theoretical advantages for direct, intrathrombus instillation of urokinase include direct activation of clot-bound plasminogen with minimal activation of free-circulating plasminogen, delivery of high local doses of the agent to the thrombus while minimizing systemic concentrations, reduce overall doses of the agent given, and the ability to easily monitor intrapulmonary pressures. Therefore, there is some enthusiasm for catheter-directed, intrathrombus administration of urokinase for acute PE.[51]

Several investigators have reported on the use of intrapulmonary urokinase for acute PE.[52,53] In one study, 13 patients were treated with urokinase for angiographically proven PE within 14 days of major surgery.[52] The catheter was positioned in the pulmonary artery clot and 2,200 IU/kg was injected directly into the clot. This was followed by a continuous infusion of urokinase at 2,200 IU/kg/hr until the clot lysed or up to a maximum of 24 hr. Concomitant heparin was also administered at a rate of 500 U/hr. The serum fibrinogen level was monitored every 6 hr and maintained at no less than 200 mg/dl. Follow-up pulmonary angiography at 24 hr revealed that 98% of the clots had completely disappeared from the pulmonary vasculature. No deaths or bleeding complications occurred. Two patients received an inferior vena cava filter. In another series, 16 patients with massive PE were given a bolus of 500,000 IU of urokinase directly into the clot, followed by an attempt to break up the clot using the tip of the catheter.[53] An infusion of 1,000,000 IU of urokinase was then given into the right atrium over a 12-hr period. No concomitant heparin was administered. Cardiac output, total pulmonary vascular resistance, and mean pulmonary artery pressures all improved following the thrombolytic therapy. The mean improvement for each parameter studied was statistically significant ($p < 0.001$). All patients survived, and in no case did the urokinase therapy fail. One patient did suffer a severe bleeding complication.

Based upon the above studies and our experience with thrombolysis of peripheral arterial bypass grafts, we have made an attempt to be more aggressive in treatment of acute PE, even in the presence of a relative contraindication (Figures 2.1 and 2.2). Pa-

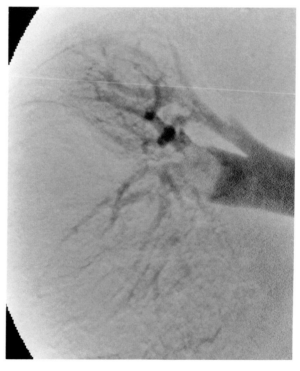

A

Figure 2.1 A 27-yr-old female on estrogen and status-post bone marrow transplant for Hodgkin's disease developed the acute onset of shortness of breath after a 6-hr airplane trip. **A.** The diagnostic arteriogram revealed large emboli in the interlobar and the apical segmental arteries on the right. The left pulmonary artery was free of embolic disease. The patient had known upper lobe fibrosis from radiation therapy. She also had received chemotherapy known to induce pulmonary fibrosis. It was elected to undertake thrombolytic therapy. She was hemodynamically stable, although she did have a resting heart rate of 120 bpm. Her mean pulmonary artery pressure was 15 mm Hg. The patient's platelet count was 100,000 mm³. **B.** Following page.

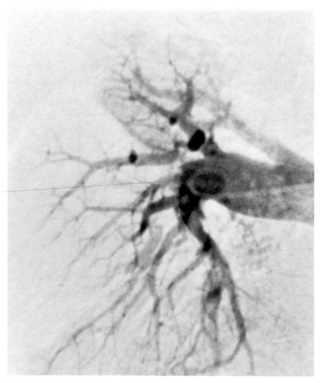

B

Figure 2.1 B. After 10 hr of urokinase infusion at 100,000 IU/hr directly into the clot with a pigtail catheter, follow-up angiography showed significant improvement in the right lower lobe perfusion. Systemic heparin was also given throughout the urokinase therapy. Symptoms improved and the urokinase infusion was terminated.

tients are carefully screened for an absolute contraindication for thrombolytic therapy. Pulmonary angiography is performed to document the presence and distribution of PE and to measure pulmonary arterial and right heart pressures. If the patient is unable to lay supine, the pulmonary angiogram is performed from a basilic vein approach. Otherwise, the study is usually performed from the femoral vein approach. If there is a large volume of central clot or an asymmetric amount of thrombus involving one lung in association with either right ventricular dysfunction, compromised hemodynamics (hypotension or tachycardia), or persistent hypoxemia despite anticoagulation, catheter-directed intrapulmonary thrombolytic therapy is initiated.

The diagnostic pulmonary arterial catheter is removed over a guidewire, maintaining access in the pulmonary artery. An appropriate-size introducer sheath (usually 6-Fr or 7-Fr) is inserted into the femoral or basilic vein and sutured in place. This is connected to a heparinized saline flush (4,000 IU heparin/1,000 cc normal saline), which is infused at 30 cc/hr. A 5- or 6-Fr pigtail catheter is then advanced over the guidewire and embedded into the clot. Next, 250,000 U of urokinase are mixed with 3,000 U of heparin and given as a bolus into the clot. A continuous urokinase infusion is then given through the pulmonary arterial catheter at a rate of 80,000–200,000 IU/hr. The infusion rate depends upon the size of the patient and the risk factors for bleeding. Systemic heparin is also administered to maintain the partial thromboplastin time at 1.5 to 2.5 times the upper limits of normal. Fibrinogen levels are monitored at 4 to 6-hr intervals. If there is a rapid decrease in the systemic fibrinogen level, the urokinase infusion rate is decreased. If the fibrinogen level falls to less than 100 mg/dl, the urokinase infusion is terminated. We have encountered one patient in whom the

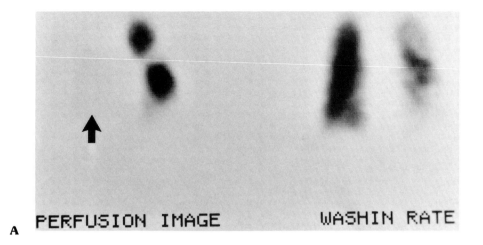

A

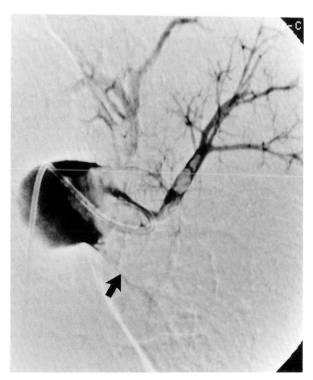

B

Figure 2.2 A 65-yr-old male presented with an acutely threatened left lower extremity secondary to peripheral vascular disease. Three days after a successful in situ saphenous vein bypass graft from the left common femoral artery to the posterior tibial artery, the patient developed acute shortness of breath, hypotension, and a near-syncopal episode. **A.** A ventilation/perfusion lung scan in the posterior projection revealed no perfusion to the left lung (arrow) with relatively normal ventilation (right-hand side of figure). There are also some perfusion abnormalities involving the right lung. Despite the initiation of anticoagulation, the patient remained unstable. His oxygen saturation was 91% on a 100% nonrebreather mask. **B.** A digital substraction pulmonary angiogram using a hand injection of nonionic contrast demonstrated a large embolus (arrow) in the left main pulmonary artery. The mean pulmonary artery pressure was 40 mm Hg. An inferior vena cava filter was placed and then a pigtail catheter was embedded into the PE. Following a 250,000 IU bolus of urokinase, an infusion was initiated at 100,000 IU/hr. The patient was systemically heparinized. **C.** Following page.

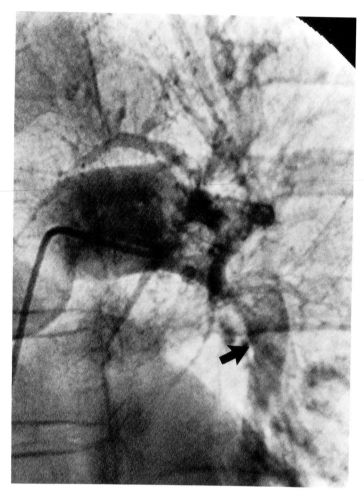

C

Figure 2.2 C. After 16 hr of urokinase infusion, a repeat angiogram showed improved flow to the left lower lobe (arrow). The mean pulmonary pressure decreased to 30 mm Hg. Oxygen saturation increased to 95% on a 60% nonrebreather mask. Urokinase therapy was terminated. The supplemental oxygen was rapidly tapered over a 2-day period.

clot was relatively resistant to lysis. In this patient, use of a multisidehole, pulse-spray catheter and manual pulse-spraying resulted in further clot lysis (Figure 2.3).

The bleeding rates that were reported from the thrombolytic trials in the 1970s are not currently applicable. A better understanding of the mechanism of action of thrombolysis, improved catheter and guidewire technology, the greater use of intravascular sheaths, and the knowledge to minimize invasive procedures and vascular punctures has decreased the incidence of significant bleeding complications.[38] The argument that most patients with acute PE will have a contraindication for thrombolytic therapy is not supported by a large patient survey which revealed that 50% of patients with high-probability lung scans or pulmonary angiographic evidence for PE are acceptable candidates for treatment with thrombolysis.[54] Since the mortality rate associated with acute PE has not changed in the past 30 yr, widespread use of thrombolysis should be strongly considered. However, when diffuse bilateral pulmonary emboli are present, intravenous administration of the thrombolytic agent is probably just as beneficial as catheter-directed lysis.[43]

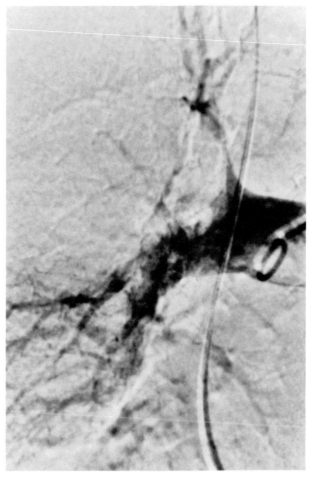

A

Figure 2.3 A 71-yr-old female presented with the acute onset of shortness of breath, hypotension, and marked hypoxemia despite supplemental oxygen. A. A digital subtraction angiogram performed from a right basilic vein approach demonstrated a large clot occluding the majority of the right truncus anterior and a portion of the right lower and middle lobe vessels. B, C, and D. Following pages.

Surgical Embolectomy

Patients with massive central PE can have markedly compromised hemodynamics and develop irreversible cardiocirculatory shock. If they are too unstable to undergo or have a contraindication to thrombolytic therapy, the only remaining therapeutic options for these patients are percutaneous or surgical embolectomy or clot fragmentation. Traditionally, surgical embolectomy has been associated with a high perioperative mortality rate. With improvements in anesthesia and cardiopulmonary bypass technology, 30-day survival rates after surgical pulmonary embolectomy have been reported to be as high as 62.5–84.3% at centers specializing in the treatment of thromboembolic disease.[55,56]

Yet, surgical embolectomy is still associated with significant morbidity and mortality and very few centers in the United States have extensive experience with this type

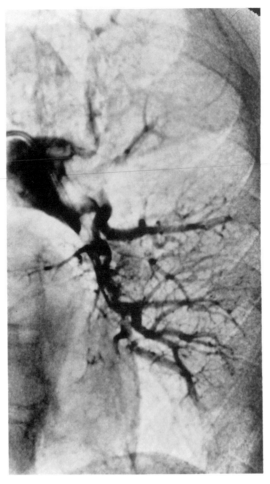

B

Figure 2.3 B. A large volume of clot was also present in the left main pulmonary artery. The mean pulmonary artery pressure increased from 27 to 45 mm Hg after two hand injections of nonionic contrast. An inferior vena cava filter was placed. Subsequently, a pigtail catheter was embedded into the left pulmonary artery clot. A 250,000 IU bolus of urokinase was given and an infusion was initiated at 100,000 IU/hr. The patient was also systemically heparinized. C and D. Following pages.

of surgery. Therefore, percutaneous transvenous devices designed to remove or fragment centrally obstructing PE are being developed. Of all the devices that have been used or tested in this setting, the Greenfield suction embolectomy device is the only one that is currently FDA-approved.

Percutaneous Embolectomy

Greenfield Embolectomy Device

The Greenfield device (Boston Scientific, Natick, MA) is a 10-F braided catheter with an 0.045-inch internal diameter (ID). The tip of the catheter has threads on it that allow the use of either a 5-mm or 7-mm-diameter plastic cup (Figure 2.4). The catheter is maneuvered by using a large control handle, and is designed for insertion via a femoral or jugular venotomy. More recently, 16F sheaths with hemostatic valves (Cook Inc, Bloomington, In) have become available and allow advancement and withdrawal

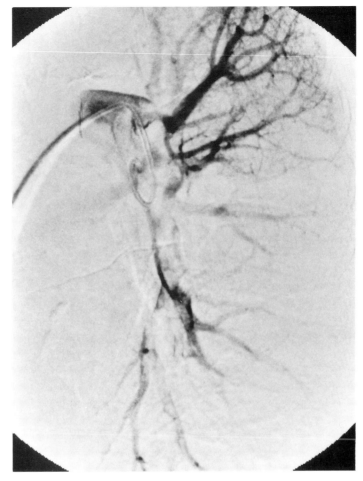

C

Figure 2.3 C. After 18 hr of urokinase infusion, there was slight improvement to left lower lobe perfusion. Because of the slow progression of clot lysis, using a multisidehole catheter, urokinase was either pulse-sprayed or drip-infused directly into the clot. **D.** Following page.

of the catheter with a 5 mm cup on it. Once the cup on the catheter tip comes in contact with the embolic material, manual suction is generated via a side port on the control handle. The catheter and the clot are then removed as a unit through the venotomy site or a vascular sheath. Multiple passes with the catheter may be required. Dr. Greenfield and his colleagues have reported on their experience using this device in 46 patients over a 22-yr period.[57] Emboli were extracted in 35 (76%) of 46 patients. There was an average reduction in mean pulmonary artery pressure of 8 mm Hg and a significant increase in mean cardiac output after embolectomy. The 30-day mortality rate was 30%. When subgroups of patients were analyzed, embolectomy was most successful for major and submassive PE, and least likely to be helpful in patients with chronic, recurrent PE. Timsit et al. also reported on their experience with the Greenfield device.[58] The procedure was considered unsuccessful in 7 of 18 patients. Three (43%) of these 7 patients died during their hospitalization. The remaining 11 (61%) patients immediately improved, but 2 (18%) of these 11 patients did not survive their hospital stay.

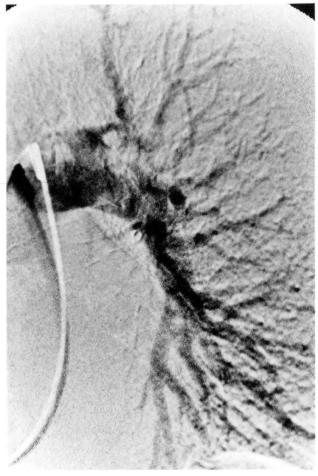

D

Figure 2.3 D. A repeat arteriogram at 51 hr showed further improvement. The patient's mean pulmonary artery pressure decreased to 27 mm Hg and did not increase after injection of contrast material. Urokinase infusion was terminated. The patient's dyspnea was markedly improved. The supplemental oxygen was rapidly tapered and discontinued. The patient was discharged following full oral anticoagulation.

Other than the two reported series described above, experience with the Greenfield suction embolectomy catheter has been relatively small. The device is somewhat bulky, requires familiarity with the control handle, and is primarily designed for insertion via a surgical venotomy. There are no standard introducer sheaths that are currently available for use with the 7-mm suction cup.

Several other percutaneous devices are currently being evaluated for possible application in the treatment of acute PE. Most of these devices incorporate concepts of mechanical fragmentation or hydrodynamic maceration and aspiration.

Hydrodynamic Thrombectomy (Hydrolyser) Catheter

The Hydrolyser catheter (Cordis Europa, Roden, Netherlands) is a straight, 7-Fr double-lumen catheter, 65 cm in length, with a 6-mm-diameter oval sidehole located 4 mm from its distal tip.[59] The catheter is made of nylon and has a relatively stiff body. The distal, rounded tip was initially closed, but in its newest version, it is open to al-

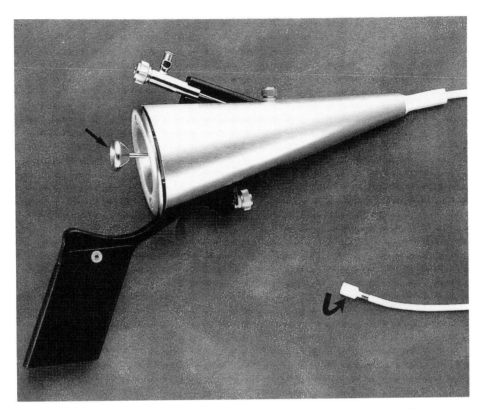

Figure 2.4 The Greenfield suction embolectomy device consists of a large handle with a "joy stick" (straight arrow) which is used to control the steerable catheter. A 5-mm cup (curved arrow) is seen on the end of the catheter.

low passage of an 0.025-inch guidewire. The catheter is designed to be introduced through a 7-Fr sheath. One of the two lumens consists of a narrow (0.6 mm) injection channel with its distal tip oriented 180° opposite the tip of the catheter. Saline is injected through the small injection channel at a constant flow rate of 3 cc per second, up to a maximum pressure of 750 psi using a standard contrast injector (Medrad, Pittsburgh, PA). The saline exits the catheter as a high-velocity (150 km/hr) saline jet in a retrograde direction, directed over the sidehole near the tip of the catheter. This effect results in a lower pressure in the sidehole (Venturi effect). Because of the pressure gradient, the thrombotic material is drawn into the sidehole, where it is fragmented by the saline jet. The debris is removed through the second lumen, a larger (1.0 mm) efferent channel. The efferent lumen is connected to a collection bag (Figure 2.5). No suction is required. The removed volume of fluid is equal to the injected volume plus an admixture of fragmented clot and blood. The total output in the collection bag usually does not exceed the saline input by more than 20%.[59]

The thrombus suction technique using the Hydrolyser catheter has been demonstrated to be effective at removing clots in peripheral arteries and veins, as well as dialysis fistulas.[59-61] It is designed for use in vessels 5–9 mm in diameter. When used in larger vessels, the device tends to open a defined tract within the clot, but it does not promote removal of the entire clot burden. Application of the Hydrolyser catheter in the pulmonary arterial circulation appears to be limited at this time.

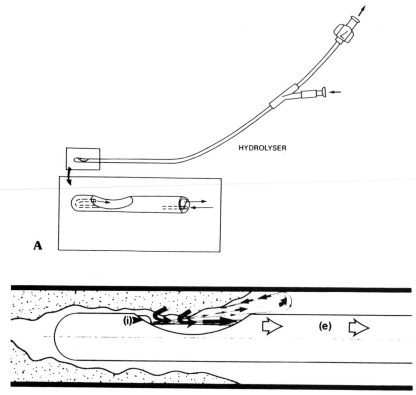

Figure 2.5 The Hydrolyser catheter is a 7-Fr double-lumen catheter with a blunt end. **A.** An injection channel is oriented 180° opposite the tip of the catheter. The fluid jet is directed across an oval sidehole into the discharge collection channel. (Reprinted with permission from van Ommen et al.[60]) **B.** A drawing of the Hydrolyser catheter in a blood vessel shows the fluid jet (large straight arrow) originating from the injection channel (i) and directed across the open hole at the distal tip of the catheter. The Venturi effect is created (smaller arrows). Thrombotic material is drawn in the sidehole where it is fragmented by the saline jet and discharged via the efferent collection channel (e).

Rheolytic Thrombectomy Catheter

The Rheolytic Thrombectomy Catheter uses high-velocity saline jets to macerate thrombus, while allowing withdrawal of the resulting debris via the same catheter. It is a double-lumen catheter that is made in several diameters (4 to 6 Fr). The smaller lumen is made from a tiny stainless steel tube which allows the injection of saline at pressures up to 30,000 psi. The small lumen also communicates with a latex balloon. The balloon is inflated to help center the catheter and occlude vessel flow during operation. The larger lumen is used to evacuate the debris that is generated, but it can also be used as an injection or guidewire port. The stainless steel tubing at the catheter tip has 4 to 8 jet orifices 25–50 μm in diameter. One of the jets is directed into the catheter orifice to facilitate evacuation of the clot debris. The remaining jets are oriented in a retrograde fashion, but angled to avoid direct impact on the vessel wall, while providing the necessary mechanical forces to effect clot maceration and breakdown. A positive displacement pump provides the power for the saline jets and is activated by a foot switch by the operator.[62] Fluid is removed through the exhaust lumen at the same rate that it is infused (Figure 2.6).

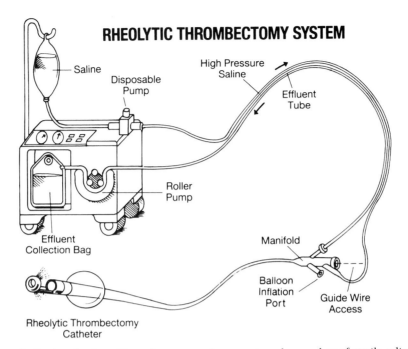

Figure 2.6 The Rheolytic Thrombectomy catheter system shows a bag of sterile saline supplying a disposable pump. The pump pressurizes the system to allow saline injection under high pressure. The balloon inflation port and the guidewire lumen are shown. A nondisposable unit drives the disposable high-pressure pump and the roller pump is used to limit the flow of thrombus debris in the exhaust fluid. The thrombus debris is transported through the efferent channel of the catheter to a disposable collection bag. (Reprinted with permission from Drasler et al.[62])

The Rheolytic catheter can be inserted over a wire through an appropriate-size introducer sheath. The device has been used in vitro and in vivo with some success, although the high-velocity jets could potentially cause endothelial damage.[63] Although its application in the setting of PE has been entertained, the Rheolytic catheter has yet to be used in this clinical setting.

Impeller-Basket Device

The Impeller-Basket Device consists of a small impeller 2.5 mm in length and 2.3 mm in diameter, which is mounted on a flexible shaft and fixed between two revolving bearings within the center of a self-expandable basket (Figure 2.7). The basket consists of four spiral-shaped wires mounted on the tip of a 7-Fr catheter. The basket has a 20-mm floppy tip. The impeller is driven by a 0.5-mm rotating wire and is connected to an external electric motor drive which can produce rotational speeds up to 100,000 rpm. The expanded basket centers the impeller within the vessel lumen, in theory, minimizing trauma to the vessel wall. The rotation of the impeller creates a hydrodynamic vortex which pulls thrombotic material into the basket, fragmenting the clot material (Figure 2.8). The device is designed to be inserted through a 7-Fr sheath that is long enough to be placed into the pulmonary arteries.[64]

The Impeller-Basket has been tested in vitro and in vivo. In vitro, 5-day-old clots were treated in a glass model. More than 90% of the particles generated with the Impeller Device were smaller than 10 μm, while 5.5% of the particles were larger than 1,000 μm.[65] In animal experiments, 7 of 9 artificially created emboli were completely

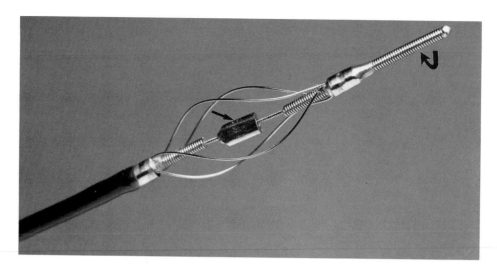

Figure 2.7 The Impeller-Basket Device is shown. The central impeller (straight arrow) can rotate up to 100,000 rpm. A vortex is created that draws the clot material through the wire basket, causing fragmentation of the clot. There is a flexible tip on the catheter (curved arrow).

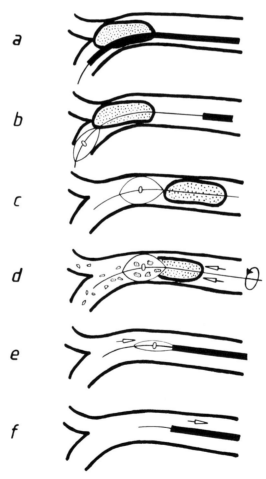

Figure 2.8 The Impeller-Basket Device is designed to be inserted through a 7-Fr guiding sheath beyond the embolus (a). Once the Device is advanced through the sheath beyond the embolus, the guiding catheter is retracted to expose the basket (b). The clot can then be retracted into a larger, central vessel (c). The impeller is then activated and clot fragmentation occurs (d). Following clot fragmentation, the guiding sheath is advanced over the basket (e) and the guiding catheter and basket are removed as a unit (f). (Reprinted with permission from Schmitz-Rode et al.[65])

fragmented in less than 10 sec (Figure 2.9). Free plasma hemoglobin levels did not increase in the animals after treatment.[64] Autopsy evaluation did not show any macroscopic or microscopic wall damage to the vessel at the impeller site in any of the animals. The limitation of the device is its relative stiffness and lack of steerability. In addition, subsegmental occlusions remained in the animal models following treatment, indicating that not all the resulting fragments are as small as the in vitro tests suggest.[65]

Thrombolizer and Modified Impeller Catheter

The Thrombolizer and modified Impeller are two high-speed, rotating catheters which are similar in design and operation. They are both designed to be used through a vascular sheath. The Thrombolizer is a thrombectomy catheter that is commercially available in Europe (Cordis, Europa). The Thrombolizer system consists of an 8-Fr outer catheter with an inner 5-Fr catheter that protrudes 7 cm from the tip of the 8-Fr outer catheter. The inner 5-Fr catheter has four, longitudinal slits, each 15 mm in length, in its distal portion. The inner catheter is designed to rotate relative to the 8-Fr, outer catheter. The four bands in the distal portion of the 5-Fr catheter are flat when the 5-Fr catheter is not rotating. When the inner catheter begins to rotate, the centrifugal forces cause the flat bands to open into a basketlike shape to a diameter that is dependent upon the rotational speed (Figure 2.10). The device has a central 0.035-inch lumen.

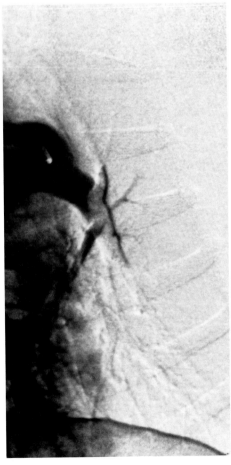

A

Figure 2.9 A. Experimentally induced pulmonary embolism in an animal is seen in the left main pulmonary artery. B. Following page.

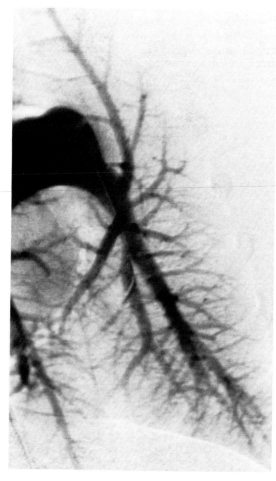

B

Figure 2.9 B. Following percutaneous Impeller-Basket fragmentation of the embolus, there is significant improvement to the left lung perfusion.

The Impeller catheter is an over-the-wire system and is modified from the previously described Impeller-Basket device. The Impeller catheter is made of Teflon, with an outer 8-Fr catheter and inner, rotating 5-Fr catheter. It is designed to track over an 0.035-inch guidewire. The outer catheter opens to a 10-mm-diameter protective basket, once its exits the introducer sheath. The inner catheter can rotate independently of the outer catheter and opens to a basket 5 mm in diameter. The diameter of the inner basket is independent of the rotational speed.

Both the Thrombolizer and Impeller catheter systems are driven by an automatic turbine which can rotate the inner catheters at speeds of 100,000 to 150,000 rpm. At rapid rotational speeds, a strong vortex is created by the rotating baskets, exerting a suction effect on the surrounding thrombotic material. The clot is then fragmented into small pieces by the spinning baskets.[66]

Both of these devices have been tested in animals with artificially induced PE. The Thrombolizer did not rotate properly with its original automatic drive and required a significant modification to work effectively. The Thrombolizer was effective in only 1 of 5 animals. In one animal, despite moderate recanalization on one side, the tip of the Thrombolizer catheter broke off when attempting to treat the other side. The Impeller catheter demonstrated more reliable rotational function in all treatment sessions. In the majority of animals, moderate to complete recanalization was achieved with this

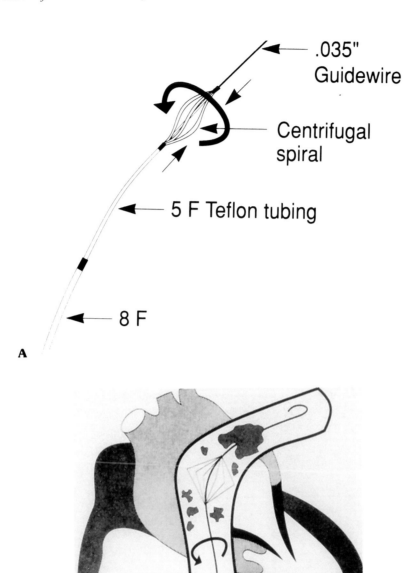

Figure 2.10 A. A drawing of the Thrombolizer catheter demonstrates the 5-Fr Teflon tubing with four slits in its distal aspect. There is a guidewire lumen. With activation of the rotational motor, the four flat bands in the distal catheter assume a more basket-like shape due to the centrifugal forces. B. The drawing demonstrates the theoretical application of the Thrombolizer catheter for PE. With rapid rotation, the Thrombolizer catheter opens up and mechanically fragments clot.

device. Although both fragmentation catheters were able to clear occluded main pulmonary arteries in several instances, side branches were partly obstructed by the resulting fragments. In the cases in which some successful fragmentation occurred, there was a statistically significant decrease in pulmonary artery pressures. Histologic evaluation at the sites of treatment showed considerable periarterial and peribronchial hemorrhage, more prominent in the animals treated with the Thrombolizer catheter.

There are no reports of these devices being used in humans for the treatment of PE. Localized vascular trauma to the pulmonary arterial circulation may limit their clinical application.

Rotatable Pigtail Catheter

The Rotatable Pigtail Catheter is a custom-made modification of a high-torque 5-Fr pigtail catheter. It is 110 cm in length and has 10 sideholes for contrast injection. It also has a radiopaque tip (Figure 2.11). At the outer curvature of the pigtail loop, an oval sidehole is present along the axis of the catheter shaft. The catheter is introduced into a flexible 5.5-Fr sheath with a radiopaque marker at its tip, a valve for hemostasis, and a sideport at its proximal end. The catheter is designed to be used over an 0.035-inch movable-core J wire. An electrical motor is connected to the Luer-lock adapter on the proximal end of the catheter and can generate rotational speeds up to 500 rpm. The pigtail catheter is designed to rotate within the sheath with a guidewire exiting through the distal sidehole. The sheath prevents precessing of the catheter shaft, thereby minimizing damage along the venous access route. The wire serves as a rigid central access for pigtail rotation. During activation of the electrical motor, the catheter can be advanced and pulled back over the wire. The catheter can also be used for follow-up angiograms after clot fragmentation.[67]

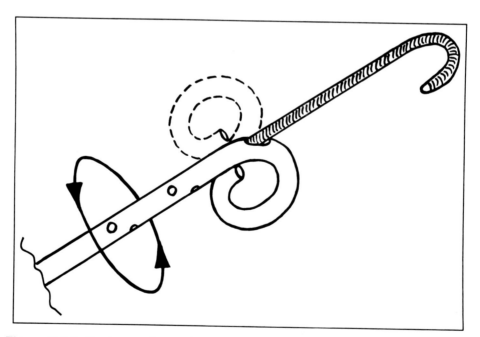

Figure 2.11 The drawing depicts the rotation of the pigtail catheter about the axis of a stationary guidewire. Emboli are fragmented by the mechanical action of the rotating catheter loop. During rotation, the pigtail catheter can be advanced or withdrawn over the guidewire. Sideholes are present within the catheter to allow contrast injection after the fragmentation procedure. (Reprinted with permission from Schmitz-Rode et al.[67])

The rotational movement of the pigtail portion of the catheter acts directly upon the clots in the pulmonary arteries, causing fragmentation and distal migration of the smaller fragments. The volume of the peripheral pulmonary arteries is approximately 2 times that of the central pulmonary arteries. Therefore, redistribution of a large, central clot may acutely improve cardiopulmonary hemodynamics. Clots located in a more distal location can also be managed by advancing the catheter and manually rotating the pigtail catheter with the handle, while closely observing the shape of the pigtail tip. When the pigtail shape is deformed by the size of the vessel, the rotation is stopped. No damage to the tip of the catheter is generally observed.

Although experience with the Rotatable Pigtail Catheter is still preliminary and experimental, a few unreported clinical cases from Germany have been encouraging.

Amplatz Thrombectomy Device

The Amplatz Thrombectomy Device (ATD) (Microvena, White Bear Lake, MN) consists of a 120-cm-long, 8-Fr, polyurethane catheter with an impeller mounted on a drive shaft inside a metal cap 5 mm in length. The metal cap has three sideports which are used for recirculation of clot particles (Figure 2.12). An air turbine can generate up to 150,000 rpm at 50 psi.[68–70] The high speed of the impeller creates a vortex that recirculates and pulverizes acute clot, creating a fluid with very small, suspended particles (95% smaller than 13 μm).[71] There are two sideports in the distal catheter that allow for high-pressure infusion of saline to reduce friction and cool the system or to inject contrast medium to facilitate visualization during fluoroscopic manipulation.[68–70,72,73] This device is currently FDA-approved for use in thrombosed dialysis fistulas.

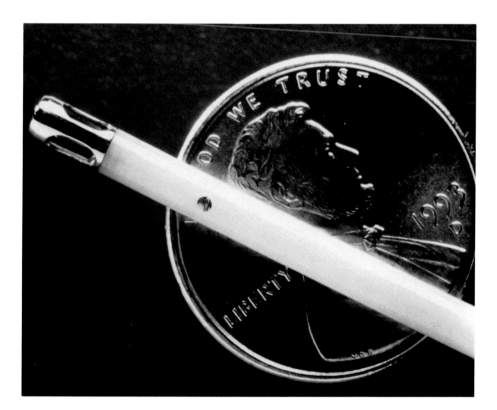

A

Figure 2.12 A. The Amplatz thrombectomy device (ATD) is shown with a penny as a reference for size.

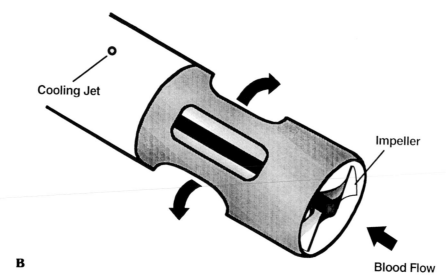

B

Figure 2.12 B. A drawing of the distal tip of the ATD shows a recessed impeller within a 5-mm metal capsule. Thrombus is aspirated, liquefied, and then expelled through the sideports (curved arrows).

Access into the pulmonary artery is achieved using standard angiographic techniques from a percutaneous femoral vein approach. Pressure measurements and pulmonary angiography are performed, and the extent of PE determined. An 0.038-inch exchange length wire (260 cm) is used to exchange the diagnostic catheter for a multipurpose 10-Fr guiding catheter that is 95 cm in length (Cordis, Miami, FL). The guiding catheter is positioned into the clot and the ATD is introduced through the guiding catheter. To avoid bends and kinks, the device should be introduced and advanced very carefully through the guiding catheter. Any bend or kink may produce breakage of the metal shaft inside the ATD catheter, necessitating its replacement. Mechanical thrombectomy is initiated with the ATD activated at full speed. The device is advanced in a slow, back-and-forth motion. The multipurpose configuration of the guiding catheter allows for some degree of steerability of the device inside the pulmonary artery. After thrombectomy with the ATD, some of the resulting fluid may be aspirated through the guiding catheter. Contrast medium can be injected through the guiding catheter to visualize the amount of residual clot. If there is persistent occlusion of the main pulmonary artery or a large pulmonary artery branch, the guiding catheter is advanced over a guidewire into the clot. The ATD is again advanced into the residual clot and activated. At the end of the procedure, pulmonary arterial pressures are measured, and a repeat pulmonary arteriogram is performed.

One of the authors of this chapter (R.U.) has treated five patients with massive PE using the ATD.[73] All patients were treated on a compassionate-use basis for life-threatening disease, and signed a special informed consent approved by the institutional review board (IRB). There were 4 males and 1 female, ranging in age from 25 to 64 yr (mean = 45 yr). All patients presented with some combination of anxiety, hypoxia, dyspnea, chest pain, metabolic acidosis, and a widened arterial to alveolar oxygen gradient (>15 mm Hg). Three of the five patients presented with moderate to severe hypotension. One patient presented with syncope. Two patients had symptoms of deep venous thrombosis and two patients had prior histories of PE. Two of the patients had a major surgical procedure performed 4 days (neurosurgery) and 2 months (heart

TABLE 2.2 Demographics and Information About the Patients With Massive PE Treated with the Amplatz Thrombectomy Device

Patient No.	Age	Sex	Risk Factors	Symptoms and Signs	Duration of Symptoms
1	40	M	Heart surgery, IV drug abuse, PPE	CP, A, D, H	Started 2 months before current symptoms, worsening over last 9 days
2	62	M	Neurosurgery, DVT	CP, A, D, H	4 days
3	25	M	Alcoholic cardiomyopathy	H, C, seizures, respiratory and cardiac arrest	2 days
4	35	F	DVT, PPE	A, D H	1 day
5	64	M	Diabetes, myocardial infarction, coronary angioplasty	CP, D, H, S tachycardia, metabolic acidosis	1 day

Abbreviations: CP = chest pain; D = dyspnea; H = hypotension; S = syncope; PPE = previous pulmonary embolism; DVT = deep vein thrombosis; C = cyanosis; A = anxiety.

surgery) before the embolic event. One patient was diabetic and had a myocardial infarction 12 months before the PE. Another patient with alcohol-induced cardiomyopathy presented with an enlarged heart and seizures, followed by a respiratory and cardiac arrest 8 hr before the procedure (Table 2.2).

Nuclear medicine lung scans provided strong evidence of massive PE in all patients. Massive PE was confirmed by pulmonary angiography in all patients (Table 2.3). Following mechanical thrombectomy with the 8-Fr ATD, repeat angiography and nuclear medicine scanning demonstrated good improvement in pulmonary perfusion in one patient and moderate improvement in three patients (Table 2.3). One patient developed a fatal complication shortly after the procedure and follow-up angiography and nuclear medicine lung scanning were not performed.

In the four surviving patients, there was immediate clinical improvement after the procedure, with reduction of dyspnea and resolution of hypotension and chest pain. However, there was no statistically significantly improvement in pulmonary artery pressures. In three patients, pulmonary artery pressures actually increased after mechanical thrombectomy. Improvement in arterial oxygenation and arterial–alveolar oxygen gradients were also not consistent (Table 2.4). All surviving patients were discharged within 8 days (3, 5, 4, and 8 days, respectively) after the thrombectomy treatment. Clinical follow-up at 7, 7, 14, and 18 months, respectively, showed improvement of exertional dyspnea in all four patients.

Mild arrhythmias occurred in all patients when the guiding catheter for the ATD was exchanged over the wire. Two major complications were observed following mechanical thrombectomy in two patients. Patient number 5 presented with massive hemoptysis at the end of the thrombectomy procedure. Postthrombectomy arteriography did not show any signs of extravasation, dissection, or vessel damage. It is believed that hemoptysis in such cases may be caused by the sudden reperfusion of high-pressure blood flow to an infarcted pulmonary artery territory.[74] Although the patient was intubated for a period of 12 hr for precautionary reasons, bleeding subsided spontaneously over several minutes, and no additional treatment was required. The patient was discharged 6 days after the event. In the one patient who died in the periprocedural period, thrombectomy had been completed and the device removed. During preparation for pressure measurements and a repeat arteriogram, the patient became restless, suffered a major seizure, and had a respiratory

TABLE 2.3 Quantitative Assessment of Pulmonary Circulation in Massive Pulmonary Embolism Before and After Mechanical Thrombectomy, According to The Miller's Index[32]

| | Before MT % Obstruction of Pulmonary Circulation | | | | After MT % Obstruction of Pulmonary Circulation | | | |
| | Right | | Left | | Right | | Left | |
Patient No.	Pulmonary Arteriography	V/Q scan	Pulmonary Arteriography	V/Q Scan	Pulmonary Arteriography	VQ scan	Pulmonary Arteriography	VQ scan
1	0	0	100	100	0	0	70	70
2	10	20	80	80	10	20	40	50
3	80	90	30	50	N/A	N/A	N/A	N/A
4	60	60	90	60	40	50	70	70
5	80	60	60	70	50	40	50	50

MT = mechanical thrombectomy; V/Q scan = ventilation/perfusion scan.

TABLE 2.4 Physiologic Parameters Before and After Mechanical Thrombectomy for Massive Pulmonary Embolism

Patient No.	Before MT			After MT			Clinical Outcome (Complications)
	BP (mm Hg)	PAP (mean)	$D_{A\text{-}a}\,O_2$ (mm Hg)	BP (mm Hg)	PAP (mean)	$D_{A\text{-}a}\,O_2$ (mm Hg)	
1	115/70	N/A	65	130/75	N/A	37	Moderate improvement
2	130/65	74/40 (52)	57	140/80	69/38 (46)	555	Marked improvement
3	120/60	70/40 (51)	91	130/75	119/52 (74)	N/A	Death (irreversible respiratory/cardiac arrest)
4	125/65	89/37 (59)	177	182/102	104/42 (64)	531	Moderate improvement
5	118/77	44/12 (25)	56	136/99	56/22 (37)	6	Moderate improvement (hemoptysis)

Abbreviations: BP = systemic blood pressure; PAP = pulmonary artery pressure; $D_{A\text{-}a}\,O_2$ = arterial–alveolar O_2 gradient; MT = mechanical thrombectomy.

and cardiac arrest. Emergency resuscitation was unsuccessful. Permission for necropsy was refused.

Free plasma hemoglobin increased above 50 mg/dl in all patients after the procedure, but dropped to a normal level within 24 hr. The ATD has a definite, but transient hemolytic effect.[75] Free plasma hemoglobin promotes intranephronal cast formation and can cause acute renal failure. Therefore, use of the ATD should be given careful consideration in patients with compromised renal function. However, no renal failure developed in this group of patients or in other patients treated with the ATD.[69,70] If the device is used in patients with borderline renal function, the activation time should probably be restricted to less than 5 min.[72]

Of note, the Thrombolizer, Impeller-Basket Device, Impeller Catheter, and Rotatable Pigtail Catheter may also cause hemolysis, although it has not been well documented in the literature. Other devices such as the Rheolytic catheter and the Hydrolyser do not appear to cause significant hemolysis. However, with the Rheolytic catheter and the Hydrolyser device, larger volumes of blood may be aspirated during the hydrolytic maceration process and possibly cause significant blood loss.

Based on the history, angiographic findings, results, and follow-up of patients un-

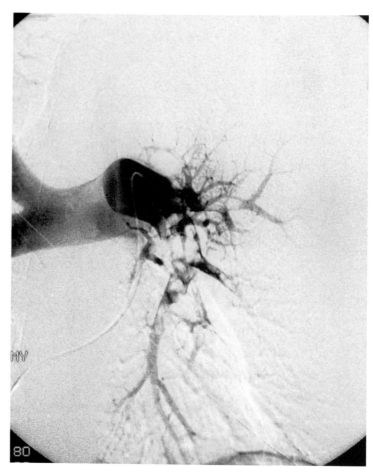

A

Figure 2.13 A 62-yr-old man with a history of high blood pressure and diabetes underwent surgery for an advanced acoustic neuroma. On the fourth postoperative day, he suffered a massive PE. **A.** A pulmonary angiogram revealed PE occluding the left main pulmonary artery. Due to the recent surgery, the use of fibrinolytic therapy was contraindicated. The angiographic catheter was exchanged for a 10-Fr guiding catheter and mechanical thrombectomy using the ATD was performed. Activation time was only 20 secs. **B, C,** and **D.** Following pages.

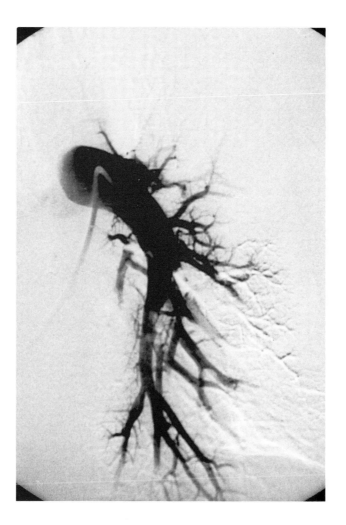

B

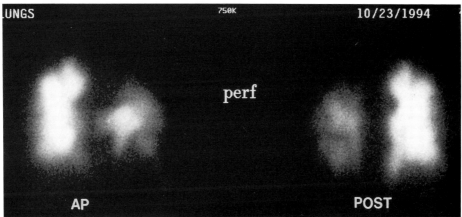

C

Figure 2.13 B. The postthrombectomy study showed improved pulmonary perfusion. C. The pretreatment perfusion lung scan demonstrated bilateral PE, greatest on the left side. **D.** Following page.

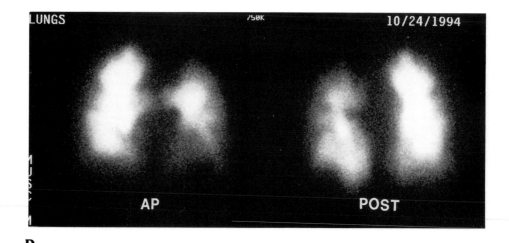

D

Figure 2.13 D. After thrombectomy, a repeat scan showed improved perfusion to the left lung.

dergoing mechanical thrombectomy with the ATD, three subgroups of patients with PE can be identified. Type I patients with fresh clots that have recently embolized appear to respond well to mechanical thrombectomy (Figure 2.13). In Type II patients with old, organized clots that have recently embolized, mechanical thrombectomy with the ATD is less effective (Figure 2.14). Type III patients with a history of old, organized chronic PE with recent worsening secondary to recurrent PE respond least to the effects of mechanical thrombectomy (Figure 2.15).

Text continues on page 57

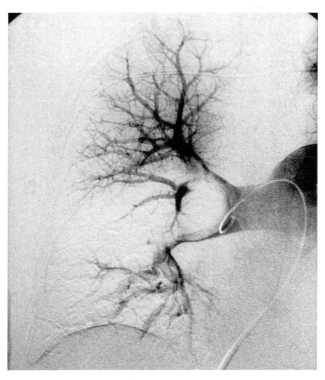

A

Figure 2.14 A 64-yr-old man with a history of diabetes and a prior myocardial infarction, and 1 yr status postcoronary angioplasty, was admitted with the acute onset of dyspnea, chest pain, tachycardia, hypotension, metabolic acidosis, and hypoxemia. A. A pulmonary arteriogram shows massive PE in the main right pulmonary artery, **B, C, D, E, F, G,** and **H.** Following pages.

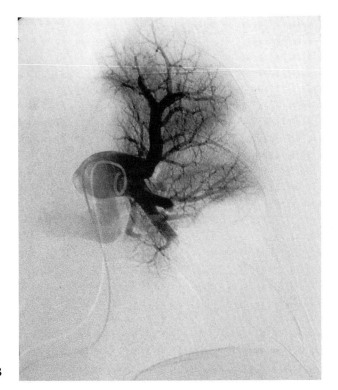

B

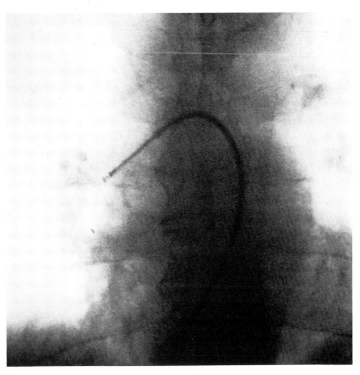

C

Figure 2.14 B. and a large filling defect within the main left pulmonary artery. C. and D. The diagnostic catheter was exchanged for a 10-Fr guiding catheter and the ATD was used to debulk the PE on both sides. Total activation time was 8 min 11 sec. D, E, F, G, and H. Following pages.

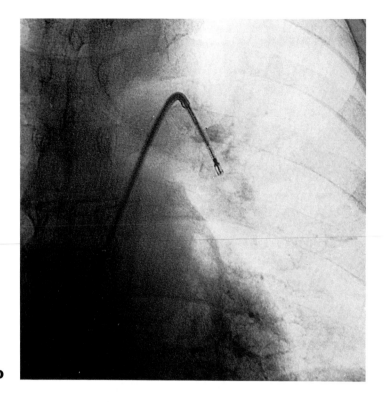

D

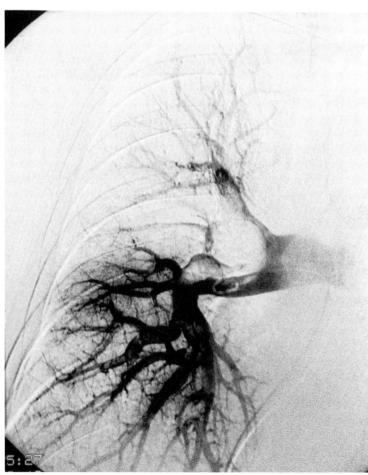

E

Figure 2.14 E. After thrombectomy, there is improved perfusion to the right lower lobe. F, G, and H. Following pages.

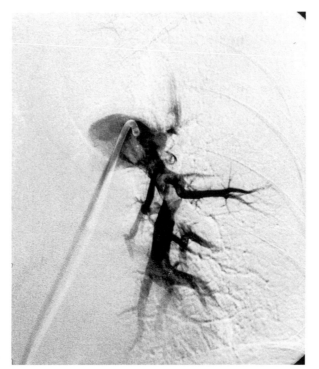

F

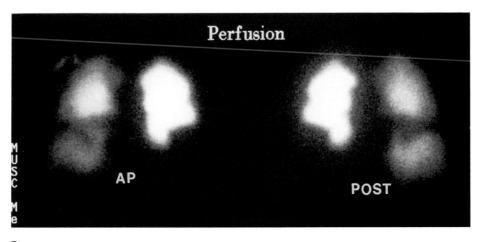

G

Figure 2.14 F. After the thrombectomy on the left side, the patient experienced severe hemoptysis (approximately 900 cc). The post-thrombectomy pulmonary arteriogram revealed better perfusion to the left lower lobe and no extravasation of contrast media. Persistent large filling defects remained. G. The prethrombectomy perfusion lung scan showed reduced perfusion to both lungs consistent with massive PE. H. Following page.

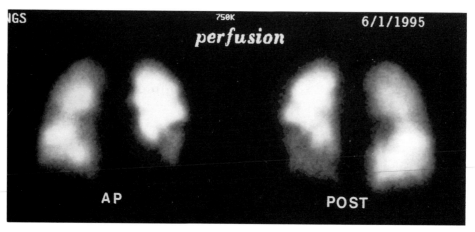

H

Figure 2.14 H. A follow-up perfusion lung scan 12 hr after the procedure showed improved pulmonary perfusion.

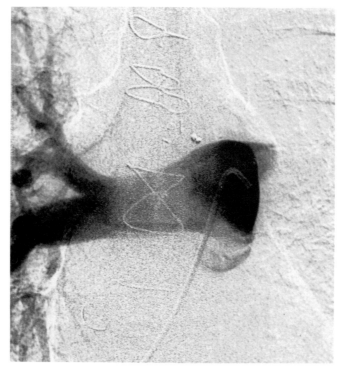

A

Figure 2.15 A 40-yr-old male with a prior history of PE and a past history of drug abuse, multiple lung abscesses requiring surgical treatment, and surgery for tricuspid valve endocarditis 2 yr earlier, presented with a 2-month history of progressive shortness of breath and chest pain, with recent worsening over the past 9 days. A. A pulmonary arteriogram showed complete obstruction of the left pulmonary artery. B, C, D, E, and F. Following pages.

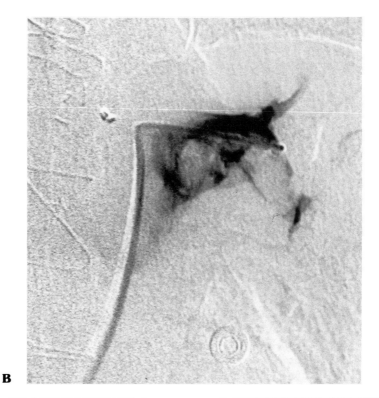

B

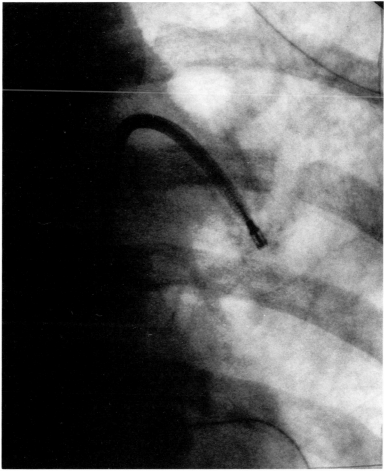

C

Figure 2.15 B. The catheter was left in place in contact with the clot, and an infusion of urokinase at 60,000 IU/h for 6 hr and 100,000 IU/h for 18 hr was performed. Follow-up angiography showed minimal interval change in the total occlusion of the left pulmonary artery. C. The angiographic catheter was then exchanged over a guidewire for a 10-Fr guiding catheter and mechanical thrombectomy with the ATD was performed. Total activation time was 7 min 58 sec. D, E, and F. Following pages.

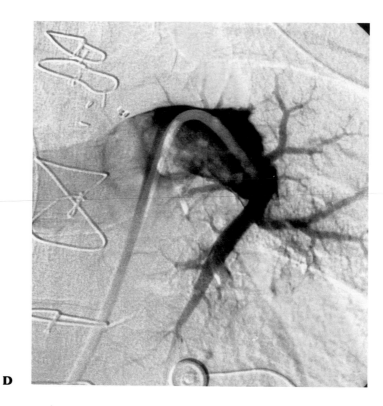

D

E

Figure 2.15 D. Repeat angiography revealed partial resolution of the large thrombus in the left main pulmonary artery with some peripheral fragments. Following completion of the mechanical thrombectomy, infusion of urokinase was restarted at 100,000 IU/hr for an additional 24 hr. A follow-up angiogram demonstrated no significant change in the appearance, indicating organized pulmonary emboli. E. Initial perfusion scan shows no perfusion to the left lung. F. Following page.

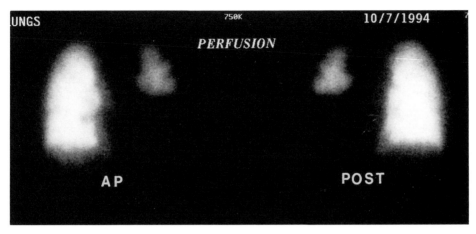

F

Figure 2.15 F. Follow-up perfusion scan 4 months after the mechanical thrombectomy shows some perfusion to the left upper lobe, but no significant change in the left lower lobe.

SUMMARY

Critical factors affecting the natural course of acute PE are the age of the embolic material, the effectiveness of in vivo fibrinolysis, and the occurrence of in situ fragmentation and redistribution of the clot material.[1] Although older, organized thrombotic material is more likely to be adherent to the venous wall and less likely to embolize, when it does embolize, it tends to pass unaltered into the heart and pulmonary circulation, and frequently gets stuck in the main pulmonary artery.[74] When acute or fresh thrombi embolize, they tend to dissipate or fragment into pieces on passage through the right ventricle, causing more peripheral, less compact emboli. It is easy to understand why an older clot that has embolized is more difficult to fragment and dissolve with fibrinolysis, but it is still unclear why some acute emboli do not resolve in some patients. It is possible that an acute embolus can occasionally follow an aberrant path of organization and recanalization, and leave endothelial residua that obstruct or significantly narrow major pulmonary arteries.[74] Other factors that affect the degree of resolution of acute PE are related to the size of the embolus, the presence of existing cardiopulmonary disease, the status of the endogenous fibrinolytic/coagulation system, and the type of treatment used.

Once the diagnosis of acute PE has been established, therapy should be initiated as soon as possible to minimize the morbidity and mortality associated with the embolic event, and to enhance the chances for vascular recanalization. Patients who do not have any underlying cardiopulmonary disease and are not compromised by their acute embolic event can usually be treated with a 3- to 6-month course of anticoagulation. Patients who have a moderate volume of clot (>1 lobe) and are hemodynamically compromised (tachycardia, systemic hypotension, right ventricle dysfunction, and/or pulmonary hypertension), or persistently hypoxemic despite appropriate anticoagulation and supplemental oxygen administration should be considered for more aggressive intervention.

Thrombolytic therapy appears to be useful in rapidly restoring more normal hemodynamics and may prove to be useful in reducing the sequelae of chronic pulmonary hypertension. With a greater understanding of the risks associated with fibrinolysis, bleeding complications can be reduced to a minimum. Direct intrathrombus infusion of lower doses of the thrombolytic agent may also reduce bleeding complications without decreasing the beneficial fibrinolytic affect.

Although percutaneous embolectomy and fragmentation techniques are intriguing, most of the devices are not widely available. Despite the lack of availability of these percutaneous devices, simple catheter techniques, occasionally coupled with thrombolytic administration, have resulted in dramatic improvements in patients with massive, acute PE.[76,77] Yet, older, more organized thrombus may be refractory to thrombolysis and mechanical fragmentation and require surgical intervention.

Identifying patients who are most likely to benefit from percutaneous mechanical fragmentation/thrombectomy and/or thrombolytic therapy versus surgical embolectomy appears to be extremely important in critically ill patients with a large volume of clot. Since fresh clots are rich in activated platelets, it may be possible to identify patients with acute PE using radiolabeled polypeptides specific for activated platelets. Indeed, there are clinical trials testing polypeptide agents that bind specifically to platelet receptors IIB/IIIA.[78] These platelet receptors become activated during the process of acute clot formation. In short, when we are better able to define the nature of the embolic material, it will be easier to determine which patients with PE will benefit from nonsurgical methods of vascular recanalization.

The authors would like to acknowledge Ms. Tammy Amos for her expert help in preparing this manuscript.

REFERENCES

1. Dalen JE, Alpert JS: Natural history of pulmonary embolism. *Prog Cardiovasc Dis* 17:259–270, 1975.
2. Hermann RE, Davis JH, Holden WD: Pulmonary embolism: a clinical and pathologic study with emphasis on the effect of prophylactic therapy with anticoagulants. *Am J Surg* 102:19–28, 1961.
3. Barritt DW, Jordan SE: Anticoagulant drugs in the treatment of pulmonary embolism: a controlled trial. *Lancet* 1:1309–1312, 1960.
4. Lindblad B, Sternby NH, Bergqvist D: Incidence of venous thromboembolism verified by necropsy over 30 years. *Brit Med J* 302:709–711, 1991.
5. Oster G, Tuden L, Colditz G: A cost-effective analysis of prophylaxis against deep-vein thrombosis in major orthopedic surgery. *JAMA* 257:203–209, 1987.
6. Jones TK, Barnes RW, Greenfield LJ: Greenfield vena cava filter: rationale and current indications. *Ann Thorac Surg* 42:S48–S55, 1986.
7. Carson JL, Kelley MA, Duff A, et al: The clinical course of pulmonary embolism. *N Engl J Med* 326:1240–1245, 1992.
8. Hull RD, Raskob GE, Hirsh J, et al: Continuous intravenous heparin compared with intermittent subcutaneous heparin in the initial treatment of proximal-vein thrombosis. *N Engl J Med* 315:1109–1114, 1986.
9. Hull RD, Raskob GE, Rosenbloom D, et al: Heparin for 5 days is compared with 10 days in the initial treatment of proximal venous thrombosis. *N Engl J Med* 322:1260–1265, 1990.
10. Levine MN, Hirsh J, Kelton JG: Heparin-induced bleeding. In Lane DA, Lindauhl U (eds): *Heparin Chemical and Biological Properties, and Clinical Applications.* London, Edward Arnold, 1989, pp 517–532.
11. King DJ, Kelton JG: Heparin-associated thrombocytopenia. *Ann Intern Med* 100:535–540, 1984.
12. Ginsberg JS, Kowalchuk G, Hirsh J, et al: Heparin effect on bone density. *Thromb Haemost* 64:286–289, 1990.
13. White PW, Sadd JR, Nensel RE: Thrombotic complications of heparin therapy: including 6 cases of heparin-induced skin necrosis. *Ann Surg* 190:595–608, 1979.
14. Jacques LB: Heparins: anionic polyelectrolyte drugs. *Pharm Rev* 31:99–166, 1979.
15. Curry N, Bardana EJ, Pirofsky B: Heparin sensitivity: report of a case. *Arch Intern Med* 132:744–745, 1973.
16. Enoxaparin—a low molecular weight heparin. *The Medical Letter* 35:75–76, 1993.

17. Albada J, Nieuwenhuis HK, Sixma JJ: Treatment of acute venous thromboembolism with low-molecular-weight heparin (Fragmin): results of a double-blind randomized study. *Circulation* 80:935–940, 1989.

18. Holmgren K, Andersson G, Fagrell B, et al: One-month versus six-month therapy with oral anticoagulants after symptomatic deep vein thrombosis. *Acta Med Scand* 218:279–284, 1985.

19. Gallus A, Jackaman J, Tillett J, et al: Safety and efficacy of warfarin started early after submassive venous thrombosis or pulmonary embolism. *Lancet* 2:1293–96, 1986.

20. Hull R, Hirsh J, Jay R, et al: Different intensities of oral anticoagulant therapy in the treatment of proximal-vein thrombosis. *N Engl J Med* 307:1676–81, 1982.

21. Chesebro JH, Fuster V, Elveback LR, et al: Trial of combined warfarin plus dipyridamole or aspirin therapy and prosthetic heart valve replacement: risk of aspirin compared with dipyridamole. *Am J Cardiol* 51:1537–41, 1983.

22. Benotti JR, Dalen JE: The natural history of pulmonary embolism. *Clin Chest Med* 5:403–10, 1984.

23. Raschke RA, Reilly BM, Guidry JR, et al: The weight-based heparin dosing nomogram compared with a "standard care" nomogram: a randomized controlled trial. *Ann Intern Med* 119:874–81, 1993.

24. Dalen JE, Banas JS Jr., Brooks HA, et al: Resolution rate of acute pulmonary embolism in man. *N Engl J Med* 280:1194–99, 1969.

25. Tow DE, Wagner HN: Recovery of pulmonary arterial blood flow in patients with pulmonary embolism. *N Engl J Med* 176:1053–59, 1967.

26. Urokinase pulmonary embolism trial study group: Urokinase pulmonary embolism trial: Phase 1 results. *JAMA* 214:2163–72, 1970.

27. Urokinase-streptokinase pulmonary embolism trial study group: Urokinase-streptokinase pulmonary embolism trial: Phase 2 results. *Jama* 229:1606–1613, 1974.

28. Sharma GVRK, Burleson VA, Sasahara AA: Effective thrombolytic therapy on pulmonary-capillary blood volume in patients with pulmonary embolism. *N Engl J Med* 303:1842–1845, 1990.

29. Sharma GVRK, Folland ED, McIntyre KM, et al: Long-term hemodynamic benefit of thrombolytic therapy in pulmonary embolic disease (abstract). *J Am Coll Cardiol* 15:65a, 1990.

30. Schwarz F, Stehr H, Zimmerman R, et al: Sustained improvement of pulmonary hemodynamics in patients at rest and during exercise after thrombolytic therapy of massive pulmonary embolism. *Circulation* 71:117–123, 1985.

31. deSoyza NDB, Murphy ML: Persistent post-embolic pulmonary hypertension. *Chest* 62:665–668, 1972.

32. Anderson DR, Levine MN: Thrombolytic therapy for the treatment of acute pulmonary embolism. *Can Med Assoc J* 146:1317–1324, 1992.

33. Sherry S: Thrombolytic therapy for noncoronary diseases. *Ann Emerg Med* 20:396–404, 1991.

34. National Institutes of Health Consensus Panel: Thrombolytic therapy and thrombosis: A National Institutes of Health consensus development conference. *Ann Intern Med* 93:141–144, 1980.

35. Wolfe MW, Lee RT, Feldstein ML, et al: Prognostic significance of right ventricle hypokinesis and perfusion lung scan defects in pulmonary embolism. *Am Heart J* 127:1371–1375, 1994.

36. Goldhaber SZ: Thrombolysis for pulmonary embolism. *Prog Cardiovasc Dis* 34:113–134, 1991.

37. Hirsch DR, Goldhaber SZ: Laboratory parameters to monitor safety and efficacy during thrombolytic therapy. *Chest* 99:113S–120S, 1991.

38. UKEP Study Research Group: The UKEP Study: multicenter clinical trial on two local regimens of urokinase in massive pulmonary embolism. *Europ Heart J* 8:2–10, 1987.

39. Sane DC, Kaliff RM, Topol EJ, et al: Bleeding during thrombolytic therapy for acute myocardial infarction: mechanisms and management. *Ann Intern Med* 111:1010–1022, 1989.

40. Matsumoto AH, Selby JB Jr, Tegtmeyer CJ, et al: Recent development of rigors during infusion of urokinase: Is it related to an endotoxin? *JVIR* 15:433–438, 1994.

41. Goldhaber SZ, Heit JA, Sharma GVRK, et al: Randomized control trial of recombinant tissue plasminogen activator versus urokinase in the treatment of pulmonary embolism. *Lancet* 2:293–298, 1988.

42. Goldhaber SZ, Kessler CM, Heit JA, et al: Recombinant tissue-type plasminogen activator versus a novel dosing regimen of urokinase in acute pulmonary embolism: a randomized controlled multicenter trial. *J Am Coll Cardiol* 20:24–30, 1992.

43. Verstraete M, Miller GAH, Bounameaux H, et al: Intravenous and intrapulmonary recombinant tissue-type plasminogen activator in the treatment of acute massive pulmonary embolism. *Circulation* 77:353–360, 1988.

44. Dotter CT, Rosch J, Seaman AJ: Selective clot lysis with low-dose streptokinase. *Radiology* 11:31–36, 1974.

45. Katzen BT, van Breda A: Low dose streptokinase in the treatment of arterial occlusions. *Am J Roentgenol* 136:1171–1178, 181.

46. Kandarpa K: Technical determinants of success in catheter-directed thrombolysis for peripheral arterial occlusions. *JVIR* 6:55S–61S, 1995.

47. Shortell C, Ouriel K: Thrombolysis in acute peripheral arterial occlusion: predictors of immediate success. *Ann Vasc Surg* 8:59–65, 1994.

48. van Breda A, Robison J, Feldman L, et al: Local thrombolysis in the treatment of arteriographic occlusions. *J Vasc Surg* 1:103–112, 1984.

49. van Breda A, Katzen BT, Deutsch A: Urokinase versus streptokinase in local thrombolysis. *Radiology* 165:109–111, 1987.

50. van Breda A, Graor R, Katzen BT, et al: Relative cost-effectiveness of urokinase versus streptokinase in the treatment of peripheral vascular disease. *JVIR* 2:77–87, 1991.

51. Schmitz-Rode T, Günther RW: Pulmonary arterial flow alterations in massive pulmonary embolism: significance for selective intrapulmonary thrombolysis (abstract). *Radiology* (Suppl)197(P):284, 1995.

52. Molina JE, Hunter DW, Yedlick JW, et al: Thrombolytic therapy for postoperative pulmonary embolism. *Am J Surg* 163:375–381, 1992.

53. Gonzalez-Juanatey JR, Valdes L, Amaro A, et al: Treatment of massive pulmonary thromboembolism with low intrapulmonary dosages of urokinase: short-term angiographic and hemodynamic evolution. *Chest* 102:341–346, 1992.

54. Terrin M, Goldhaber SZ, Thompson B, et al: Selection of patients with acute pulmonary embolism for thrombolytic therapy: the thrombolysis in pulmonary embolism (TIPE) patient survey. *Chest* 95:279S–281S, 1989.

55. Myer G, Tamisier D, Sors H, et al: Pulmonary embolectomy: a 20-year experience at one center. *Ann Thorac Surg* 51:232–236, 1991.

56. Kieny R, Sharpentier A, Kieny MT: What is the place of pulmonary embolectomy today? *J Cardiovasc Surg* 32:549–554, 1991.

57. Greenfield LJ, Proctor MC, Williams DM, et al: Long-term experience with transvenous catheter pulmonary embolectomy. *J Vasc Surg* 18:450–458, 1993.

58. Timsit JF, Reynaud P, Meyer G, et al: Pulmonary embolectomy by catheter device in massive pulmonary embolism. *Chest* 100:655–658, 1991.

59. Reekers J, Kromhout J, van der Waal K: Catheter for percutaneous thrombectomy: first clinical experience. *Radiology* 188:871–874, 1993.

60. van Ommen V, van der Ven FH, Daemen MJ, et al: In vivo evaluation of the Hydrolyser Hydrodynamic Thrombectomy Catheter. *JVIR* 5:823–826, 1994.

61. Vorwerk D, Sohn M, Schurmann K, et al: Hydrodynamic thrombectomy of hemodialysis fistulas: first clinical results. *JVIR* 5:813–821, 1994.

62. Drasler WJ, Jenson ML, Wilson GJ, et al: Rheolytic catheter for percutaneous removal of thrombus. *Radiology* 182:263–267, 1992.

63. Cela MC, Amplatz K: Nonsurgical pulmonary embolectomy. In Cope C (ed): *Current Techniques in Interventional Radiology.* Philadelphia, Current Medicine, 1994, pp 12.2–12.12.

64. Schmitz-Rode T, Vorwerk D, Günther RW, et al: Percutaneous fragmentation of pulmonary emboli in dogs with the Impeller-Basket Catheter. *Cardiovasc Intervent Radiol* 16.239–242, 1993.

65. Schmitz-Rode T, Günther RW: New device for percutaneous fragmentation of pulmonary emboli. *Radiology* 180:135–137, 1991.

66. Schmitz-Rode T, Adam G, Kilbingr M, et al: Fragmentation of pulmonary emboli: in vivo experimental evaluation of 2 high-speed rotating catheters. *Cardiovasc Intervent Radiol* 19:165–169, 1996.

67. Schmitz-Rode T, Günther RW, Pfeffer JG, et al: Acute massive pulmonary embolism: use of a rotatable pigtail catheter for diagnosis and fragmentation therapy. *Radiology* 197:157–162, 1995.

68. Blidsoe MC, Morabian GP, Hunter DW, et al: Mechanical clot dissolution: new concept. *Radiology* 171:231–233, 1989.

69. Coleman CC, Krendel C, Dietz CA, et al: Mechanical thrombectomy: results of early experience. *Radiology* 189:803–805, 1993.

70. Tadavarthy SM, Murray PD, Inanpudi S, et al: Mechanical thrombectomy with the Amplatz device: human experience. *JVIR* 5:715–724, 1994.

71. Yesui K, Qian V, Nazarian GK, et al: Recirculation-type Amplatz clot macerater: determination of particle size and distribution. *JVIR* 4:275–278, 1993.

72. Uflacker R, Rajagopalan P, Vujic B, et al: Treatment of thrombosed dialysis access grafts: randomized trial of surgical thrombectomy versus mechanical thrombectomy with the Amplatz device. *JVIR* 7:185–192, 1996.

73. Uflacker R, Strange C, Vujic B: Massive pulmonary embolism: preliminary results of treatment with the Amplatz thrombectomy device. *JVIR* 7:519–528, 1996.

74. Widimsky J: Prognosis of pulmonary embolism. In Morpurgo M (ed): *Pulmonary Embolism.* New York, Marcel Dekker, 1994, pp 96–105.

75. Nazarian GK, Qian Z, Coleman CC, et al: Hemolytic effect of the amplatz thrombectomy device. *JVIR* 5:155–160, 1994.

76. Brady AJB, Crake T, Oakley CM: Percutaneous catheter fragmentation and distal disbursing of proximal pulmonary embolus. *Lancet* 338:1186–1189, 1991.

77. Essop MR, Middlemost S, Skoularigis J, et al: Simultaneous mechanical clot fragmentation and pharmacologic thrombolysis in acute massive pulmonary embolism. *Am J Cardiol* 69:427–430, 1992.

78. Clinical Protocol: Phase III clinical trial evaluating the safety and efficacy of Tc-99m P280 in the detection and localization of disorders and conditions characterized by activated platelet involvement; specifically, evaluation of acute venous thrombosis by gamma scintigraphy. Protocol: 103. Londonderry, NH, Diatide, Inc., 1995–96.

C H A P T E R
3

Hemoptysis: Transcatheter Embolotherapy

Matthew A. Mauro
Nancy Keaton

Hemoptysis may be the presenting sign of a variety of cardiopulmonary diseases. The clinical course of hemoptysis is often unpredictable; a small bleed can quickly develop into a massive and potentially fatal hemorrhage. Most institutions define massive hemoptysis as 300–600 ml in a 24-hr period.[1–4] Death is most commonly from asphyxiation secondary to flooding of the alveoli with blood.[3–5] Exsanguination may occur but is uncommon. The risk of death is directly related to the amount of blood expectorated, the rate of bleeding, the amount aspirated, and the underlying pulmonary reserve.[1,2,4] Conservative therapy for severe hemoptysis carries a 50–80% mortality. Understandably, episodes of massive hemoptysis are now managed more aggressively.

Surgical resection of an isolated bleeding source is the initial therapeutic choice and may be curative. However, many patients with hemoptysis have diffuse chronic lung disease with limited pulmonary reserve and are unacceptable surgical candidates.[6,7] In addition, surgical mortality rates may be lowered by arresting the hemorrhage preoperatively in those patients who are actively bleeding.

CLINICAL CONSIDERATIONS

Severe hemoptysis requiring radiologic intervention is most often encountered in patients with a history of chronic inflammatory disease. Tuberculosis, bronchiectasis, mycetomas, sarcoidosis, and cystic fibrosis are the most common etiologies. Lung abscess, mitral stenosis, congenital heart disease with pulmonary outflow obstruction, carcinoma, and vascular anomalies are other causes of hemoptysis. Iatrogenic causes such as bronchoscopy, transthoracic needle biopsy, and pulmonary artery rupture from Swan-Ganz catheters are being reported with increasing frequency.[4, 8–10]

In most cases, severe hemoptysis originates from the systemic bronchial artery circulation. Tuberculosis, cystic fibrosis, sarcoidosis, and bronchiectasis all lead to bronchial artery hypertrophy and enlargement of peribronchial and submucosal arteriolar vessels.[11] Anastomoses develop between the bronchial and pulmonary circulations. Bleeding results from the enlarged peribronchial and submucosal vascular plexus in areas subjected to chronic inflammation and/or infections. Hemoptysis occurs in 50–90% of patients who develop mycetomas in preexisting pulmonary cavities.[4] Mechanical irritation, *Aspergillus*-associated endotoxin, *Aspergillus*-related proteolytic activity and hypersensitivity reactions have all been proposed as causes for bleeding.[4,12]

Although massive hemoptysis is the primary indication for transcatheter embolotherapy, recurrent episodes of moderate hemoptysis (loss of 100 ml of blood three times or more per day within a week) are also considered significant. These patients require urgent therapy due to the threat of airway obstruction, asphyxiation, hypotension, anemia, chemical pneumonitis, and/or exacerbation of underlying pulmonary disease.[13,14]

Recurrent hemorrhage is not uncommon even after successful transcatheter embolization. Extensive anastomoses exist between mediastinal and pleural structures and the bronchial artery circulation so that bleeding may arise from hypertrophied nonbronchial systemic collateral arteries. Occasionally, previously embolized vessels may recanalize. Therefore, patients who have undergone embolotherapy should not be denied subsequent transcatheter procedures to arrest recurrent hemoptysis.

It is imperative to define the source of bleeding and differentiate hemoptysis from bleeding originating from the upper airway or upper gastrointestinal tract. True hemoptysis tends to be bright red blood mixed with frothy sputum, whereas hematemesis is dark (from oxidation) and mixed with food.[4] The possibility of an aspirated foreign body should always be entertained. If a pulmonary infection is suspected, sputum cultures are required (including mycobacteria and fungi).[14]

After stabilization and diagnosis, the bleeding site must be localized. A chest x-ray should be obtained primarily to search for cardiopulmonary abnormalities or other potential sources of bleeding, such as foreign bodies or mycetoma. Physical examination and chest film findings are not helpful in locating the site of bleeding in 55–60% of patients.[4] Bronchoscopy is the initial procedure of choice, and its yield is significantly higher if it is performed early.[15] Computed tomography (CT) is sensitive for detecting lung cancer and bronchiectasis and is of value prior to bronchoscopy in patients with mild to moderate hemoptysis. It is less helpful in patients with severe or massive hemoptysis due to aspiration of blood into unaffected areas. When patients are admitted for severe hemoptysis, a pulmonologist, thoracic surgeon, and interventional radiologist should be called upon to coordinate therapy.

All drugs that interfere with coagulation should be discontinued and any coagulation defects corrected. Blood should be typed and crossmatched so that it can be readily administered if the need arises. Inhaled irritants should also be discontinued.[14] To prevent contamination of nonbleeding lung segments, placing the bleeding lung segment in a dependent position whenever possible may be of benefit. The patient should be encouraged to clear blood and other secretions from the airway. Administration of intravenous conjugated estrogen and vasopressin may control hemorrhage by increasing platelet aggregation and producing arteriolar smooth muscle contraction, respectively.[16,17]

Various endobronchial therapies that are now available include bronchial irrigation with iced saline, topical thrombin or epinephrine therapy, balloon catheter tamponade, direct airway tamponade with Gelfoam (Upjohn Corp., Kalamazoo, MI) pledgets, and selective single- or dual-lumen intubation.[4,14,18,19] Surgery is offered for localized abnormalities in stable patients who are not bleeding as a definitive long-term solution, or actively bleeding patients who are unresponsive to all other therapies. Patients with hypoxemia, CO_2 retention, marginal pulmonary reserve, and diffuse disease can rarely tolerate surgery and should be referred for urgent angiography and embolotherapy soon after diagnostic bronchoscopy and endobronchial therapies.[1,4,20]

INTERVENTIONAL RADIOLOGIC TECHNIQUES

Bronchial Artery Embolization (BAE)

Bronchial artery embolization (BAE) is a well-established means of managing hemoptysis.[8,13,21–28] The indications for BAE include: (1) major hemoptysis (greater than 300 ml of blood in a 24-hr period); (2) recurrent episodes of moderate hemoptysis (three or more bouts of 100 ml of blood per day within a week); and (3) chronic or slowly increasing episodes of hemoptysis.[29] The availability of lung transplantation has also stimulated a more aggressive approach to hemorrhage control in surgical candidates. Whenever possible, patients should undergo the procedure during a quiescent phase.

Arterial Anatomy

Several anatomic variations in the origins of bronchial arteries must be considered during initial selective diagnostic arteriography. The majority (90%) of bronchial arteries originate from the descending thoracic aorta between T5-T7.[30] In many individuals, a single right bronchial artery originates from a common intercosto-bronchial trunk (Figure 3.1). This common trunk usually arises from the right lateral or posterolateral surface of the aorta (Figure 3.2). On the left, multiple bronchial arteries are more common and usually originate directly from the anterior or anterolateral aspect of the aorta[31] (Figure 3.3). Variations are commonly encountered and should be expected. Both the left and right bronchial arteries can originate from a common trunk on the anterior surface of the descending aorta. There can be multiple bronchial arteries on the right and a single artery on the left. Fifteen percent of left bronchial arteries originate from the concavity of the aortic arch.

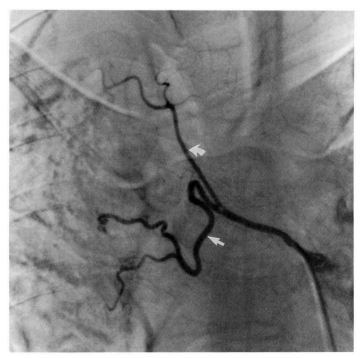

A

Figure 3.1 Right bronchial–superior intercostal trunk. **A.** Selective injection shows a common right bronchial–superior intercostal trunk. Note characteristic courses of the bronchial artery (straight arrow) following the mainstem bronchus and the intercostal artery (curved arrow) which initially ascends then follows the undersurface of the rib. **B.** Following page.

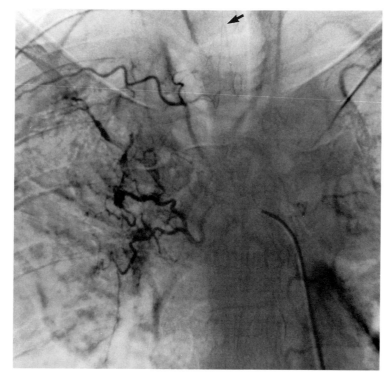

B

Figure 3.1 B. Note spinal artery branch with its characteristic hairpin turn (arrow) originating from the superior intercostal artery. In this case, a microcatheter was placed distal to the origin of the intercostal artery and an uneventful embolization was performed.

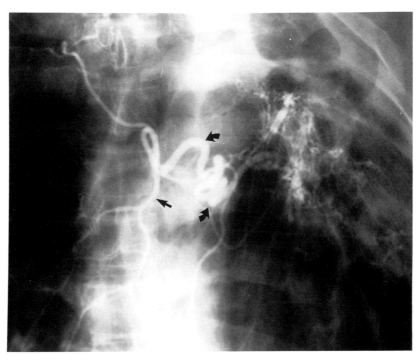

Figure 3.2 Common bronchial trunk. Both left and right bronchial arteries as well as the right superior intercostal artery arise from a common trunk. Compare relatively normal-appearing right bronchial artery (straight arrow) with the enlarged and tortuous left bronchial artery (curved arrows). In this case, the left bronchial artery was superselectively catheterized and embolized with polyvinyl alcohol (PVA) particles.

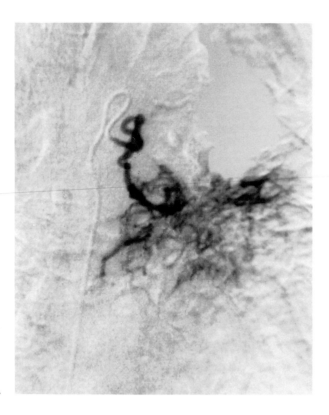

A

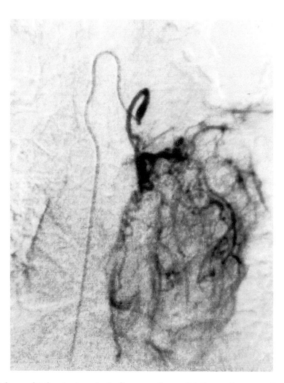

B

Figure 3.3 Two left bronchial arteries. A. Left upper bronchial arteriogram showing hypervascularity and tortuosity. B. Slightly inferior, a second bronchial artery is catheterized and shows marked hypervascularity. Both arteries require embolization to successfully arrest bleeding.

Cauldwell et al. studied bronchial artery anatomy in 150 cadavers.[32] Four anatomic variations constituted 93% of the cases: Type I (41%): two left and one right bronchial artery; Type II (21%): one left and one right bronchial artery; Type III (21%): two left and two right bronchial arteries arising separately or as common trunks from the aorta; and Type IV (10%): one left and two right bronchial arteries. More recently, an angiographic investigation by Uflacker and colleagues reported similar variations but a much higher incidence (43%) of common bronchial trunks.[21]

Normal bronchial arteries are usually 2–3 mm in diameter and extend only to the medial one-half of the lung field.[31] With chronic inflammation, these bronchial arteries enlarge and become tortuous (Figure 3.4). Bronchial arteries are the nutrient supply to the bronchi, trachea, subcarinal lymph nodes, middle one-third of the esophagus, posterior mediastinum, and vagus nerve. Bronchial arteries anastomose with the pulmonary arterial circulation at the level of the respiratory bronchiole. This bronchopulmonary anastomosis becomes very significant in situations of chronic inflammation or pulmonary hypertension[23] (Figure 3.5).

Transpleural systemic arterial collaterals are frequently seen arising from the subclavian, axillary, internal mammary, phrenic, thyrocervical, and intercostal arteries[33,34] (Figure 3.6). Nonbronchial systemic collateral arteries and/or aberrantly located bronchial arteries are often the source(s) of hemoptysis in patients who have undergone previous BAE. In a study of patients with cystic fibrosis, Cohen et al. found a significantly higher incidence of aberrant bronchial arteries (35% versus 2%) and spinal radicular arterial branches from the bronchial arteries (55% versus 5%) than the general population.[8]

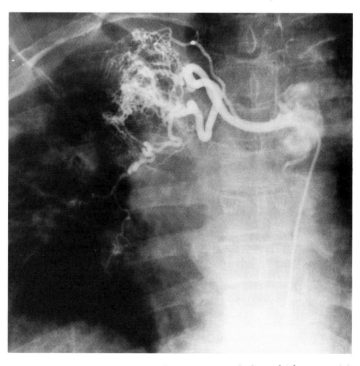

Figure 3.4 Bronchial artery in chronic inflammation. Right bronchial artery arising near aortic knob shows characteristic hypervascularity and tortuosity indicative of chronic inflammation.

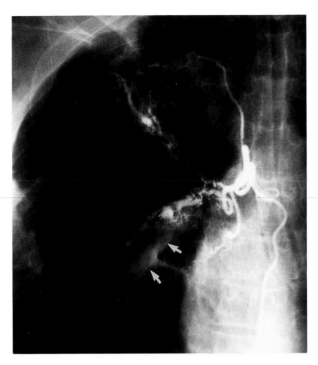

Figure 3.5 Systemic to pulmonary shunting. Right bronchial arteriogram shows obvious bronchial artery to pulmonary artery shunting (arrow).

Although exceedingly rare, inadvertent embolization of the spinal artery branch is a dreaded complication of BAE. Therefore, the anatomic relationship of the bronchial and intercostal arteries with the anterior spinal artery must be clearly understood. The major blood supply to the spinal cord is the anterior spinal artery which derives flow from the intracerebral portion of the vertebral arteries and the anterior radiculomedullary branches of the intercostal, lumbar, and/or bronchial arteries.[35] In the adult, there are usually 6–8 anterior radiculomedullary arteries that arise at different locations.[36] They all have a characteristic "hairpin-loop" configuration as the vessel enters the anterior sulcus of the spinal cord (Figure 3.1). The largest of these arteries, the artery of Adamkiewcz, can arise from the T6-L5 level. In 5% of patients, this artery arises or receives a large contribution from the right intercostobronchial trunk.

Angiography

High-quality diagnostic angiography is imperative prior to embolization. A brief neurologic examination is performed before the angiographic study. The neurologic status of the patient should be monitored throughout the course of the embolization procedure. Monitoring somatosensory evoked potentials to detect spinal cord ischemia has been recommended, but is far from routine.[37] An initial digital subtraction angiogram (DSA) of the descending thoracic aorta can be obtained to provide a roadmap. Because the bronchial arteries are often enlarged, we do not routinely obtain an initial aortogram in patients undergoing their first BAE procedure. A thoracic aortogram should be performed when selective catheterization is not quickly achieved, in patients who have had embolization procedures, or in patients without chronic inflammatory parenchymal disease.

Vascular access is ordinarily obtained via the common femoral artery. A high brachial artery approach is occasionally necessary for selective catheterization and embolization of collateral vessels arising from the subclavian artery (Figure 3.6B). A 6 Fr vascular sheath is placed and connected to a pressurized, heparinized saline infusion (2,000 units heparin per 1,000 cc normal saline at 30 cc/min). Use of a vascular sheath facilitates catheter exchanges. Long vascular sheaths extending into the aorta are used for obese patients or those with extremely tortuous iliac arteries to allow for better torque control of the catheters. Selective catheterization is begun with a reverse-curve catheter (Figures 3.2, 3.3, and 3.5). In patients with low aortic arches or relatively high bronchial artery origins, there may be insufficient space to allow a reverse-curve catheter to form and adequately probe the aortic wall. The apex of the catheter will lie partly in the transverse arch, making selective catheterization impossible. Conventional forward-looking, preshaped, steerable 0.038 inch endhole catheters (Cobra, H1H, RC, MPA, Berenstein, etc.) can then be used (Figures 3.1 and 3.4).

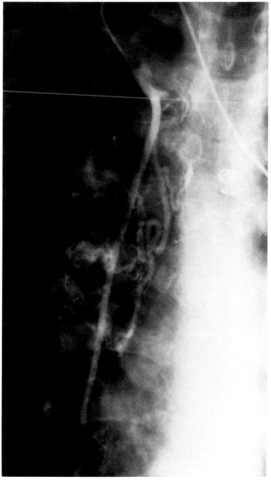

A

Figure 3.6 Nonbronchial systemic collateral arteries. Patient presents with recurrent hemoptysis following previous embolization procedures. **A.** Selective right internal mammary artery injection from femoral approach shows abnormal branches in right hila area. **B.** Following page.

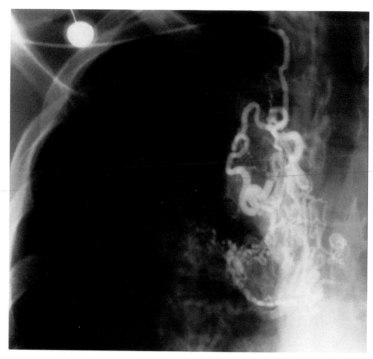

B

Figure 3.6 B. Selective catheterization of descending branch of thyrocervical trunk shows markedly enlarged and abundant collaterals in same patient. Due to vascular tortuosity, catheterization and embolization were performed via a brachial artery approach.

When selective catheterization is performed, the search should begin at the T5 to T6 level.[32] The left main stem bronchus serves as a convenient fluoroscopic landmark for locating the bronchial artery. The right lateral to posterolateral surface of the aorta is probed when searching for the right bronchial artery. An anterior to left anterolateral direction is used for left bronchial artery catheterization. The bronchial artery or intercostobronchial trunk should not be occluded during catheterization as this may cause spinal cord ischemia.

A selective DSA using low osmolar contrast media is performed for each vessel before embolization. Bronchial arteries are easily differentiated from intercostal arteries by their characteristic course, which follows the mainstem bronchi toward the hilum. Intercostal arteries have an initial cephalic course, then travel laterally along the undersurface of a rib. Use of low osmolar contrast during selective bronchial artery injections will significantly reduce the urge for the patient to cough and also the risk of causing transverse myelitis.[38,39]

When possible, DSA should be used to limit the volume of contrast and shorten the procedure. All contributions to the anterior spinal artery from the thoracic aorta have a characteristic cephalic course with a hairpin bend in the midline within the spinal canal (Figure 3.1B). Branches supplying the trachea and esophagus may also appear midline on an anteroposterior study. Oblique views may be needed to differentiate a potential spinal artery branch from other mediastinal arterial branches.

The bronchial arteries responsible for hemorrhage are almost always tortuous and enlarged. Parenchymal hypervascularity and bronchial-pulmonary vascular shunting are often present[30] (Figures 3.4 and 3.5). Bronchial artery aneurysms are occasionally seen, but frank contrast extravasation is rare[24–28,41] (Figure 3.7). If an abnormal bronchial artery is not identified in a patient undergoing their first BAE procedure, a careful and thorough search for aberrant bronchial arteries is necessary.[42]

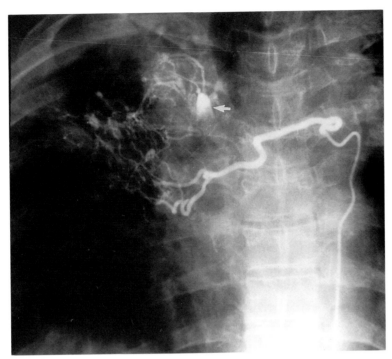

Figure 3.7 Contrast extravasation. Right bronchial arteriogram shows hypervascularity with an area of extravasation (arrow).

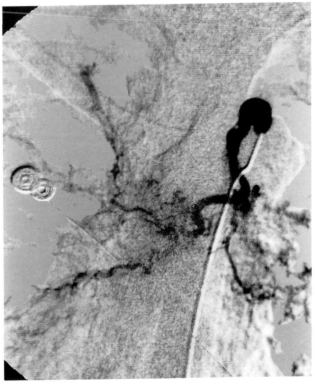

A

Figure 3.8 Continued hemoptysis. Continued hemoptysis occurred secondary to an aberrant bronchial artery and a nonbronchial systemic collateral. Patient had previous embolization of a normally located right bronchial artery just one day earlier. A. An aberrant bronchial artery with a common trunk was identified originating from the outer surface of the aortic arch. B, C, and D. Following pages.

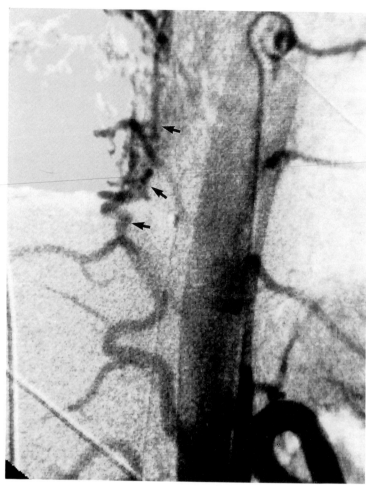

B

Figure 3.8 B. Abdominal aortogram reveals markedly enlarged right inferior phrenic artery supplying collateral branches (arrows) to the right lung. **C** and **D**. Following page.

Recurrent hemoptysis following a successful BAE is due to a bronchial artery not previously embolized (aberrant or nonaberrant), a recanalized bronchial artery, or nonbronchial systemic collaterals.[33,34,43,44] The search for aberrant bronchial arteries and nonbronchial systemic collaterals will require an arch aortogram, selective subclavian arteriogram, abdominal aortogram, and inferior phrenic arteriogram (particularly in patients with lower lobe disease)[45] (Figure 3.8). The presence of pleural thickening increases the likelihood of nonbronchial systemic collaterals as a source for hemoptysis and decreases the overall effectiveness of embolotherapy.[46]

If a systemic (bronchial or nonbronchial) arterial source of bleeding is not identified, selective pulmonary arteriography must be performed.[24,25,47–50] Chronic cavitary tuberculosis can erode into an adjacent pulmonary arterial branch, producing a pulmonary artery pseudoaneurysm (Rasmussen aneurysm). Plessinger and Jolly reported 56 cases of Rasmussen aneurysms in which 49 patients (87%) died due to massive pulmonary hemorrhage.[51] In addition to tuberculosis, any destructive pulmonary process, such as a pyogenic lung abscess, can erode into an adjacent pulmonary or systemic vessel. Pseudoaneurysm bleeding should be suspected in a patient with hemoptysis when: (1) a necrotic cavity in the lung parenchyma is present; (2) the cavity is located close to a central pulmonary artery; and (3) a rapidly growing nodule or mass is noted within the cavity.[52] Pulmonary artery pseudoaneurysms can also be treated with transcatheter embolotherapy. When pulmonary artery rupture secondary to a Swan-Ganz catheter is suspected, pulmonary arteriography should also be performed.

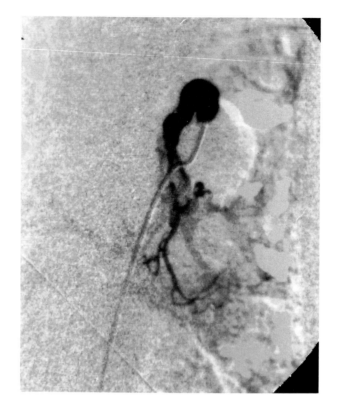

C

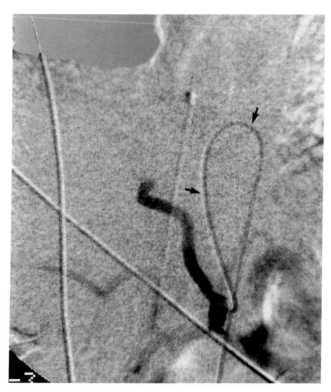

D

Figure 3.8 C. Postembolization arteriogram shows successful embolization of the right bronchial artery with PVA particles inserted through a Tracker-18 catheter. Note that the left bronchial artery was spared. **D.** Postembolization arteriogram of the right inferior phrenic artery shows occlusion following PVA embolization. In this case, selective catheterization was accomplished by using a Cobra catheter with a Waltman loop (arrows).

Embolization

Any abnormal-appearing bronchial artery supplying the region of hemorrhage should be embolized (Figure 3.3). A stable catheter position is required for embolization. Embolization of spinal artery branches should be avoided. High-quality selective DSA performed with low osmolar contrast should identify major arterial supplies to the anterior spinal artery. When a branch to the spinal artery is identified, embolization should be performed only if the catheter tip can be advanced distal to the origin of the spinal artery branch. Superselective catheterization with microcatheters is frequently possible. Frequent contrast injections during the embolization procedure are necessary. Occasionally, a branch to the spinal or coronary artery will be seen only after the resistance of the bronchial artery bed has been increased by partial distal embolization.[8,53] Some groups advocate injection of a short-acting barbiturate into the selected artery before embolization to test whether there is any significant spinal cord supply.[38,54] If there is arterial supply to the spinal cord, a transient neurologic deficit (weakness) will be produced, and the embolization should not be performed at that location. When no deficit is produced, the procedure can be performed without fear of a neurologic injury. In practice, this provocative pharmacologic test is rarely performed.

Bronchial artery embolization is very safe, particularly when particles larger than 200 μm are used. Boushy et al. found that dogs embolized with small particles (29–100 μm) developed hind limb paralysis, whereas the use of larger particles (200 μm) resulted in only transient weakness.[55] This study suggests that larger particles cannot enter small spinal branches and are safer for BAE.

When reverse-curved catheters are used, the tip is advanced deeper into the vessel by withdrawing the catheter from the groin. It is essential that the catheter does not occlude the vessel, as particulate embolization depends on brisk forward flow to propel the particles distally into the vascular bed. Arterial spasm should also be avoided by using soft-tipped catheters and guidewires and not forcing catheters into small distal vessels. If arterial spasm is present, intra-arterial vasodilators can be used.

If a stable catheter position cannot be obtained or if a distal catheter position results in spasm or flow occlusion, coaxial catheterization with a microcatheter should be performed. There are several microcatheter systems commercially available. The Tracker-18 (Target Therapeutics, Fremont, CA) is the standard and most widely used microcatheter. Other microcatheters are now available from Microvena (White Bear Lake, MN), Cook (Bloomington, IN), Medi-Tech (Watertown, MA), Cordis (Miami, FL), and Micro Interventional Systems (Sunnyvale, CA). These microcatheters have small flexible distal shafts with a highly opaque marker at the tip. They can be advanced through catheters with 0.038-inch end holes. The Tracker-325 (Target Therapeutics) has been designed primarily for peripheral applications. Unlike the Tracker-18, which tapers from 3.0 Fr to 2.2 Fr, the Tracker-325 tapers from 3.0 to 2.8 Fr and has a larger inner lumen. Although less flexible than the Tracker-18, it allows safe, distal catheterization in most peripheral arterial applications and use of larger embolic particles. All these devices permit embolization with particles (gelatin sponge, polyvinyl alcohol, microfibrillar collagen), slurry, liquids and specially designed platinum coils (Target, Cook).[8,56] These microcatheters are usually used with platinum- or gold-tipped, steerable 0.014–0.018 inch guidewires.

Embolization should be performed in the most distal site possible. With proximal occlusion, distal collaterals invariably develop, leading to recurrent bleeding. In addition, with permanent proximal occlusion, future access to the main bronchial artery will be lost. Yet, certain agents such as ethanol or very small particles (< 150 μm) should be avoided as they produce occlusion too distal, possibly leading to tissue infarction.[57] Embolization with small particles may not be possible when large bronchial artery to pulmonary artery/vein shunting is present. When large shunting is present, small particles will pass through and lodge in the pulmonary arterial bed or pass into the systemic circulation. Larger particles (greater than 500 μm) or small coils may then be required.

Materials most commonly used for BAE include Gelfoam pledgets and polyvinyl alcohol (PVA) particles.[8,9,26–28,58] The latter is our first choice for distal embolization. Polyvinyl vinyl alcohol produces relatively permanent arterial occlusion and is available in several particle sizes. Particles greater than 200 μm should be used to avoid tissue ischemia and neurologic damage.[8,55] We commonly use PVA from Biodyne, Inc. (El Cajon, CA) and begin with 200–300 μm or 300–500 μm particles, depending on the degree of shunting seen on preliminary angiograms. One vial of PVA is placed in a 20-cc syringe with the plunger removed. The plunger is replaced and 20 cc of a 1:1 mixture of nonionic contrast (300 mgI/cc) and saline is added. The syringe is manually agitated and the mixture is degassed by occluding the tip of the syringe with a finger, withdrawing the plunger, and vigorously agitating the syringe. The finger is removed from the tip of the syringe and the plunger is advanced to expel any gas. This can be repeated several times. The PVA solution is then connected to a 3-way stopcock via a short flexible high-pressure tubing with Luer-Lok attachments. This 20-cc syringe functions as a reservoir of PVA particles. A 1- or 3-cc Luer-Lok syringe is connected to the 3-way stopcock parallel to the catheter. The 3-cc syringe is used with 5 Fr or larger catheters, while the 1-cc syringe is used with microcatheters. The PVA particles are further mixed with in-and-out aspirations of the two syringes via the 3-way stopcock. A final check of catheter position is made with a contrast injection. The contrast is flushed from the catheter and the embolization apparatus (3-way stopcock and two syringes) connected to the catheter. By a simple adjustment of the direction of the 3-way stopcock, the mixture is withdrawn into the administration syringe (1 or 3 cc) from the reservoir (20-cc syringe) and slowly injected into the bronchial artery under fluoroscopic control. At regular intervals, the catheter is gently cleared with a saline injection (several 5-cc syringes of saline should be appropriately marked and available). A contrast injection is then performed to evaluate the status of the embolized vascular bed. When forward flow is markedly reduced (exaggerated pulsatile flow is seen), injections of PVA should be stopped. If needed, more proximal occlusion can then be accomplished with Gelfoam pledgets or torpedoes, placed one at a time until flow ceases.

Gelfoam (gelatin sponge) is readily available and slowly resorbed; it can be used as small pledgets, long torpedoes, or as part of a slurry mixture. Gelfoam alone may also be used for BAE. One to two-millimeter cubes are placed initially for distal occlusion followed by 3–4 mm pledgets or 3 by 7 mm torpedoes for more proximal blockade. When used for initial embolization, several cubes are placed in an empty 1- or 3-cc syringe with forceps. Dilute contrast is then drawn into the syringe so that the Gelfoam remains close to the syringe tip. The catheter is cleared of contrast. The Gelfoam is firmly injected into the catheter while the tip of the syringe is elevated (Gelfoam floats in dilute contrast). A second syringe (1 or 3 cc) of saline is then used to completely discharge the Gelfoam from the catheter. The Gelfoam particles can often be seen as filling defects in the contrast stream. The catheter has been cleared of particles when no contrast exits the catheter. Resorption of Gelfoam can lead to rapid recanalization and recurrent bleeding.[59]

A Gelfoam slurry mixture has also been successfully used for BAE. The mixture consists of Gelfoam shavings, dextrose-50, Ethiodol (Savage Labs, Melville, NY), and ε-aminocaproic acid.[60] The solution is administered in small aliquots using a 3-cc or 1-cc syringe, for standard catheters or microcatheters, respectively. The slurry is radiopaque and produces a more permanent occlusion than Gelfoam pledgets.

In general, proximal coil embolization should be avoided. Occasionally, enormous bronchial arteries with large systemic-pulmonary shunts are present, necessitating the use of coils for adequate and safe occlusion.[54,61] A stable catheter position is needed along with coils 15–25% larger than the vessel to avoid retrograde dislodgement of the coil into the aorta.[62] Some of these vessels can now be superselectively catheterized with microcatheters and deposition of large platinum coils can be safely performed. Microcoils are easily loaded into the microcatheters and can be delivered quickly to the target vessel by using a vigorous saline flush with a 1- or 3-cc syringe. The pusher wire is often not needed for coil deployment. However, permanent coil occlusion should only be used if other methods fail or are contraindicated.

Whenever possible, all vessels in the abnormal region should be embolized. A postembolization aortogram is useful to identify any previously overlooked arteries or to confirm occlusion of the embolized vessels. Once the procedure is complete, a final brief neurologic examination is performed and the sheath removed. The volume and rate of hemoptysis will decrease abruptly following a successful procedure. It may take several days for all bleeding to subside. If the bleeding has not decreased substantially in 24 hr, repeat arteriography is needed to detect additional bronchial arteries (aberrant or nonaberrant), nonbronchial systemic collaterals, and/or a pulmonary artery source (Figure 3.8). In the absence of severe cavitary lung disease, an additional systemic arterial source is likely. One must also consider a nonpulmonary source of bleeding in those patients with diffuse systemic diseases who have not responded to successful embolotherapy.

RESULTS

Bronchial artery embolization has been shown to be successful in the immediate and long-term control of hemoptysis. Approximately 75–100% of patients have prompt cessation of bleeding following BAE.[22,44,63] Patients who have a surgically correctable disease and are surgical candidates usually proceed to a definitive resection. When BAE and surgical resection are used together, BAE can both stabilize the patient and ensure maximum preservation of lung tissue.[23]

Long-term control of hemoptysis in patients treated with BAE occurs in approximately 80% of patients.[22,24,64] Approximately 20% of patients successfully embolized have recurrence of bleeding within 6 months to 1 yr. Recurrent hemoptysis is usually secondary to progression of disease, development of new systemic collaterals, recanalization of previously embolized arteries or, rarely, a pulmonary arterial source. Patients with chronic inflammatory diseases, such as cystic fibrosis, are likely to have recurrences. However, BAE in patients with cystic fibrosis has proved to be beneficial.[8,9] Recurrent bleeding is also more common in patients with aspergillomas, as these lesions tend to recruit extensive systemic collaterals through pleural adhesions. Patients with lung cancer are prone to recurrent bleeding as the tumor becomes more invasive.[47] Most of the previous studies with long-term follow-up used Gelfoam as the embolizing agent. Long-term success may improve now that PVA particles are more commonly used.

Immediate failures of the procedure occur in 10–25% of patients.[10,24,65] Death due to asphyxiation can occur in patients who are bleeding massively. Airway control with tracheal intubation may be necessary in these patients. Failure to identify or embolize all involved bronchial or nonbronchial systemic arteries will result in at least a partial failure. A technical failure will also result from the inability to obtain a sufficiently stable catheter position, therefore preventing embolization.

COMPLICATIONS

Minor adverse affects are much more common than major complications with BAE. Chest pain and dysphagia are believed to be secondary to occlusion of branches of the bronchial arteries to the posterior mediastinum and middle esophagus. A low-grade fever can occur after BAE, but usually resolves in 2–7 days. The fever is believed to be a foreign body reaction inherent to the procedure rather than a complication.

Necrosis of the mainstem bronchi has been reported following embolization with gelatin sponge powder. Infarction of the left main stem bronchus occurred in a patient after embolization with ethanol.[58] A single case of bronchoesophageal fistula formation has also been reported.[66]

Spinal cord injury is a dreaded complication of BAE. Transverse myelitis is believed to be related to the toxicity of ionic contrast media. The incidence of spinal cord complications has decreased dramatically with greater use of DSA and low-osmolar contrast agents. In fact, there were no instances of transverse myelitis in 432 patients undergoing BAE in four large recent series.[24,63,67] Should transverse myelitis develop, there is usually a partial return of function.[68] There is only one reported case of spinal cord infarction following BAE, and this involved embolization of a left intercostal artery rather than a bronchial artery.[69] Careful selective preembolization angiography and the use of particles greater than 200 μm will help to minimize the occurrence of this serious complication.

Inadvertant embolization of a nontarget artery is a potential complication of any embolization procedure. Reflux of particles has resulted in bowel ischemia and necrosis, and embolization of the anterior tibial artery.[22] In order to minimize such complications, stable catheter position or coaxial microcatheter techniques and frequent contrast injections to assess for vascular stasis are essential. Bronchial artery dissection and/or dissection of the aortic wall are also technical complications that preclude effective BAE.

PERCUTANEOUS NONVASCULAR THERAPY

Hemoptysis can also occur in patients with cavitary pulmonary aspergillomas. Massive hemoptysis is the cause of death in 5–14% of these patients. Traditional bronchial artery embolization has been successful in the short-term treatment of bleeding secondary to aspergillomas. However, these patients have the highest recurrence rate of hemoptysis and mortality rate following embolotherapy.[64,65]

Lee et al. have recently demonstrated a safe and effective percutaneous nonvascular treatment of aspergilloma cavities with daily instillations of a mixture containing amphotericin B, bromhexine, and normal saline.[70] Hemoptysis was controlled within 5 days in all patients, and complete resolution of the cavity was achieved in 75% of patients. To avoid intervening vessels, Klein and colleagues have recommended catheter placement under contrast-enhanced CT guidance.[71] Addition of 5 cc of 2% lidocaine to the amphotericin mixture helped reduce coughing during instillation. Daily afternoon saline irrigations with 50–100 cc were performed and believed to hasten resolution. Munk et al. also treated intracavitary aspergillomas effectively by the percutaneous instillation of amphotericin in a gelatin form.[72] The gelatin preparation, which was liquid at 40°C, solidified at body temperature and remained within the cavity; only one treatment was necessary. Complete resolution was documented in three of the four patients treated. Complications related to this procedure have included bleeding, pneumothorax, superinfection of the cavity, and empyema formation.

REFERENCES

1. Bobrowitz ID, Ramakrishna S, Shim Y-S; Comparison of medical vs. surgical treatment of major hemoptysis. *Arch Intern Med* 143:1343–1346, 1983.
2. Crocco JA, Rooney JJ, Fankushen DS, et al: Massive hemoptysis. *Arch Intern Med* 121:495–498, 1968.
3. Stoller JK: Diagnosis and management of massive hemoptysis: a review. *Respir Care* 37:564–581, 1992.
4. Cahill BC, Ingbar DH: Massive hemoptysis: assessment and management. *Clin Chest Med* 15:147–168, 1994.

5. Winter SM, Ingbar DH: Massive hemoptysis: pathogenesis and management. *J Intensive Care Med* 3:171–188, 1988.

6. Levitsky S, Lapey A, di Sant' Agnese PA: Pulmonary resection for life-threatening hemoptysis in cystic fibrosis. *JAMA* 213:125, 1970.

7. Porter DK, Van Every MJ, Mack JW: Emergency lobectomy for massive hemoptysis in cystic fibrosis. *J Thorac Cardiovasc Surg* 86:409, 1983.

8. Cohen AM, Doershuk CF, Stein RC: Bronchial artery embolization to control hemoptysis in cystic fibrosis. *Radiology* 175:401–405, 1990.

9. Fellows KE, Khaw KT, Schuster S, et al: Bronchial artery embolization in cystic fibrosis: technique and long-term results. *J Pediatr* 95:959–963, 1979.

10. Remy J, Arnaud A, Fardou H, et al: Treatment of hemoptysis by embolization of bronchial arteries. *Radiology* 122:33–37, 1977.

11. Deffebach ME, Charan NB, Lakshminarayan S, et al: The bronchial circulation: small, but a vital attribute of the lung. *Am Rev Respir Dis* 135:463–481, 1987.

12. Stefanini M, Marin HM, Soardi F, et al: The comparative activity in vivo of trypsin and aspergillin O (mold fibrinolysin). *Angiology* 13:254–259, 1962.

13. Tonkin ILD, Hanissian SW, Boulden TF, et al: Bronchial arteriography and embolotherapy for hemoptysis in patients with cystic fibrosis. *Cardiovasc Intervent Radiol* 14:241, 1991.

14. Schidlow DV, Taussig LM, Knowles MR: Cystic fibrosis foundation consensus conference report on pulmonary complications of cystic fibrosis. *Pediatr Pulmonol* 15:187, 1993.

15. Saumench J, Excarrabill J, Padró L, et al: Value of fiberoptic bronchoscopy and angiography for diagnosis of the bleeding site in hemoptysis. *Ann Thorac Surg* 48:272, 1989.

16. Popper J: The use of premarin IV in hemoptysis. *Dis Chest* 37:659, 1960.

17. Magee G, Williams MH Jr: Treatment of massive hemoptysis with intravenous pitressin. *Lung* 160:165, 1982.

18. Swersky RB, Chang JB, Wisoff BG, et al: Endobronchial balloon tamponade of hemoptysis in patients with cystic fibrosis. *Ann Thorac Surg* 27:262, 1979.

19. Jolliet P, Soccal P, Chevrolet JC: Control of massive hemoptysis by endobronchial tamponade with a pulmonary artery balloon catheter. *Crit Care Med* 20:1730–1732, 1992.

20. Garzon AA, Cerruti MM, Golding ME: Exsanguinating hemoptysis. *J Thorac Cardiovasc Surg* 84:829–833, 1982.

21. Uflacker R, Kaemmerer A, Picon PD, et al: Bronchial artery embolization in the management of hemoptysis: technical aspects and long-term results. *Radiology* 157:637–644, 1985.

22. Tan RT, McGahan JP, Link DP, et al: Bronchial artery embolization in management of hemoptysis. *J Intervent Radiol* 6:67–76, 1991.

23. Roberts AC: Bronchial artery embolization therapy. *J Thoracic Imaging* 5:60–72, 1990.

24. Rabkin JE, Astafjev VI, Gothman LN, et al: Transcatheter embolization in the management of pulmonary hemorrhage. *Radiology* 163:361–365, 1987.

25. Muthuswamy PP, Akbik F, Franklin C, et al: Management of major or massive hemoptysis in active pulmonary tuberculosis by bronchial artery embolization. *Chest* 92:77–82, 1987.

26. Vujic I, Pyle R, Hungerford GD, et al: Angiography and therapeutic blockage in the control of hemoptysis. *Radiology* 134:19–23, 1982.

27. Bookstein JJ, Moser KM, Kalafer ME, et al: The role of bronchial arteriography and therapeutic embolization in hemoptysis. *Chest* 72:658–661, 1977.

28. Harley JO, Killien FC, Peck AG: Massive hemoptysis controlled by transcatheter embolization of the bronchial arteries. *Am J Roentgenol* 128:303–304, 1977.

29. Stoll JF, Bettmann MA; Bronchial artery embolization to control hemoptysis: a review. *Cardiovasc Intervent Radiol* 11:263, 1988.

30. Hellekant C: Bronchial angiographie und intraarterielle chemotherapie bei bronchial-kairzinom. *Radiologe* 19:521–527, 1979.

31. Kadir S: *Diagnostic Angiography*. Philadelphia, WB Saunders, pp 162–171, 1986.

32. Cauldwell EW, Siekert RG, Lininger RE, et al: The bronchial arteries: an anatomic study of 150 human cadavers. *Surg Gynecol Obstet* 86:395–412, 1948.

33. Keller FS, Fosch J, Loflin TG, et al: Nonbronchial systemic collateral arteries: significance in percutaneous embolotherapy for hemoptysis. *Radiology* 164:687–692, 1987.

34. Jardin M, Remy J: Control of hemoptysis: systemic angiography and anastomoses of the internal mammary artery. *Radiology* 168:377–383, 1988.

35. Tveten L: Spinal cord vascularity: III. The spinal cord in man. *Acta Radiol Diagn* 17:257–273, 1976.

36. Eames FA, Roberson GH: Angiography of the spine. In Kadir S: *Diagnostic Angiography.* Philadelphia, WB Saunders, pp 496–509, 1986.
37. Scrodt JF, Becker GJ, Scott JA, et al: Bronchial artery embolization: monitoring with somatosensory evoked potentials. *Radiology* 164:135–139, 1987.
38. Doppman JL, Girton M, Oldfeld EH: Spinal Wada test. *Radiology* 161:319–321, 1986.
39. Kardjiev V, Symeonov A, Chankov I: Etiology, pathogenesis, and prevention of spinal cord lesions in selective angiography of the bronchial and intercostal arteries. *Radiology* 112:81, 1974.
40. Tanaka F, Hayakawa K, Satoh Y, et al: Evaluating bronchial drainage pathways in patients with lung disease using digital subtraction angiography. *Invest Radiol* 28:434–438, 1993.
41. Osada H, Kawada T, Ashida H, et al: Bronchial artery aneurysms. *Ann Thorac Surg* 41:440–442, 1986.
42. McPherson S, Routh WD, Nat H, et al: Anomalous origin of bronchial arteries: potential pitfall of embolotherapy for hemoptysis. *J Vasc Interv Radiol* 1:86, 1990.
43. Parke WW, Michels NA: The nonbronchial systemic arteries of the lung. *J Thorac Cardiovasc Surg* 49:694–707, 1965.
44. Moore LB, McNey RE, Vujic I: Massive hemoptysis: control by embolization of the thyrocervical trunk. *Radiology* 161:173–174, 1986.
45. Cohen AM, Antoun BW, Stern RC: Left thyrocervical trunk bronchial artery supplying right lung: source of recurrent hemoptysis in cystic fibrosis. *Am J Roentgenol* 158:1131, 1992.
46. Tamura S, Kodama T, Otsuka N, et al: Embolotherapy for persistent hemoptysis: the significance of pleural thickening. *Cardiovasc Intervent Radiol* 16:85–88, 1993.
47. Ferris EJ: Pulmonary hemorrhage: vascular evaluation and interventional therapy. *Chest* 80:710–714, 1981.
48. Remy J, Smith M, Lemaitre L, et al: Treatment of massive hemoptysis by occlusion of a Rasmussen aneurysm. *Am J Roentgenol* 135:605–606, 1980.
49. Renie WA, Rodeheffer RJ, Mitchell S, et al: Balloon embolization of a mycotic pulmonary aneurysm. *Am Rev Respir Dis* 126:1107–1110, 1982.
50. Davidoff AB, Udoff EF, Schonfeld SA: Intraaneurysmal embolization of a pulmonary artery aneurysm for control of hemoptysis. *Am J Roentgenol* 142:1010–1029, 1984.
51. Plessinger VA, Jolly TN: Rasmussen's aneurysms and fatal hemorrhage in pulmonary tuberculosis. *Am Rev Tuberc* 60:589–603, 1949.
52. Remy J, Lemaitre L, Lafitte JJ, et al: Massive hemoptysis of pulmonary arterial origin: diagnosis and treatment. *Am J Roentgenol* 143:963–969, 1984.
53. Miyazono N, Inoue H, Hori A, et al: Visualization of left bronchial-to-coronary artery communication after distal bronchial artery embolization for bronchiectasis. *Cardiovasc Intervent Radiol* 17:36–37, 1994.
54. Lois JF, Gomes AS, Smith DC, et al: Systemic-to-pulmonary collateral vessels and shunts: treatment with embolization. *Radiology* 169:671–676, 1988.
55. Boushy SF, Helgason AH, North LB: Occlusion of the bronchial arteries by glass microspheres. *Am Rev Respir Dis* 102:249–263, 1971.
56. Matsumoto AH, Suhocki PV, Barth KH: Superselective Gelfoam embolotherapy using a highly visible small caliber catheter. *Cardiovasc Intervent Radiol* 11:303–306, 1988.
57. Ivanick MJ, Thorworth W, Donahue J, et al: Infarction of the left main-stem bronchus: a complication of bronchial artery embolization. *Am J Roentgenol* 141:535–537, 1983.
58. Wholey MH, Chamorro HA, Rao G, et al: Bronchial artery embolization for massive hemoptysis. *JAMA* 236:2501–2505, 1976.
59. Fairfax AJ, Ball J, Batten JC, et al: A pathological study following bronchial artery embolization for haemoptysis in cystic fibrosis. *Br J Dis Chest* 74:345–352, 1980.
60. Mauro MA, Jaques PF: Transcatheter embolization with a Gelfoam slurry. *J Intervent Radiol* 2:157–159, 1987.
61. Fuhrman BP, Bass JC, Castaneda-Zuniga W, et al: Coil embolization of congenital thoracic vascular anomalies in infants and children. *Circulation* 70:284–289, 1984.
62. Nancarrow PA, Fellows KE, Lock JE: Stability of coil emboli: an in vitro study. *Cardiovasc Intervent Radiol* 10:226–229, 1987.
63. Magilligan DJ, Seetaramaiah R, Zayat P: Massive hemoptysis: control by transcatheter BAE. *Ann Thorac Surg* 32:392–400, 1981.
64. Katoh O, Kishikawa T, Yamada H, et al: Recurrent bleeding after arterial embolization in patients with hemoptysis. *Chest* 97:541–546, 1990.

65. Uflacker R, Kaemmerer A, Neves C, et al: Management of massive hemoptysis by bronchial artery embolization. *Radiology* 146:627–634, 1983.

66. Helenon CH, Chatel A, Bigot JM, et al: Fistule oesophago-bronchique gauche agrès embolization bronchique. *Nouv Presse Med* 6:4209, 1977.

67. Hayakawa K, Tanaka F, Torizuka T: Bronchial artery embolization for hemoptysis: immediate and long-term results. *Cardiovasc Intervent Radiol* 15:154–159, 1992.

68. Feigelson HH, Ravin HA: Transverse myelitis following selective bronchial arteriography. *Radiology* 85:663–665, 1965.

69. Vujic I, Pyle R, Parker E, et al: Control of massive hemoptysis by embolization of intercostal arteries. *Radiology* 137:616–620, 1980.

70. Lee K, Kim H, Kim Y, et al: Treatment of hemoptysis in patients with cavitary aspergilloma of the lung: value of percutaneous instillation of amphotericin B. *Am J Roentgenol* 161:727–731, 1993.

71. Klein J, Fang K, Chang M: Percutaneous transcatheter treatment of an intracavitary aspergilloma. *Cardiovasc Intervent Radiol* 16:321–324, 1993.

72. Munk P, Vellet A, Rankin R, et al: Intracavitary aspergilloma: transthoracic percutaneous injection of amphotericin gelatin solution. *Radiology* 188:821–823, 1993.

CHAPTER
4

Transcatheter Management of Pulmonary Arteriovenous Malformations

Jeffrey S. Pollak

Arteriovenous malformations of the lung are congenital abnormalities in which a direct connection between a pulmonary artery and vein exists, circumventing the normal capillary bed. This abnormality was first described in 1897; however, the development of appropriate lung-conserving surgical methods required several decades.[1,2] Transcatheter closure was first reported in 1977, and quickly proved to be the treatment method of choice.[3-5]

CLINICAL BACKGROUND

While early reports indicated a 36% to 60% incidence of hereditary hemorrhagic telangiectasia (HHT) (Osler-Weber-Rendu syndrome) in patients with pulmonary arteriovenous malformation (PAVM), with intensive family screening the associated incidence rises to above 85%.[4,6,7] The remaining 15% of PAVM appear to be isolated events, unrelated to any other disorder.

The classic findings of HHT are telangiectasias of the skin and mucous membranes, repeated nosebleeds, and an autosomal dominant pattern of inheritance.[8] The incidence is estimated at 1 to 2 per 100,000, but is probably higher because many patients escape diagnosis. The underlying disorder appears to be dilatation of a postcapillary venule, which eventually progresses to arteriolar dilatation and direct arteriovenous shunting.[9] Five organs are primarily affected: skin, nose, lung, central nervous system (CNS), and gastrointestinal (GI) tract. The papular, red, blanching, mucocutaneous telangiectasias can be subtle but generally progress with time. The skin of the face, lips, tongue, conjunctiva, and fingers, especially about the nails, should be carefully examined. Lesions are frequently not evident until after adolescence. Epistaxis is the most common symptom, occurring in 90% of patients. This generally starts by the third decade and progresses with age.[10] The risk of PAVM in patients with HHT is approximately 15%, although it rises to over one-third if another family member has PAVM.[11] Most CNS manifestations of HHT are related to paradoxical emboli, but CNS vascular malformations can also be seen. GI bleeding occurs in approximately 20% of patients.

The gene for HHT in association with PAVM has recently been identified as endoglin, on chromosome 9q3.[12,13] This gene produces a binding protein for transforming growth factor-β that is present on endothelial cells, permitting cellular response to this growth factor. Abnormalities of this gene do not appear to be present in HHT families without PAVM, indicating genetic heterogeneity to the syndrome. Different mutations of this gene also appear to be present in different families, indicating that a simple genetic test will not be forthcoming in the near future.

Symptoms and signs related to PAVM are due to right-to-left shunting or bleeding secondary to rupture of a component of the PAVM. Right-to-left shunting leads to hypoxemia and permits paradoxical emboli to occur. Dyspnea and fatigue occur in over 70% of patients with PAVM, but in our personal experience, stroke, transient ischemic attacks (TIA), and brain abscesses from paradoxical emboli are more common modes of clinical presentation in the unscreened population. Overall, 55% of patients described a history of stroke or TIA, while another 9% had abscesses. Signs may include cyanosis, digital clubbing, and murmur. Other manifestations include hemoptysis (13%) and hemothorax (9%), which can occasionally be massive and life-threatening.[14] Enlargement of and massive bleeding from PAVMs during pregnancy has also been reported.[15] High output heart failure is unusual, but has been described as a mode of presentation in neonates.[16] Other entities that have uncommonly been found in association with PAVM include secondary hypertrophic osteoarthropathy and juvenile polyposis.[17]

Laboratory evaluation of patients with PAVMs may reveal polycythemia; however, this is infrequent, since even relatively small shunts bring patients to clinical attention due to their CNS sequelae. Anemia can also be seen secondary to recurrent nasal bleeding. Arterial blood gases (ABGs) will indicate a shunt by showing hypoxemia on room air and an inadequate rise in oxygen saturation on 100% O_2. Hypoxemia is usually worse in the erect position since PAVMs have a predilection for the lower lobes. This is the basis for the use of supine and erect pulse oximetry to screen patients.[18]

PATHOLOGY

Pulmonary arteriovenous malformations range in size from microscopic to several centimeters in diameter. Simple PAVMs account for 80% of macroscopic lesions and are characterized by an enlarged single feeding artery, an enlarged single draining vein, and an aneurysm connecting the two (Figure 4.1). The remainder of PAVMs are complex, resembling systemic arteriovenous malformations, with numerous arteries and veins and a complex nidus (Figure 4.2). Rarely, connections with systemic vessels may be seen.[19]

The lesions are usually subpleural in location. They are frequently multiple (up to 58%) and bilateral (up to 42%), and occur predominantly in the lower lobes (55% to 84%).[2] (Figure 4.3). Rarely, a diffuse pattern is present with numerous lesions densely distributed within a region of lung. Multiplicity is more common with HHT. In addition to any macroscopic PAVMs, microscopic lesions should be assumed to present in patients with HHT.

DIAGNOSTIC WORKUP

The evaluation of patients with suspected PAVM consists of confirming the diagnosis in symptomatic patients, screening asymptomatic patients, and determining whether the lesion warrants therapy. Chest radiography and ABGs are preliminary steps in this

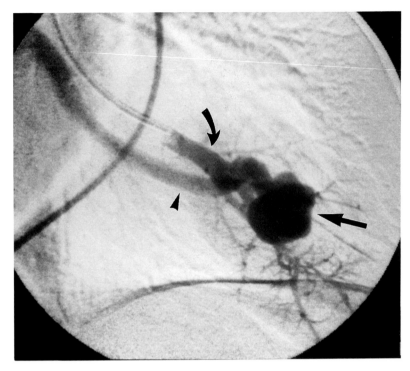

Figure 4.1 Selective angiogram of a simple PAVM in the left lower lobe. There is a single feeding artery (curved arrow), single draining vein (arrowhead), and connecting aneurysm (straight arrow). The artery to the lesion also gives off branches to normal lung which are partly superimposed on the malformation.

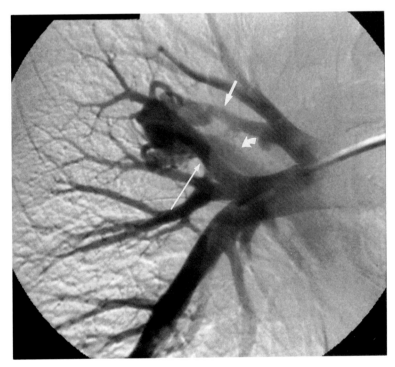

A

Figure 4.2 A. Digital subtraction angiogram in a right anterior oblique projection of a complex malformation in the right lung. Several feeding arteries are seen from the upper branch to the superior segment of the lower lobe (long straight arrow) and the posterior segment of the upper lobe (short straight arrow). The major draining vein parallels the superior segmental artery (short curved arrow). **B.** Following page.

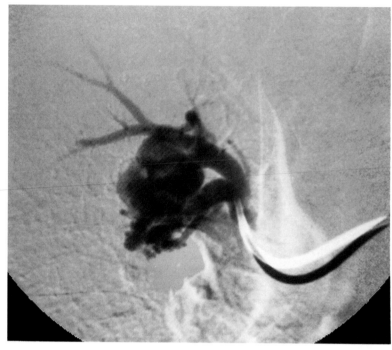

B

Figure 4.2 B. The complex, septated malformation is better visualized on a selective injection of the upper branch of the superior segmental artery.

process. These two studies should uncover any significant shunt that could place even an asymptomatic patient at risk for major embolic complications.

Chest Radiographs

Plain films of the chest classically demonstrate the lobular soft tissue mass of the aneurysmal arteriovenous communication, the feeding artery coursing from the hilum, and the draining vein passing into the left atrium (Figure 4.4). While the aneurysm of simple lesions is frequently seen, the vessels often are not. Complex malformations can appear multilobulated and may have less well-defined margins. The plain film findings of PAVM are not reliably present, due to the relatively small size of many significant lesions and the masking by normal structures, such as the diaphragms. A negative chest radiograph in the presence of a positive ABG should not deter further investigation.

Computed Tomography

Conventional computed tomographic (CT) scanning has a high sensitivity in diagnosing and localizing PAVM.[20] Findings are a noncalcified nodule or serpiginous mass with feeding arteries and draining veins (Figure 4.5). Contrast enhancement occurs, but contrast administration is not essential if the proper morphology is present. False-positive studies can occur from other lesions that enhance with contrast, such as vascular metastases.[21] Improved identification and characterization of lesions as simple or complex is possible with helical CT and three-dimensional techniques.[22]

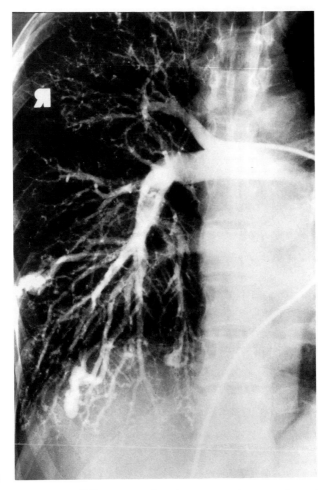

A

Figure 4.3 A (above) and B (following page). Pulmonary angiograms of a patient with HHT and hypoxemia. Multiple, bilateral, varyingly sized malformations are seen, most in the lower lobes. Several tiny lesions in the right lateral costophrenic angle are too small to warrant occlusion.

While the aneurysm or nidus of a lesion appears to be accurately assessed by CT, it is less clear how accurate CT is for measuring the minimum size of the feeding arteries. This is an important factor in deciding whether to treat asymptomatic patients. Nevertheless, it seems possible that current generation CT scanning may be able to replace invasive ABGs in the screening process and permit more direct angiography at the time of embolization. Computed tomography also is of value in following patients after therapy.

Contrast Echocardiography

Intravenous injection of agitated saline to produce echogenic microbubbles during echocardiography has proved to be a useful method for detecting right-to-left shunts in the heart. Normally, none of the echogenic bubbles should enter the left cardiac chambers since they are filtered by the pulmonary circulation. In the presence of cardiac defects or pulmonary arteriovenous shunts, the echogenic bubbles will appear on the left side. The lack of any demonstrable structural anomalies of the heart with visu-

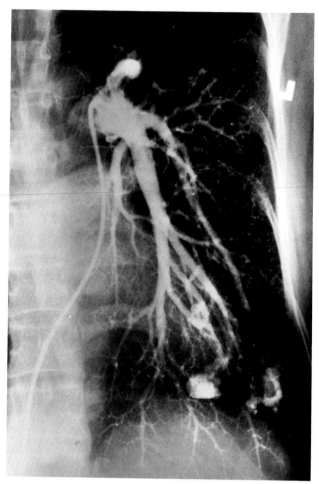

B

Figure 4.3 *(Continued.)*

alization of left atrial echoes increases the specificity of the test. While very sensitive, contrast echocardiography is unable to determine the location, size, and number of PAVMs.[23]

Radionuclide Shunt Studies

Technetium-99m albumin microspheres or macroaggregates used for lung scanning can demonstrate right-to-left shunting due to abnormal entry of these particles into the systemic circulation. Quantification of the shunt is also possible, but at rest and during exercise.[24,25] Although a radionuclide shunt study has the advantage of being noninvasive, the location, size, and number of PAVMs cannot be determined.

Pulmonary Angiography

The gold standard for diagnosing a PAVM is pulmonary angiography (Figures 4.1, 4.2, and 4.3). Selective injections of both pulmonary arteries are necessary with filming in at least two projections. The frontal view is generally acquired using conventional cut-film technique, whereas oblique views can be acquired by digital imaging. A careful search for multiple lesions should be performed and supplemental views may be nec-

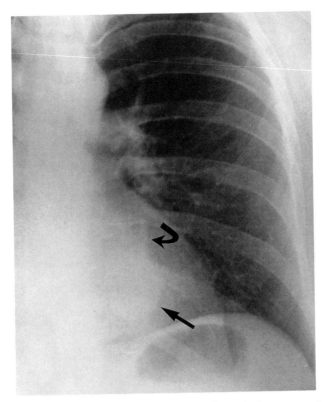

Figure 4.4 Chest radiograph of a 47-yr-old woman with HHT who presented with a brain abscess. A large mass is seen in the left lower lobe (straight arrow) with a vessel from the hilum leading to it (curved arrow) representing the artery. The vein is not well visualized.

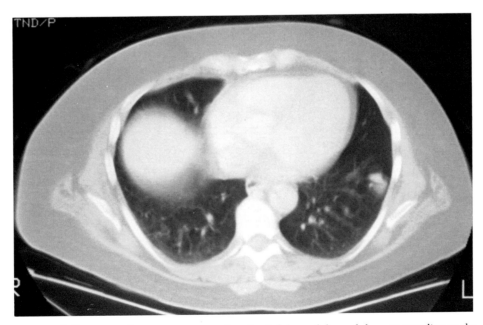

Figure 4.5 CT scan demonstrating an enhancing left lower lobe nodule corresponding to the simple PAVM shown in Figure 5.1. The vascular channels are not well seen as they pass out of the plane of this image.

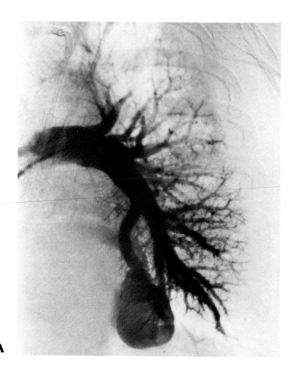

A

B

Figure 4.6 A. Left pulmonary angiogram of patient shown in Figure 5.4 depicts a large simple-appearing lesion in the left lower lobe. B. Selective angiography of the arterial trunk to this region shows two adjacent simple malformations (arrows). C. Following page.

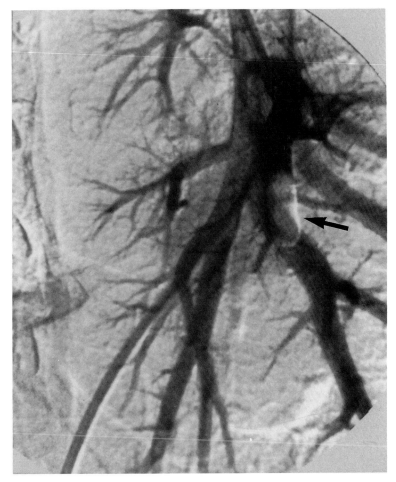

C

Figure 4.6 C. A detachable silicone balloon was used to occlude the vessel feeding these two PAVMs (arrow).

essary if there are any suspicious areas. It is possible that preangiographic CT may be able to limit the lung regions that need to be studied.

Simple malformations will have a single feeding artery, an intervening aneurysm, and a single draining vein (Figure 4.1). Complex lesions have several arteries and veins with an irregular, frequently septated, connecting nidus (Figure 4.2). Patients with multiple lesions can have both types. Furthermore, there is a continuum between these two extremes. Lesions that initially appear simple can subsequently be found to have more than one artery entering the aneurysm on selective contrast injections, or multiple simple-appearing lesions may be found adjacent to one another (Figure 4.6).

Lesions can vary in size and distribution (Figure 4.3). Rarely, diffuse involvement of a region of the lung by numerous lesions can occur. Multiple tiny lesions, below the threshold of angiography, should be assumed to be present in patients with HHT. Therefore, the risk of paradoxical bacterial emboli still remains even after therapy.

THERAPY

Treatment of PAVM is indicated to alleviate symptoms and signs of the right-to-left shunt and as prophylaxis against paradoxical embolization. Conservative therapy carries an unacceptably high rate of complications, with significant morbidity reaching 33% and mortality as high as 29%.[2] The goal of therapy is to eliminate all individual shunts in which the feeding artery is 3 mm or larger as even lesions this small can increase the risk of a stroke.[26] Smaller lesions may require therapy when they are numerous enough to cause significant hypoxemia.

Surgery

Surgical treatment of PAVM has evolved toward lung-conserving procedures such as local excision or segmentectomy.[6,7,27] Ligation of the feeding arteries is often difficult. Although surgical mortality is generally low (0 to 6%),[2] a lobectomy or pneumonectomy will sacrifice large volumes of potentially normal lung. Disadvantages of surgery include the discomfort, risk, and recuperative period associated with a thoracotomy, the associated loss of normal lung tissue, and the problems presented by multiple, bilateral PAVMs.

Embolotherapy

Porstmann first described embolization of PAVMs in 1977.[3] This description was quickly followed by other case reports using coils and detachable balloons (DBs).[28,29] Further experience has shown its effectiveness and advantages over surgery, making it the preferred method of treatment.[4,5]

On a day preceding the embolization, a complete, bilateral diagnostic pulmonary angiogram is done through one of the femoral veins to determine the number, location, and architecture of the lesions. The best projection for visualizing the arterial supply is also determined. On the day of the embolization, the contralateral femoral vein is used. An 8-Fr sheath is placed, and 3,000 to 5,000 units of heparin are administered. A 7-Fr multipurpose catheter (Cordis, Miami, FL or Cook, Inc., Bloomington, IN) or another similar catheter is advanced into the pulmonary circulation in conjunction with a Bentson wire (Cook, Inc.). This catheter is usually capable of selecting most branches, especially in the lower and upper lobes. A Headhunter-shape catheter (Cook, Inc.) is also effective for selecting lower lobe branches. An internal mammary shape catheter (Cook, Inc.) is occasionally useful for right middle lobe and lingular branches. A 5-Fr Berenstein catheter (Medi-Tech, Watertown, MA) can be used in conjunction with an 8-Fr nontapered guiding catheter (Interventional Therapeutics Corp., South San Francisco, CA or Nycomed-Ingenor Laboratories, Paris, France) (Figure 4.7). The guiding catheter gives the support necessary to maintain a stable position across the heart, while the more flexible 5-Fr catheter permits easy advancement into a superselective position.

The optimal site to occlude in a feeding artery is the narrowest segment distal to any significant supply to normal lung. Since there is frequently dilatation of the artery immediately before it enters the aneurysm, the optimal site may lie several centimeters proximal to the arteriovenous connection. Unlike complex systemic vascular malformations, occlusion of the nidus is not necessary, and indeed risks rupture. Effective control of PAVMs is achieved by occlusion of the feeding arteries alone. This can be achieved with either embolization coils or DBs.

Due to the lack of FDA-approved DBs, coil emboli are currently the primary agents used for transcatheter occlusion of PAVMs. These devices are helices of stainless steel wire covered with polyester fibers to make them moderately thrombogenic. Forming a "nest" with several coils is usually necessary to produce occlusion, especially with larger vessels. This can be accomplished by placing several large coils followed by placement of progressively smaller coils to effect complete vessel occlusion. Conventional 0.035–0.038 inch Gianturco coils (Cook, Inc.) are commercially available in outer diameters measuring 2–15 mm. The proper coil diameter to use is approxi-

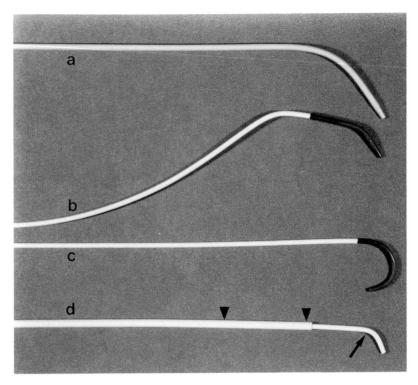

Figure 4.7 Different shape catheters frequently used for PAVM embolization. **A.** 7.2-Fr multipurpose-shape catheter, **B.** 5-Fr H1 cerebral-shape catheter, **C.** 5-Fr Rösch Inferior Mesenteric (RIM) catheter, and **D.** 8-Fr nontapered guiding catheter (arrowheads) which can be shaped with steam, with an inner 5-Fr Berenstein catheter (arrow).

mately 20% larger than the expected true vessel diameter. If the coil is too small, it can potentially migrate through the PAVM. If the coil is too large in diameter, it will elongate and displace itself and the tip of the catheter from the target vessel.

The coils are available in a variety of lengths. The longer the coil, the more stainless steel and polyester there is to induce vessel thrombosis; however, the longer the coil, the greater the tendency to displace the catheter tip from the target vessel during deployment of the coil.[30] This underscores the importance of stable catheter positioning during the procedure. If catheter stability is in doubt, test passage of a guidewire can be performed prior to coil insertion. Use of shorter coils and a floppy guidewire to push the coil is also less likely to cause the catheter tip to recoil and dislodge from the target vessel. Delivering coils through an occlusion balloon catheter (Medi-Tech/Boston Scientific) is helpful when embolizing high-flow malformations or lesions in which it is difficult to maintain stable catheter position (Figure 4.8). The use of an adjacent occlusion balloon may also be important for embolizing high-flow lesions with a DB, to prevent excessive drag on the balloon and its premature detachment. Following embolization, a control angiogram is performed to confirm occlusion of the PAVM and to look for any residual feeding arteries or previously undetected malformations.

Gianturco coils are designed to be pushed through appropriately sized polyethylene catheters. The coils can become "stuck" in catheters made from polyurethane, polyvinyl chloride, or some of the newer hydrophilic materials (Glidecatheter, Medi-Tech/Boston Scientific).

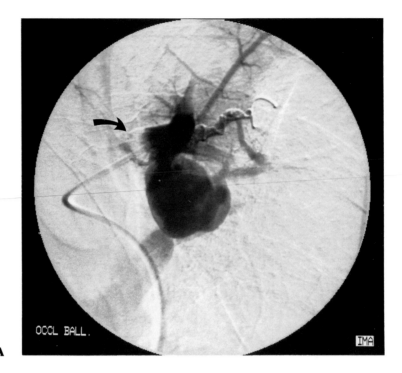

Figure 4.8 A. The feeding artery to the left upper lobe PAVM in Figure 5.4 was relatively short, not permitting a stable position for the selective catheter. After coils were placed in the distal portion of the complex lesion, an occlusion balloon was placed proximally in the vessel (arrow). Further coil embolization was now possible. B. Final angiogram shows a tight nest of proximal coils and no residual malformation.

In rare instances, use of platinum microcoils (Cook, Inc., and Target Therapeutics, San Jose, CA)[31] may be necessary. These coils are designed to be delivered through 3-Fr microcatheters with inner diameters of 0.018–0.025 inch. Microcoils are available in a variety of shapes, lengths, and diameters. Although some polyester fibers are attached to these coils, they are not nearly as thrombogenic as Gianturco coils. Large quantities and dense packing of microcoils are usually required to induce vessel thrombosis. Microcoils also cost 3 times more (per coil) than Gianturco coils. Therefore, the only reason to use microcoils is to embolize vessels that are difficult to access using standard 5-Fr catheters.

Two DBs have been used extensively in the neurovascular system and, in a limited fashion, in the periphery: the Detachable Silicone Balloon (Interventional Therapeutics Corp.) and the latex Goldvalve Balloon (Nycomed-Ingenor Laboratories. Maximum inflated balloon sizes range from 6 to 15 mm in diameter and 8 to 30 mm in length.[30] The larger balloons have correspondingly larger uninflated diameters that require larger introducers/guiding catheters.

Detachable balloons (DBs) consist of a shell of compliant silicone or latex and a self-sealing valve or ligature to maintain inflation. The DBs are mounted on a thin, flexible delivery-inflation catheter. An outer, coaxial, detachment catheter is frequently used in conjunction with the delivery catheter to hold the DB in place during release. Traction of the inflated balloon against the vessel wall as the delivery catheter is retracted may be sufficient to obviate the need for a detachment catheter. The balloon, its delivery catheter, and its detachment catheter are advanced into the desired vessel through a nontapered guiding catheter.

After the target vessel is selected, the guiding catheter is introduced using an exchange wire. After the DB is advanced into position (Figure 4.9) and test inflated, con-

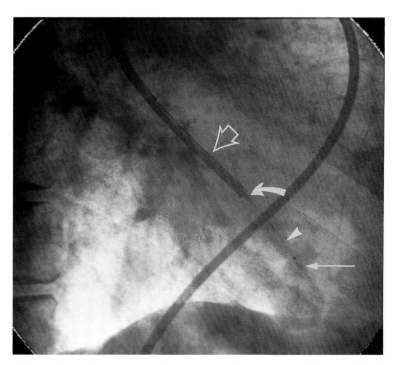

Figure 4.9 A detachable silicone balloon in a simple PAVM is well outlined by the aerated lung. The system consists of the uninflated balloon (straight arrow), a 2-Fr deliver catheter (arrowhead), 4.2-Fr detachment catheter (curved arrow), and 8-Fr introducer (open arrow). The balloon is slightly too distal in location in this image and was retracted approximately 1 cm before inflation and release.

trast is injected through a Y-adapter to confirm an appropriate occlusion. If acceptable, the balloon is released (Figure 4.6C). Goldvalve balloons will usually remain inflated for a minimum of 1 month, while detachable silicone balloons appear to remain inflated longer. After 3 wks, permanent vessel obliteration is nearly always present, even if the DB deflates.[33]

Coils have several advantages over DBs embolic agents. They are readily available, relatively inexpensive, easily placed through most diagnostic catheters, and FDA-approved. On the other hand, DBs permit test occlusion, repositioning, cross-sectional mechanical vessel obstruction with a single device, and, occasionally, flow-direction into a vessel that could not otherwise be catheterized. Unfortunately, there are no available DBs that are FDA-approved.

Complications

Major clinical complications of embolotherapy appear to be quite rare.[4,5,34] In reviewing our experience, paradoxical air embolization was seen in approximately 5% of patients undergoing embolotherapy. As the geometry of pulmonary arteries changes with respiratory excursions, catheters tend to become wedged and air can be introduced. This wedging should be prevented by careful attention to backflow prior to injection. Furthermore, all peripheral intravenous lines should be cleared of air. The most common symptoms caused by air embolization are angina and bradycardia. These symptoms occur when air enters the right coronary artery, the ostium of which is anterior and nondependent in the supine patient. The symptoms usually resolve several minutes after atropine and/or nitroglycerin therapy. Paradoxical migration of embolization devices has been noted in fewer than 1% of procedures and has been associated with no adverse sequela. Loss of a device elsewhere in the lung is also rare. Procedurally induced paradoxical thromboembolism has not been seen, perhaps due to routine heparinization. Local thrombosis at the venipuncture site has occurred in one patient with polycythemia who had multiple catheterizations of the same vein. Phlebotomy should be done at the start of the procedure in patients with elevated hematocrits in order to minimize thrombotic complications. The two femoral veins should be punctured alternately, and excessively long catheterization times should be avoided. Rupture of a malformation with hemorrhage was seen in one patient in whom intra-aneurysmal embolization was required due to a short feeding artery. Completion of the occlusion controlled the hemorrhage.

After embolization, patients are instructed to use an incentive spirometer for several days to prevent atelectasis. Pleuritic chest pain with occasional fevers occurs in over 20% of patients. This is probably due to pulmonary infarction. Acetaminophen or non-steroidal anti-inflammatory agents can be described to control this self-limited problem.

Results

Occlusion of nearly all significant lesions can be achieved, although several catheterizations may be necessary.[4,5] Dyspnea and fatigue improve and patients are protected against macroscopic paradoxical emboli. Complex lesions and diffuse involvement of a region of the lung present the greatest challenges. Several therapeutic sessions may be necessary to occlude the numerous channels present in these lesions. The diffuse variety may also necessitate sacrifice of substantial amounts of normal lung tissue.

Persistence or recurrence of a malformation occurs in fewer than 10% of cases and is usually due to an unembolized artery or, rarely, recanalization. Deflation of DBs was noted in 6% of PAVMs, but only one that deflated in less than 3 wks resulted in recanalization.[35] The DB appears to be more prone to deflate when placed adjacent to a coil. Recanalization through coils can occur as well.

FOLLOW-UP

After therapy, patients should have repeat chest radiographs (Figure 4.10), ABGs, and clinical assessment at 1 day, 1 month, and then every 3 to 5 yr to look for new, persistent, and/or recurrent, malformations. Slow growth of PAVMs has also been documented.[36] It is likely that helical CT scanning will play an important role in follow-up, possibly replacing ABGs.[20] Persistence of the aneurysm or nidus without significant reduction in size probably indicates continued perfusion.

Patients with HHT must be assumed to have microscopic PAVMs. To protect against brain abscess, these patients, and those with sporadic lesions that are incompletely embolized, should take prophylactic antibiotics before all procedures capable of causing bacteremia.

ACQUIRED PAVM OR PULMONARY FISTULA

An acquired pulmonary arteriovenous fistula is uncommon and can usually be treated like a PAVM. Acquired fistulas have been described in association with Glenn or Fontan shunts for congenital heart disease, schistosomiasis, actinomycosis, metastatic thyroid carcinoma, cirrhosis, amyloidosis, and erosion of an aneurysm into a

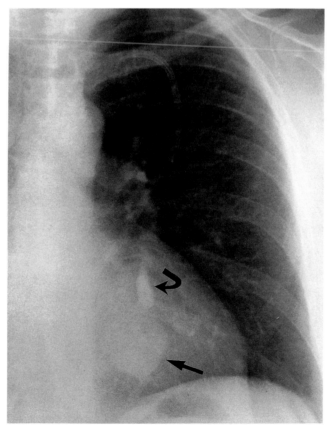

A

Figure 4.10 A. Chest radiograph 1 day after embolization of the malformation shown in Figures 5.4 and 5.6. The aneurysm remains visible at this early date (arrow), with the detachable balloon in the feeding artery (curved arrow). **B**. Following page.

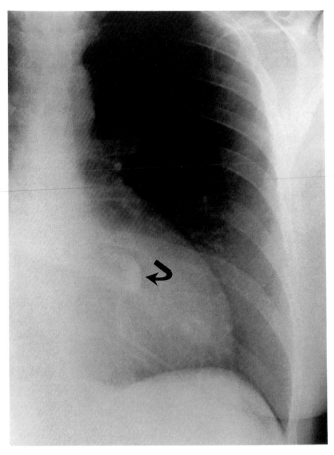

B

Figure 4.10 B. Two years later, the balloon remains inflated (curved arrow), but the malformation has disappeared.

vein.[2,37–40] Clinical manifestations, akin to those of congenital PAVMs, can include dyspnea, fatigue, and paradoxical emboli. Embolotherapy offers an effective method for relieving most of these lesions.

ACKNOWLEDGMENT

The guidance, pioneering work, and rich resource material generously shared by Robert I. White, Jr., M.D., is deeply appreciated.

REFERENCES

1. Churton T: Multiple aneurysms of pulmonary artery. *Br Med J* 1:1223, 1897.
2. Burke CM, Safai D, Nelson DP, et al: Pulmonary arteriovenous malformations: a critical update. *Am Rev Respir Dis* 134:334–339, 1986.
3. Porstmann W: Therapeutic embolization of arteriovenous pulmonary fistula by catheter technique. In Kelop O: *Current Concepts in Pediatric Radiology.* Berlin, Springer, 1977, pp 23–31.
4. White RI Jr, Lynch-Nyhan A, Terry P, et al: Pulmonary arteriovenous malformations: techniques and long-term outcome of embolotherapy. *Radiology* 169:663–669, 1988.
5. Chilvers ER, Whyte MKB, Jackson JE, et al: Effect of percutaneous transcatheter embolization on pulmonary function, right-to-left shunt, and arterial oxygenation in patients with pulmonary arteriovenous malformations. *Am Rev Respir Dis* 142:420–425, 1990.

6. Dines DE, Arms RA, Bernatz PE, et al: Pulmonary arteriovenous fistula. *Mayo Clin Proc* 49:460–465, 1974.

7. Dines DE, Seward JB, Bernatz PE: Pulmonary arteriovenous fistula. *Mayo Clin Proc* 58:176–181, 1983.

8. Perry WH: Clinical spectrum of hereditary hemorrhagic telangiectasia (Osler-Weber-Rendu disease). *Am J Med* 82:989–997, 1987.

9. Braverman IM, Keh A, Jacobson BS: Ultrastructure and three-dimensional organization of the telangiectasias of hereditary hemorrhagic telangiectasia. *J Invest Dermatol* 95:422–427, 1990.

10. Aassar OS, Friedman CM, White RI Jr: The natural history of epistaxis in hereditary hemorrhagic telangiectasia. *Laryngoscope* 101:977–980, 1991.

11. Hodgson CH, Burchell HB, Good CA, et al: Hereditary hemorrhagic telangiectasia and pulmonary arteriovenous fistula: study of a large family. *N Engl J Med* 261:625–636, 1959.

12. McAllister KA, Grogg KM, Johnson DW, et al: Endoglin, a TGF-β binding protein of endothelial cells, is the gene for hereditary haemorrhagic telangiectasis type 1. *Nature Genetics* 8:345–351, 1994.

13. Shovlin CL, Hughes JMB, Tuddenham EGD, et al: A gene for hereditary haemorrhagic telangiectasia maps to chromosome 9q3. *Nature Genetics* 6:205–209, 1994.

14. Ferrence BA, Shannon TM, White RI Jr, et al: Life-threatening pulmonary hemorrhage with pulmonary arteriovenous malformations and hereditary hemorrhagic telangiectasia. *Chest* 106:1387–1390, 1994.

15. Laroche CM, Wells F, Shneerson J: Massive hemothorax due to enlarging arteriovenous fistula in pregnancy. *Chest* 101:1452–1454, 1992.

16. Allen SW, Whitfield JM, Clarke DR, et al: Pulmonary arteriovenous malformation in the newborn: a familial case. *Pediatr Cardiol* 14:58–61, 1993.

17. Baert AL, Casteels-van Daele M, Broeckx J, et al: Generalized juvenile polyposis with pulmonary arteriovenous malformation. *Am J Roentgenol* 141:661–662, 1983.

18. Ueki J, Hughes JMB, Peters AM, et al: Oxygen and 99mTc-MAA shunt estimations in patients with pulmonary arteriovenous malformations: effects or changes in posture and lung volume. *Thorax* 49:327–331, 1994.

19. Laffey KJ, Thomashow B, Jaretzki A III, et al: Systemic supply to a pulmonary arteriovenous malformation: a relative contraindication to surgery. *Am J Roentgenol* 145:720–722, 1985.

20. Remy J, Remy-Jardin M, Wattinne L, et al: Pulmonary arteriovenous malformations: evaluation with CT of the chest before and after treatment. *Radiology* 182:809–816, 1992.

21. Cirimelli KM, Colletti PM, Beck S: Metastatic choriocarcinoma simulating an arteriovenous malformation on chest radiography and dynamic CT. *J Comput Assist Tomogr* 12:317–319, 1988.

22. Remy J, Remy-Jardin M, Giraud F, et al: Angioarchitecture of pulmonary arteriovenous malformations: clinical utility of three-dimensional helical CT. *Radiology* 191:657–664, 1994.

23. Barzilai B, Waggoner AD, Spessert C, et al: Two-dimensional contrast echocardiography in the detection and follow-up of congenital pulmonary arteriovenous malformations. *Am J Cardiol* 68:1507–1510, 1991.

24. Chilvers ER, Peters AM, George P, et al: Quantification of right to left shunt through pulmonary arteriovenous malformations using 99m-Tc albumin microspheres. *Clin Radiol* 39:611–614, 1988.

25. Whyte MKB, Peters AM, Hughes JMB, et al: Quantification of right to left shunt at rest and during exercise in patients with pulmonary arteriovenous malformations. *Thorax* 47:790–796, 1992.

26. Rosenblatt M, Pollak JS, Fayad PB, et al: Pulmonary arteriovenous malformations: what size should be treated to prevent embolic stroke? *Radiology* 186:937, 1993.

27. Puskas JD, Allen MS, Moncure AC, et al: Pulmonary arteriovenous malformations: therapeutic options. *Ann Thorac Surg* 56:253–258, 1993.

28. Taylor BG, Cockerill EM, Manfredi F, et al: Therapeutic embolization of the pulmonary artery in pulmonary arteriovenous fistula. *Am J Med* 64:360–365, 1978.

29. Terry BG, Barth KH, Kaufman SL, et al: Balloon embolization for the treatment of pulmonary arteriovenous fistulas. *N Engl J Med* 302:1189–1190, 1980.

30. Chuang VP, Wallace S, Gianturco C, et al: Complications of coil embolization: prevention and management. *Am J Roentgenol* 137:809–813, 1981.

31. Morse SS, Clark RA, Puffenbarger A: Platinum microcoils for therapeutic embolization: non-neuroradiologic applications. *Am J Roentgenol* 155:401–403, 1990.

32. Matsumoto AH, Selby JB Jr, Tegtmeyer CJ: Detachable balloons as peripheral vascular agents. *Sem Intervent Radiol* 9:62–71, 1992.

33. Kaufman SL, Strandberg JD, Barth KH: Therapeutic embolization with detachable silicone balloons: long-term effects in swine. *Invest Radiol* 14:156–161, 1979.

34. Remy-Jardin M, Wattine L, Remy J: Transcatheter occlusion of pulmonary arterial circulation and collateral supply: failures, incidents, and complications. *Radiology* 180:699–705, 1991.

35. Pollak JS, Egglin GTE, Rosenblatt MM, et al: Clinical results of transvenous systemic embolotherapy with a neuroradiologic detachable balloon. *Radiology* 191:477–482, 1994.

36. Teragaki M, Akioka K, Yasuda M, et al: Case report: hereditary hemorrhagic telangiectasia with growing pulmonary arteriovenous fistulas followed for 24 years. *Am J Med Sci* 295:545–547, 1988.

37. Kopf GS, Laks H, Stansel HC, et al: Thirty-year follow-up of superior vena cava–pulmonary artery (Glenn) shunts. *J Thorac Cardiovasc Surg* 100:662–671, 1990.

38. Kamei K, Kusumoto K, Suzuki T: Pulmonary amyloidosis with pulmonary arteriovenous fistula. *Chest* 96:1435–1436, 1989.

39. Lundell C, Finck C: Arteriovenous fistulas originating from Rasmussen aneurysms. *Am J Roentgenol* 140:687–688, 1983.

40. Lange PA, Stoller JK: The hepatopulmonary syndrome. *Ann Intern Med* 122:521–529, 1995.

Insertion and Care of Long-Term Central Venous Catheters

William E. Campbell, Jr.
Matthew A. Mauro
Paul F. Jaques

Traditionally, devices such as cuffed catheters and subcutaneous ports have been placed by surgeons in the operating room. However, in recent years, the radiologist's role has expanded from occasional manipulation of malpositioned catheters or retrieval of catheter fragments to a role as a primary operator in the placement and management of these devices.[1,2] Advances in catheter and guidewire design and in imaging technology now allow the interventional radiologist to provide central venous access via alternate routes, particularly in complicated cases where conventional access routes have been exhausted or in patients with unusual venous anatomy or venous occlusion. Percutaneous placement of these devices by interventional radiologists using ultrasound and/or fluoroscopic guidance has been shown to be cost-effective and safe.[3–10] Both procedural and late complication rates are similar to, and in some instances lower than, those associated with surgical placement.

In recent years, there has been a rapid expansion of industry centered on venous access devices and outpatient therapy. Long-term central venous catheters have allowed individuals requiring hemodialysis, plasmapheresis, chemotherapy, long-term antibiotic therapy or analgesic administration, and parenteral nutrition to obtain these treatments as outpatients. These devices have been particularly useful for those patients receiving hospice or home health nursing.

TYPES OF CENTRAL VENOUS CATHETERS

A variety of devices are available for long-term central venous access. Contemporary devices consist of a silicone or polyurethane catheter attached to an external connector or implantable subcutaneous port. Catheters are available in single-, dual-, and triple-lumen designs that commonly range from 4 to 13 Fr diameter for adults and 2 to 7 Fr diameter for children. In addition, external catheters are available in both nontunneled and tunneled designs. Nontunneled catheters are preferred for short-term use of days to weeks. Tunneled catheters and subcutaneous ports are preferred for long-term central venous access of months to years.

Nontunneled Catheters

Nontunneled catheters are available in both tapered and nontapered designs. The standard triple-lumen catheter has a tapered tip and is typically placed by house staff at

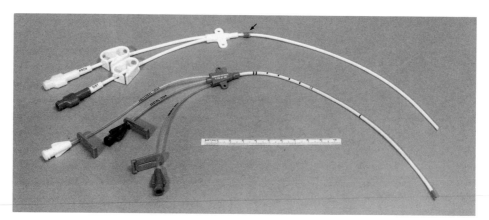

Figure 5.1 Nontunneled catheters. *Top:* Dual-lumen Hohn catheter with VitaCuff (arrow). *Bottom:* Standard polyethylene triple-lumen catheter.

the patient's bedside. However, the interventional radiologist may be consulted for triple-lumen placement in cases of difficult access or coagulopathy.

The Hohn catheter (Bard Access Systems, Salt Lake City, UT) is a 5-Fr single-lumen or 7-Fr dual-lumen nontapered fixed-length silicone catheter intended for intermediate term use of several weeks to several months (Figure 5.1). Because of the blunt nontapered tip on this catheter, a 6- or 8-Fr peel-away sheath is often needed for placement. The Hohn catheter has a silver-impregnated collagen cuff (Vitacuff; Vitaphore, Menlo Park, CA) which is positioned immediately within the skin exit site and serves as a temporary antimicrobial barrier. The silver-impregnated collagen cuff slowly dissolves over 6 wks. Both triple-lumen and Hohn catheters are secured by external sutures.

Peripherally inserted central catheters (PICC) are venous access devices designed for extremity placement. These 4–6 Fr (for adults) and 2–5 Fr (for children) silicone or polyurethane catheters are most frequently inserted into an antecubital vein and advanced into the superior vena cava (SVC). However, they may also be placed in veins in the forearm or upper arm. The PICC lines are generally not tunneled and carry a low procedure risk when compared with more centrally placed devices. Disadvantages include small lumen size with restricted flow rates and the need for intact upper extremity venous anatomy for placement. In many institutions, these catheters are placed by trained nurses or house staff. However, in patients with venous occlusions, blind placement of PICC lines is frequently unsuccessful. In such instances, ultrasound and fluoroscopic guidance with on-table venography may give the interventional radiologist a higher rate of successful central placement.[11–13]

Tunneled Catheters

Catheters requiring a subcutaneous tunnel are intended for long-term use of months to years. These catheters are single and multilumen devices available with an end-hole (Hickman, Broviac, and Leonard; Bard Access Systems) or with a tip-occluded valved catheter (Groshong; Bard Access Systems) (Figure 5.2). The slit-like valve of the Groshong catheter is designed to allow both aspiration of blood and infusion of fluid while theoretically preventing reflux of blood into the catheter when it is not in use, thereby decreasing the rate of catheter thrombosis and eliminating the need for heparinization.

Subcutaneous tunneling of catheters provides greater mechanical stability and protection against endovascular infection. Tunneled catheters typically have a circumferential Dacron (E.I. Dupont de Nemours, Wilmington, DE) cuff, which when placed in

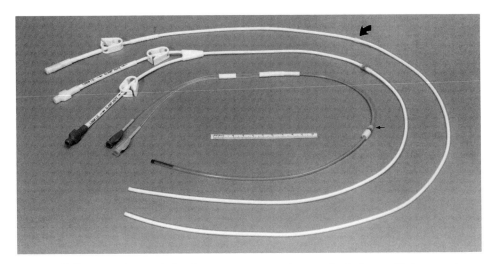

Figure 5.2 External tunneled catheters. *From top to bottom:* Single-lumen Hickman catheter with Dacron cuff (curved arrow); dual-lumen Leonard catheter with both Dacron cuff and VitaCuff; Groshong catheter with Dacron cuff and VitaCuff (straight arrow).

the subcutaneous tract, allows ingrowth of fibrous tissue 4 to 6 wk after placement, thus securing the catheter within the tract and creating a barrier to infection. Various catheters are also available with a second cuff composed of silver-impregnated collagen (VitaCuff), which serves as an additional antimicrobial barrier. As previously noted, this cuff is positioned immediately within the skin exit site.

Dialysis catheters are available in both cuffed (tunneled) and noncuffed (nontunneled) designs (Figure 5.3). These catheters are typically large, dual-lumen, high-flow devices with staggered tips and are manufactured in fixed lengths, based on the average adult and pediatric patient, for subclavian vein (SCV) or internal jugular vein

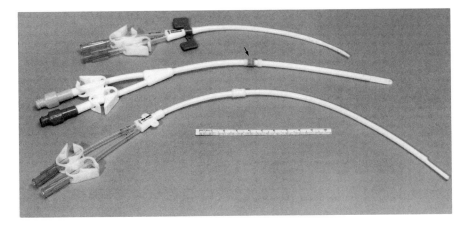

Figure 5.3 Dialysis/phresis catheters. *From top to bottom:* Tapered (nontunneled) 10.8-Fr dual-lumen Vas-Cath (Bard Access Systems); staggered tip 13.5-Fr Hickman dual-lumen dialysis/pheresis catheter with VitaCuff (arrow) and Dacron cuff; Vas-Cath soft-cell dialysis catheter with Dacron cuff.

(IJV) placement. A variety of longer lengths are now available for unconventional access sites (left IJV, inferior vena cava). Internal jugular vein placement is preferred to avoid subclavian vein stenosis and the associated complications following dialysis graft placement in the ipsilateral upper extremity.[14]

Ports

Implantable subcutaneous ports consist of stainless steel, titanium, or plastic surrounding a compressed silicone disk designed for access with a noncoring needle (Huber needle: American Medical Inc., New Bedford, MA) (Figure 5.4). The plastic and titanium ports are compatible with magnetic resonance imaging. The disks of standard chest wall ports are designed for 1,000–2,000 accesses, whereas those of small extremity ports are designed for 400–500 accesses. These devices are available in single- or dual-lumen designs connected to an end-hole or valved-tip catheter. Catheter sizes vary from 5 to 10 Fr for single-lumen devices and from 10 to 13 Fr for dual-lumen designs. Standard ports are designed for central placement in average and large adults. Extremity ports (PAS Port; Pharmacia Deltec, St. Paul, MN) (R-Port; Medi-Tech, Watertown, MA) are very low profile devices designed primarily for placement in the upper extremities (Figure 5.5). However, extremity ports may also be placed centrally in very thin adults and children. Some catheters are designed with either preattached or attachable (separate port and catheter require attachment) ports.

Central ports are placed within a subcutaneous pocket over the upper pectoral region, with the attached catheter tunneled to the venous entry site. The catheter may be introduced to the distal SVC or proximal right atrium by either percutaneous or cut-down techniques into the subclavian, jugular, axillary, brachial, basilic, or cephalic veins. Subcutaneous ports are most frequently placed in those patients requiring chemotherapy or other intermittent access regimens.

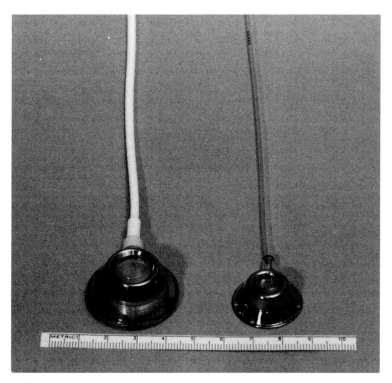

Figure 5.4 Implantable subcutaneous ports. *Left:* Standard titanium port. *Right:* Small, low-profile, titanium port.

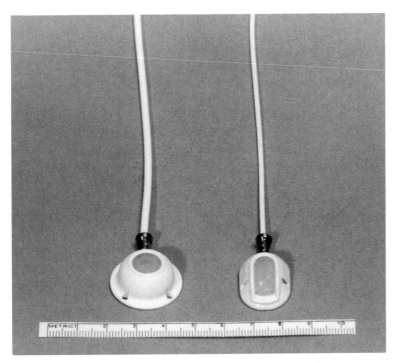

Figure 5.5 Small subcutaneous ports. *Left: Plastic low-profile port. Right:* Extremity R-port.

Port catheters have no external components when not in use and therefore are more cosmetically pleasing to the patient. Implanted subcutaneous devices are less prone to damage and infection than external catheters. Studies suggest that the intact skin protects the device when not in use.[15–20] Subcutaneous ports also require significantly less maintenance when not in use, needing only one flush per month. By comparison, most tunnelled catheters require more frequent flushing to maintain catheter patency. If a patient is going to require uninterrupted, continuous intravenous infusions, or at minimum daily infusions, the advantages of a port catheter over a tunneled catheter are less clear. When used for a continuous period of time, port needles should be changed at least once a week. With uninterrupted use, infection rates and catheter care regimens are quite similar for port and tunneled venous access systems. Therefore, the primary situation in which a port catheter seems to be advantageous is when intermittent, but reliable, venous access is needed for more than 6 months.

Dialysis Catheters

Dialysis catheters are manufactured in fixed lengths. Noncuffed dialysis catheters are available for short-term access, whereas cuffed catheters are available for prolonged dialysis access. We prefer the IJV for dialysis catheter placement to minimize the risk of developing SCV stenosis complicating upper extremity shunt placement.[14]

Noncuffed tapered dialysis catheters are placed using standard Seldinger techniques. Long-term cuffed catheters are not tapered and require a peel-away sheath for venous placement. In some cases, catheter length can be chosen such that the cuff is placed immediately within the subcutaneous space at the venous access site. However, most catheters require a subcutaneous tunnel for appropriate placement. All catheters should be heparinized according to the manufacturer's recommendations; the volume of heparin solution varies with catheter length.

PROCEDURAL TECHNIQUES

Percutaneous placement of long-term central venous access devices requires ten procedural steps: (1) choice of access device, (2) choice of access site, (3) venous access, (4) measurement of intravenous catheter length, (5) formation of subcutaneous tunnel or pocket, (6) insertion of catheter into tunnel or pocket, (7) insertion of catheter into central venous system, (8) closure of dermatotomies, (9) application of sterile dressing, and (10) routine catheter care.

Choice of Access Device

Primary factors influencing the choice of a specific device include the availability of access sites, the indications for central venous access, number of lumens needed, frequency of use, and patient preference. Common indications for a long-term central venous line include a need for chemotherapy, antibiotic therapy, parenteral alimentation, and/or hemodialysis. Less common applications include plasmapheresis and long-term transfusion requirements. A single lumen device is sufficient for most applications. However, when multiple agents are incompatible or simultaneous infusions are needed, a multilumen catheter may be required. Multilumen lines sacrifice lumen size and flow rates and are more susceptible to catheter-related infection due to the increased handling of these devices.

Ultimately patient preference should be strongly considered. While repeated needle sticks for subcutaneous ports may be intolerable for some, external catheters may be too restrictive for others. Although some patients may find a subcutaneous port cosmetically preferable, when frequent use is anticipated, external catheters are often preferred over subcutaneous ports. Ultimately, the most suitable device is the one that permits normal lifestyle and recreational activities, while fulfilling the demands of the therapy required.

Choice of Access Site

Choosing an access site depends on several factors: the type of device to be placed, venous patency, existing access, and patient preference. Both tunneled and nontunneled devices are routinely placed via a SCV or IJV approach. When fluoroscopic guidance is not available, we prefer to use an IJV approach due to the straighter course for the catheter into the right atrium and the decreased likelihood of a malpositioned catheter. For the placement of dialysis catheters, an IJV access is also preferred so that the subclavian veins can be preserved and the stenotic complications following upper extremity shunt or fistula placement can be minimized.[14]

We routinely perform a preliminary ultrasound examination to assess venous patency and detect aberrant venous anatomy prior to any line placement. When extensive venous occlusion or difficulty passing the guidewire is encountered, on-table venography may be helpful. Inferior vena cava (IVC) access via the translumbar or transhepatic route may be chosen when no other routes for central access are available.

It is not uncommon for a patient to present with an existing access device. A new access site on the contralateral side is generally preferred due to the increased risk of infection when an existing site is used. However, when it is difficult to gain access into a different site, the existing one may be used.

Most patients prefer the nondominant side or the side contralateral to prior surgery or radiation therapy for subclavian or upper extremity access. Some patients prefer to have their subcutaneous ports placed in the upper extremity for cosmetic reasons. However, it should be noted that extremity ports are more difficult to access.

Venous Access

Subclavian Vein

The standard technique for SCV access involves advancing an entry needle medially along a horizontal plane toward the suprasternal notch, under the medial two-thirds of the clavicle. Alternatively, direct puncture of the SCV or axillary vein can be performed under fluoroscopic guidance during contrast administration through an extremity vein. Guidewire placement via the antecubital or transfemoral route may also be used for fluoroscopic guidance.

Ultrasound guidance using a 5-MHz or 7-MHz linear array transducer is our preferred method for subclavian or axillary vein access. Ultrasound-guided access allows accurate venous entry lateral to the clavicle/first rib space, thus avoiding the potential problem of catheter compression and the "pinch-off" syndrome at the thoracic inlet.[21,22] By puncturing the SCV in a lateral, extrapleural location, the risk of causing a pneumothorax is also reduced. The lateral subclavian vein is located slightly anterior and caudal to the subclavian artery. The vein is identified immediately caudal to the lateral half of the clavicle and is differentiated from the artery by its position, easy compressibility, and respiratory variation. The artery can be distinguished by its slightly more cephalad and posterior location, as well as its characteristic pulsations.

When ultrasound guidance is used, the ultrasound transducer is oriented transversely with the medial edge against the midclavicle. This orientation allows longitudinal visualization of the SCV/axillary vein segment. A small dermatotomy is made at the lateral edge of the transducer and a 7-cm, 21-gauge needle is advanced at a 30–60° angle along the plane of the transducer during real-time imaging until the needle tip contacts the anterior venous wall. A short thrust is then necessary to puncture the vein. Once free return of blood is obtained, contrast injection may be used to confirm an intravenous position, although this is not usually necessary. The course of the 0.018-inch guidewire passed through the 21-gauge needle to the right atrium is usually sufficient to confirm venous placement.

When ultrasound guidance is unavailable or does not clearly delineate the vascular anatomy, the SCV can be directly entered using fluoroscopic guidance and bony landmarks. The SCV maintains a relatively constant position as it crosses the anterior first rib (Figure 5.6). Using the most lateral point of the first rib as 90° from vertical, the SCV crosses the first rib between 85–104° in 82% of patients (Figure 5.7). A skin nick is made at the lateral margin of the second rib, and a 21-gauge needle is passed obliquely from the skin nick onto the anterior first rib immediately caudal to the most lateral extent of the first rib. Once the tip of the needle reaches the lateral margin of the first rib, the needle is angled steeply posterior and advanced assertively onto the first rib. The needle is then slowly withdrawn as suction is applied. Upon blood return, an intravenous position of the needle tip can be confirmed by contrast injection or guidewire placement. If the needle did not enter the SCV, the procedure is repeated with the needle tip directly slightly more cranially or caudally. Using this method, inadvertent arterial punctures are uncommon. However, when they do occur, there have been no adverse sequelae related to the use of a small gauge needle.

Internal Jugular Vein

The standard techniques for puncturing the IJV are well described. The most commonly used technique is based on anatomic landmarks. The technique consists of retracting the carotid artery medially while a needle is advanced at a 30–60° angle from a point midway between the angle of the mandible and clavicle toward the ipsilateral nipple. Ultrasound guidance is another method for puncturing the IJV. With experience, successful entry into the IJV on the first pass is achieved in most ultrasound-guided cases. The 7.5-MHz transducer is oriented in the transverse plane 1–2 cm above the clavicle, allowing the com-

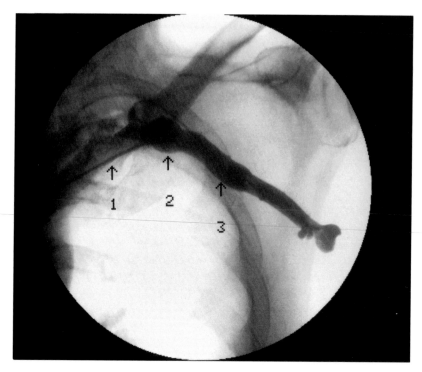

Figure 5.6 Subclavian venogram showing normal course of vein with respect to bony landmarks. Arrows indicate usual venous entry site: (1) Standard access technique using bony landmarks. (2) Fluoroscopic first rib technique. (3) Ultrasound guidance.

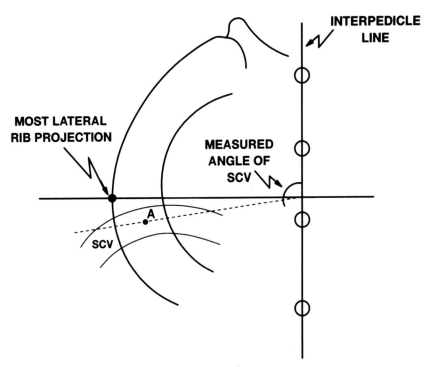

A

Figure 5.7 Relationship of subclavian vein and first rib. A. Typical angular position of SCV in relation to first rib. B. Following page.

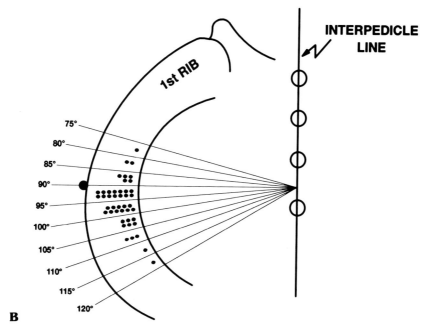

Figure 5.7 B. Frequency of positional variance of SCV central lumen.

mon carotid artery and IJV to be seen side by side, with the vein lateral to the artery. This low insertion site in the space between the sternal and clavicular heads of the sternocleidomastoid muscle avoids transversing the muscle, but does not lead to a higher pneumothorax rate because ultrasound guidance is used. Depending on transducer orientation, the IJV may be seen anterior to the artery. By adjusting the orientation of the transducer, a real-time image in which the IJV is oriented in a side by side fashion with the carotid artery can be generated, thereby minimizing the chance for inadvertent carotid puncture. A dermatotomy is made immediately cephalad to the transducer over the IJV and a 4-cm, 21- or 18-gauge needle is used to enter the IJV during real-time imaging. Once the anterior wall of the vein has been indented by the needle tip, a short, brisk thrust of the needle is required to enter the vein. Needle position is confirmed with blood aspiration, and a guidewire is then advanced into the right atrium.

Extremity

Venous access in the upper extremity may be obtained in any of the superficial veins of the forearm, but is usually via the basilic, cephalic, or brachial vein. Palpation may suffice when antecubital or forearm veins are used. However, access into veins of the upper arm frequently requires ultrasound or fluoroscopic guidance. If ultrasound guidance is used, a venogram must be obtained following venous entry to ensure a continuous pathway to the heart. If fluoroscopic guidance is used, a preliminary venogram is performed to confirm patency and select an appropriate site for venous entry. The vein is punctured during a contrast injection. In either case, punctures are made with 21-gauge needles and followed by insertion of 0.018-inch guidewires. Nitroglycerin can be given intravenously to reduce the incidence of venospasm.

Inferior Vena Cava (IVC)

When central venous access via the SCV is not possible, access via the IVC can be obtained via the translumbar or transhepatic routes.[23-28] Transfemoral access is generally not suitable due to the increased rates of infection, catheter kinking, and interference with ambulation.

Measurement of Catheter Length

Once the needle tip is positioned within the vein, the 0.018-inch guidewire is advanced in the right atrium and the needle is removed. The transition dilator (6.3 Fr) is advanced over the 0.018 guidewire. The guidewire is then positioned within the proximal right atrium so that the tip of the wire corresponds to the subsequent desired position of the catheter tip. The guidewire is then kinked at the hub of the dilator and withdrawn until the tip is positioned at the skin entry site, as marked by an opaque instrument. The wire is again kinked at the dilator hub. The distance between the two kinks corresponds to the expected catheter length needed from the venous entry site to the intended position of the catheter tip. This measured distance does not represent the overall length of the catheter, but rather, is used to cut the chosen end-hole catheter to length or to choose the appropriate fixed-length catheter (dialysis and pheresis catheters). These catheters are optimally placed at the junction of the SCV with the right atrium. Placement within the proximal SCV or mid-distal right atrium should be avoided due to increased rates of catheter malfunction and arrhythmias, respectively.

Tunnel Formation and Catheter Placement

If a tunneled catheter has been chosen, attention is then turned to the formation of the subcutaneous tunnel. This step of the procedure varies slightly depending on whether an end-hole or valved-tip catheter is to be placed. The distal tip of the end-hole catheter must be trimmed to the appropriate length before venous placement; the valved-tip catheter is cut to length proximally and attached to the external connector after central venous placement.

End-hole Catheter

For a tunneled end-hole catheter, the subcutaneous tunnel is formed after venous access has been accomplished. The skin exit site (where the catheter exits the subcutaneous tunnel) should be placed at a position accessible to the patient for catheter maintenance. A parasternal location is generally chosen for catheters placed via the axillary, subclavian, or internal jugular vein. Care should be taken to ensure that the catheter exit site does not interfere with undergarments.

After administering local anesthesia, a small dermatotomy is made at the skin exit site using a #11 blade. The entire subcutaneous tract from skin exit site to venous entry site is then anesthetized with 1% lidocaine (usually with epinephrine) administered through a 15-cm 22-gauge needle. In patients with sickle cell disease, the presence of epinephrine in lidocaine can compromise tissue perfusion, leading to skin necrosis. Therefore, lidocaine with epinephrine should be used with extreme caution in this patient population. For end-hole catheters, the blunt plastic tunneling tool supplied in the catheter kit is negotiated subcutaneously from the skin exit to the venous entry site (Figure 5.8). The catheter is connected to the end of the tunneling device and is pulled through the subcutaneous tract until the Dacron cuff is approximately 1 to 2 cm inside the skin exit site. When present, the VitaCuff is positioned immediately within the skin exit site. Next, the catheter length from the venous entry site to its desired distal intravascular position is measured against the previously kinked 0.018-inch guidewire. The catheter is then cut to the appropriate length. An 0.038-inch guidewire is then placed through the transition dilator to the right atrium. In most instances, this guidewire can be placed into the IVC to provide added stability and avoid inadvertent advancement into the right ventricle. The dilator is removed and an appropriately sized peel-away sheath (usually supplied in the kit) is placed over the guidewire. The dilator and guidewire are removed, and the catheter is immediately in-

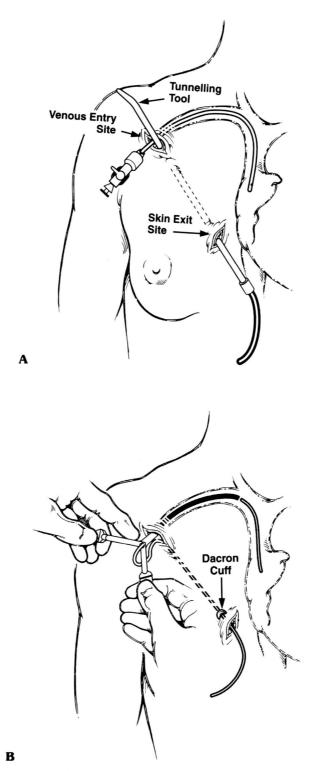

Figure 5.8 Percutaneous placement of an end-hole catheter. A. Tunneling device placed from skin exit site to venous entry site following initial SCV access. B. Catheter placed through peel-away sheath.

serted through the sheath. The patient should be carefully instructed to suspend respiration during this step of the procedure to minimize the risk of air embolism. In patients unable to cooperate, pinching the sheath between the fingers during this step may help. When the distal catheter position is satisfactory, the sheath is removed.

Occasionally, the catheter prefers to enter the internal jugular or contralateral innominate vein.[29,30] Rotation of a beveled catheter tip may help guide the catheter into the SVC. Alternatively, a forceful injection of saline may recoil the catheter tip into the appropriate position.[33] If these maneuvers fail, a hydrophilic guidewire may be used to facilitate passage of the catheter into the SVC. Refractory cases may require placement of a long sheath or femoral vein access to snare the catheter. If kinking of the introducer sheath obstructs catheter insertion (most commonly encountered in right SCV access), a hydrophilic guidewire may be placed through the catheter and sheath into the right atrium. While forward pressure on the catheter and guidewire is maintained, the sheath is slowly withdrawn until the kink is removed and the catheter is easily advanced. The sheath must not be withdrawn out of the venous system until the catheter tip has been satisfactorily positioned. If this maneuver fails to straighten the sheath and allow catheter placement, a new sheath can be placed over the guidewire and the maneuver repeated.

When catheter placement is completed and the introducer sheath removed, a single 3-0 nonabsorbable suture or steri-strip (3M, St. Paul, MN) is applied to the venous entry site. A 3-0 nonabsorbable suture is placed at the catheter exit site. This suture should be gently wrapped around the catheter for added stability. The catheter is then appropriately heparinized, and an external dressing is applied.

Valved-tip Catheter

When a valved-tip (Groshong) catheter is chosen, the peel-away sheath is placed immediately after placement of the transition dilator. There is no need for catheter length measurements. The Groshong catheter is placed into position and the sheath is removed. The valved tip does not allow back bleeding. The subcutaneous tunnel is now created from the venous entry site to the catheter exit site. The length of the tunnel is gauged from the position of the Dacron cuff on the catheter when the tip of the catheter is in its final location. After the catheter is carried through the tunnel, it is trimmed at its proximal end and the hub attached. The catheter is then secured, flushed with saline, and externally dressed.

Pocket Formation and Port Placement

For subcutaneous port placement, a cutdown tray with the necessary surgical tools is required. A site with ample subcutaneous tissue caudal and medial to the venous access site is chosen for placement in the upper chest wall. Following infiltration with 1% lidocaine (usually with epinephrine), a #15 blade is used to make a straight 5-cm skin incision either cranial or caudal to the expected position of the subcutaneous pocket. The incision is made into the subcutaneous space. Using blunt dissection, a subcutaneous pocket is formed just large enough to allow insertion of the port without excessive tension on the opposed margins of the skin incision. A pocket that is too large may allow torsion or migration of the port. Once created, the pocket is inspected visually, and gauze pads are placed within the pocket to ensure that there is no bleeding. Persistent bleeding sites may require cauterization or suture placement.

Once the pocket is ready for port placement, a short tunnel is created connecting the pocket to the venous entry site. As with tunneled catheters, the direction of the tunnel is determined by the type of catheter to be placed and whether or not the catheter is preattached to the port.[15] A small malleable tunneling tool is tunneled through the subcutaneous tissues in the appropriate direction to connect the pocket and venous entry site. The catheter is then pulled through the tunnel, using the tunneling device.

When preattached ports with end-hole catheters are used, the blunt surgical probe is tunneled from the subcutaneous pocket to the venous entry site and the catheter is pulled through. The port is then positioned within the pocket and 3-0 nonabsorbable or absorbable sutures are used to secure the port to the deep fascia. The previously kinked 0.018-inch guidewire is used for measurement and the catheter is cut to the appropriate length and inserted through a peel-away sheath into the final central venous position. A noncoring Huber needle is used to access the port. Once blood is aspirated, the port is flushed with sterile saline and heparin.

If a port with an attachable end-hole or valved-tip catheter is chosen, the proximal end of the catheter is pulled through the tunnel from the venous entry site to the pocket. The distal tip of the catheter is then placed through a peel-away sheath and appropriately positioned. The proximal end of the catheter is cut to length and attached to the subcutaneous port. Alternatively, an attachable end-hole catheter can be assembled and treated as a preassembled device. Again, the port is sutured to the deep fascia.

The pocket incision is then closed with interrupted 3-0 absorbable subcutaneous sutures and interrupted 3-0 nonabsorbable skin sutures or 4-0 absorbable sutures and steri-strips. The venous entry site is closed with a single 3-0 nonabsorbable suture or steri-strips.

Extremity ports also require the formation of a subcutaneous pocket. The location of the pocket should be carefully selected to ensure easy access without interfering with mobility of the extremity. The pocket can be placed in the forearm or upper arm and may be adjacent to or away from the venous entry site. When the pocket can be fashioned adjacent to the venous access site, the original dermatotomy is simply extended and no tunnel is required. If a distant site is selected, a tunnel is created from the venous entry site to the pocket. Following venous entry the appropriately sized sheath is placed into the vein while the pocket is formed. The catheter tip is then placed into its final central location, and the sheath removed. The catheter is brought through the tunnel (if needed), cut to length, and attached to the port. The port is then accessed, aspirated, and flushed to ensure good function. The port is placed in the pocket, sutured to the fascia, and a two-layered closure is performed.

Catheter Management and Removal

Those wishing to establish a vascular access service must also become familiar with and involved in postprocedural catheter care, patient follow-up, and management of related complications. One must also be prepared to remove catheters and ports when they are no longer needed.

A specialized nursing team for patient education and supervision of routine catheter maintenance can significantly reduce infection and catheter thrombosis rates.[32] Adherence to strict sterile technique during catheter use, daily dressing changes, and catheter heparinization cannot be overemphasized. The specialized nursing teams can also be trained to repair damaged catheters using commercially available repair kits. These repair kits are designed to replace damaged hubs or segments of a specific catheter. Radiologists placing these catheters should have such kits available and understand their use.

Removal of any venous access device is the responsibility of the service that placed it. Prior to removal of a tunneled catheter, the catheter and skin exit site are sterilely prepared and draped. The skin and subcutaneous tissues at the catheter exit site and around the catheter cuff are anesthetized using 1% lidocaine, usually with epinephrine. Tunneled catheters can occasionally be removed by simply applying steady traction. However, dissection of the Dacron cuff from the subcutaneous tissues is usually required. This blunt dissection is performed with hemostats through the skin exit site while continuous traction is applied to the catheter. Occasionally, the catheter detaches from the cuff, leaving the cuff in the subcutaneous tunnel. In this case, removal of the cuff is not usually necessary. However, a retained cuff can become a persistent source of infection, especially in cases of line sepsis or tunnel infection. Initial placement of the cuff within 1 to 2 cm of the skin exit site allows the cuff to be more easily dissected and removed. If the cuff is initially placed deeper within the subcutaneous tunnel, a short incision over the cuff parallel to the catheter may be needed to dissect and remove the cuff from the surrounding fibrous tissue.

Port removal requires a full sterile preparation and drape, a cutdown tray, and more extensive subcutaneous dissection. The previous incision site is used for cosmetic purposes. After the subcutaneous pocket has been incised, deep sutures (if present) anchoring the port are removed, allowing the port to slide free from the epithelialized surface lining the pocket. During closure of the pocket, deep sutures are often needed to eliminate any dead space that could lead to hematoma formation and an increased risk of infection. A two-layer closure is then performed using 3-0 absorbable subcutaneous sutures and 3-0 nonabsorbable cutaneous sutures.

COMPLICATIONS

Procedural Complications

Minor procedural complications include failure to gain venous access, catheter malposition, or inadvertent arterial puncture without significant hematoma. Venous access procedures with fluoroscopic or sonographic guidance result in a greater than 98% success rate for venous access, compared with a 91–95% success rate for blind placement.[5,7,33–35] Blind placement is also associated with a 1.2–2.5% incidence of catheter malposition, a complication that is immediately recognized and corrected when radiologic guidance is used.[5,35,36]

Major procedural complications include significant vascular injury, hematoma, pneumothorax, nerve injury, and air embolism. Significant injury to the mediastinal, central subclavian, or intercostal vessels may result in significant hemorrhage and a hemothorax. Specifically, inadvertent needle puncture of the subclavian artery may lead to significant hematoma formation or bleeding within the subcutaneous tunnel or pocket. However, access procedures using ultrasound guidance and a 21-gauge needle for venous puncture in a more peripheral and compressible region can virtually eliminate significant bleeding complications related to inadvertent arterial puncture.[5,7,26,34] Careful observation of the guidewire course or injection of contrast material following needle entry will easily confirm venous placement and avoid intra-arterial catheter placement. Tunnel or pocket hematomas are an infrequent complication, but are more likely to occur in patients with abnormal coagulation parameters. Therefore, coagulation and platelet abnormalities should be assessed and corrected if possible, before the procedure.

A pneumothorax resulting from a 21-gauge needle puncture is typically small and resolves within several hours. Pneumothoraces that fail to respond to conservative therapy can be evacuated using a small-bore catheter placed via the second anterior intercostal space. While blinded placement of central venous catheters is associated with a pneumothorax rate as high as 7.5%, ultrasound-guided peripheral SCV puncture is associated with a pneumothorax rate of less than 1%.[5,7,34] Following placement of the central venous catheter, a chest radiograph is obtained. If no pneumothorax is present, a follow-up chest radiograph is not routinely obtained, unless the patient develops pain or cardiopulmonary symptoms, or the catheter malfunctions.

Air embolism is a complication that may occur when a needle, catheter, or sheath used for venous access is open to the atmosphere. This complication occurs most frequently when a patient takes a deep breath while the dilator is removed from the peel-away sheath during catheter insertion. A cooperative patient should be instructed to suspend respiration during this step, or the sheath may be gently squeezed until the catheter has been placed. If an air embolism does occur, the patient should remain in the supine position to allow gradual absorption of the air while oxygen is administered and vital signs are closely monitored. In most cases, this conservative management is adequate. In cases of massive air embolus and hemodynamic instability, the placement of a pigtail angiographic catheter may be required to remove the entrapped air.

Mechanical Complications

Catheter malposition and migration into the innominate, internal jugular, or azygos veins can be managed by several techniques. An abrupt forceful injection of saline may recoil a catheter into proper position.[31] Alternatively, a hydrophilic guidewire or deflecting wire may help redirect a malpositioned catheter into the appropriate position. Refractory cases may require femoral vein access to manipulate or snare the catheter into the proper position. When malposition recurs, the intravenous catheter is usually too short and replacement of the catheter is necessary.

The incidence of catheter fragmentation has been significantly reduced since the change from needle to sheath insertion of central catheters. However, delayed fragmentation may result from compression of the catheter between the clavicle, subclavius tendon, and the first rib. This occurs when the catheter enters the vein centrally and is extravascular as it courses between the clavicle and first rib, resulting in the "pinch off" syndrome.[21,22,37] The average duration of catheter placement at the time of fragmentation is approximately 6.5 months, with equal incidence between right and left approaches.[22] Catheter entry into the SCV lateral to the clavicle/first rib space significantly reduces the risk of this complication.

The external hubs and tubing of long-term access devices may become worn or damaged with time and repeated use. Repair kits are available and should be kept in stock. Catheter repairs should be performed as soon as possible in order to minimize catheter infections.

Thrombotic Complications

Thrombotic complications occur in 3.7% to 10% of patients, despite proper catheter maintenance.[2,38,39] These complications include catheter thrombosis, venous thrombosis or both. Many of the infused chemotherapy agents and hyperalimentation fluids cause venous irritation that may result in venous thrombosis. Also, many patients requiring long-term venous access, particularly those with malignancy, are hypercoagulable. Early recognition thrombotic complications provides the best chance for successful treatment.

Catheter dysfunction is often manifested by an inability to withdraw blood and can be caused by catheter malposition, catheter thrombosis, or a pericatheter fibrin sheath. Malpositioning of the catheter may cause the tip to lodge against the venous wall, a problem that is often remedied by having the patient change the head or arm position or perform the Valsalva maneuver. If the problem persists despite these maneuvers, the catheter should be replaced.

Catheter thrombosis is effectively handled with direct installation of urokinase (Abbokinase Open-Cath; Abbott Lab, Abbott Park, IL). An amount of Abbokinase Open-Cath solution (5,000 units urokinase/cc) equal to the internal volume of the catheter is injected into the catheter lumen and allowed to remain there for 5–30 min. If the catheter cannot be aspirated after 30 min it is capped for an additional 30–60 min and aspiration is again attempted. A second dose of urokinase may be required. Overnight low-dose infusion of urokinase may be helpful in refractory cases. Low-dose warfarin prophylaxis of 1 mg daily has been shown to effectively reduce thrombotic complications without an increased risk of bleeding complications or significant change in coagulation studies.[40]

A circumferential fibrin sheath forms on all central venous catheters as early as 24 hr after insertion.[41] If this fibrin sheath extends to or around the tip of the catheter, injected fluid or contrast may track along the catheter and extravasate from the venous entry sight. Although uncommon, this can present a serious problem when cytotoxic drugs are administered. Passing a guidewire through the catheter may break the fibrin sheath at its tip and restore normal catheter function. However, successful treatment usually requires stripping the fibrin sheath from the catheter or replacement of the catheter. Fibrin sheath stripping is performed from a femoral vein approach. A nitinol goose-neck loop snare (Microvena Corp., Vadnais Heights, MN) is placed around the catheter and the fibrin sheath is stripped from the catheter (Figure 5.9). Stripping the fibrin sheath from the catheter may require several passes with the snare. A guidewire passed through the indwelling catheter into the IVC may help shorten procedure time by allowing a continued position of the snare around the catheter–guidewire combination.

Venous thrombosis associated with central venous catheters occurs in approximately 17% of autopsy patients and 70% of patients studied prospectively following placement of Hickman and Groshong catheters.[38,39] Mural thrombus can form along the catheter and venous endothelium resulting in partial or complete occlusion of the involved vein. Although nonocclusive thrombus is frequently asymptomatic, complete thrombosis may result in pain and swelling of the arm, neck, and face in 3% to 10% of patients.[38,42,43] Conservative management of thrombotic complications with anticoagulation and extremity elevation will relieve symptoms in most patients without catheter removal. Symptomatic relief can be hastened with local thrombolytic therapy or catheter removal with anticoagulation. Signs of septic thrombophlebitis are more ominous and require immediate removal of the catheter together with appropriate antibiotic coverage.

Infectious Complications

Infectious complications associated with central venous access devices arise in 10–30% of patients. Infections may occur within the soft tissues at the catheter exit site, the subcutaneous tunnel, or port pocket, or manifest systemically as catheter-related bacteremia.[44,45] Soft tissue infections present with painful induration and exudate, whereas catheter-related bacteremia presents with fever and leukocytosis. Patients who are immunosuppressed are at higher risk for catheter-related infections.

Procedural infections occurring within the first 3–5 days following catheter placement most often involve the subcutaneous tract or pocket and should be treated with appropriate oral antibiotics. More severe infections may require catheter removal. Abscess formation requires incision and drainage, antibiotics, and catheter removal. Although controversial, the use of prophylactic antibiotics at the time of catheter placement has not proven to decrease procedural infection rates significantly.

Delayed infections usually begin at the skin exit site or within the subcutaneous pocket. The majority (50–70%) of the infections are caused by skin flora and are believed to be related to improper catheter care or contamination during access. In one study, 15.4% of patients with skin exit site infections required catheter removal, compared with 69% with tunnel infections.[45] Early detection and management of superficial infections with oral antibiotics can frequently help save the access device.

Catheter-related bacteremia (CRB) should be suspected in a patient with fever and leukocytosis without any other source of infection. However, not all infections in these

Text continues on page 119

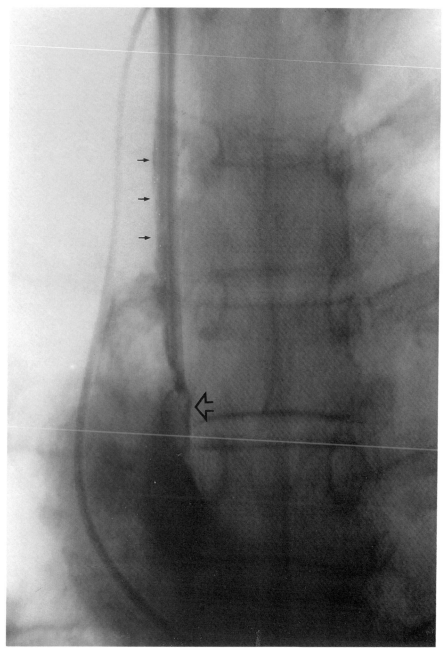

A

Figure 5.9 Stripping of fibrin sheath. **A.** Contrast injection through distal (venous) port of staggered-tip dialysis catheter demonstrates fibrin sheath (small arrows) and thrombus (open arrow) at catheter tip. **B, C,** and **D.** Following pages.

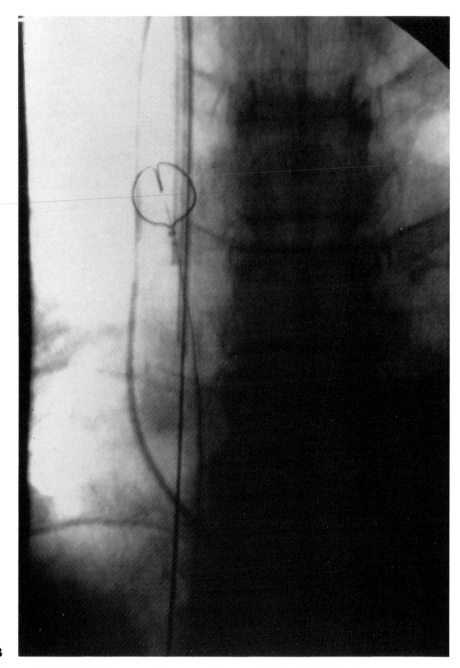

B

Figure 5.9 B. Nitinol gooseneck loop snare is engaged. C and D. Following pages.

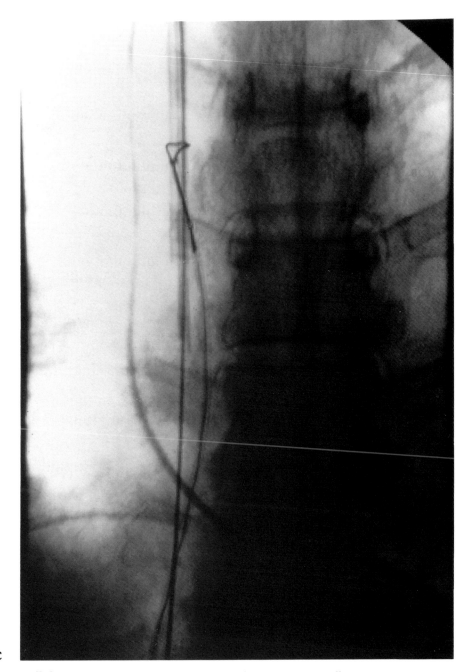

C

Figure 5.9 C. Snare is tightened around catheter for stripping. D. Following page.

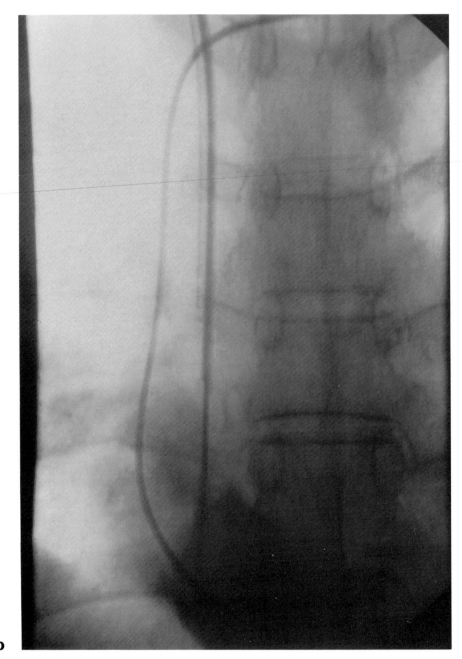

D

Figure 5.9 D. Final catheter injection showing no regional thrombus or fibrin sheath.

patients are due to the catheter. For CRB to be established, positive cultures of the same organism must be obtained from both the catheter tip and a peripheral blood sample with no other source identified. In addition, fever and leukocytosis should resolve following catheter removal. Establishing the presence of CRB without catheter removal is more difficult and requires quantitative blood cultures taken from the access device and from a peripheral site. Weightman et al. demonstrated a tenfold increase in colony counts from the catheter specimen as opposed to the peripheral specimen in those patients with CRB.[46] Most catheter-related infections can be treated successfully with a 10-day course of IV antibiotics. However, patients whose fever and leukocytosis persist or recur after 3 to 5 days of therapy should have their catheters removed. Catheter colonization with *Pseudomonas* or fungal species is particularly difficult to eradicate without catheter removal.

CONCLUSION

With economic considerations rapidly reshaping our health care system, there is a continuous effort to provide more cost-effective medical care. Long-term central venous access is rapidly becoming a service that can be provided most expeditiously and economically by the interventional radiologist. A majority of cases can be completed within 45 min, including patient preparation, procedure time, and wound dressing. Most patients require little or no postoperative recovery. Catheter-related infection and thrombosis rates for devices placed in the interventional radiology suite have been shown to be similar to those placed by surgeons in the operating room. Procedural complications can be reduced when radiologic and sonographic guidance are used.

The imaging technology available in the vascular radiology suite combined with specialized skills make the interventional radiologist particularly well suited to the role of primary operator in the placement of long-term central venous catheters. However, when establishing a venous access service, one must be prepared to devote a significant amount of time, resources, and personnel to this endeavor. Lastly, the radiologist must be willing not only to place these devices, but also to become familiar with catheter maintenance and treatment of postprocedural complications.

REFERENCES

1. Mauro MA, Jaques PF: Radiological placement of long-term central venous catheters: a review. *J Vasc Interv Radiol* 4:127–137, 1993.
2. Denny DF: Placement and management of long-term central venous access catheters and ports. *Am J Roentgenol* 161:385–393, 1993.
3. Selby JB, Tegtmeyer CJ, Amodeo C: Insertion of subclavian hemodialysis catheters in difficult cases. value of fluoroscopy and angiographic techniques. *Am J Roentgenol* 152:641–643, 1989.
4. Andrews JC, Walker-Andrews SC, William DE: Long-term central venous access with a peripherally placed subcutaneous infusion port: initial results. *Radiology* 176:45–47, 1990.
5. Lameris JS, Post PJM, Zonderland HM, et al: Percutaneous placement of Hickman catheters: comparison of sonographically guided and blind techniques. *Am J Roentgenol* 155:1097–1099, 1990.
6. Robertson LJ, Mauro MA, Jaques PF: Radiologic placement of Hickman catheters. *Radiology* 170:1007–1009, 1989.
7. Morris SL, Jaques PF, Mauro MA: Radiology-assisted placement of implantable subcutaneous infusion ports for long-term venous access. *Radiology* 184:149–151, 1992.
8. Disk L, Mauro MA, Jaques PF, et al: Radiologic insertion of Hickman catheters in HIV-positive patients: infectious complications. *J Vasc Interv Radiol* 2:327–329, 1991.
9. Openshaw KL, Picus D, Hicks ME, et al: Interventional radiologic placement of Hohn central venous catheters: results and complications in 100 consecutive patients. *J Vasc Interv Radiol* 5:111–115, 1994.

10. Cardella JF, Fox PS, Lawler JB: Interventional radiological placement of peripherally inserted central catheters. *J Vasc Interv Radiol* 4:653–660, 1993.

11. Andrews JC, Marx MV, Williams DM, et al: The upper arm approach for placement of peripherally inserted central catheters for protracted venous access. *Am J Roentgenol* 158:427–429, 1992.

12. Hovesepian DM, Bonn J, Eschelman DJ: Techniques for peripheral insertion of central venous catheters. *J Vasc Interv Radiol* 4:795–803, 1993.

13. Bonn J: Venous access: peripherally inserted central catheters. Abstract, *Society of Cardiovascular and Interventional Radiology Meeting Program*, pp 204–210, 1994.

14. Stalter KA, Stevens GF, Sterling WA: Late stenosis of the subclavian vein after hemodialysis catheter injury. *Surgery* 100:924–927, 1986.

15. Ingram J, Weitzman S, Greenberg ML, et al: Complications of indwelling venous access lines in the pediatric hematology patient: a prospective comparison of external venous catheters and subcutaneous ports. *Am J Pediatr Hematol Oncol* 13:130–136, 1991.

16. Mirro JJ, Rao BN, Stokes DC, et al: A prospective study of Hickman/Broviac catheters and implantable ports in pediatric oncology patients. *J Clin Oncol* 7:214–222, 1989.

17. Ross MN, Haase GM, Poole MA, et al: Comparison of totally implanted reservoirs with external catheters as venous access devices in pediatric oncologic patients. *Surg Gynecol Obstet* 167:141–144, 1988.

18. Mirro JJ, Rao BN, Kumar M, et al: A comparison of placement techniques and complications of externalized catheters and implantable port use in children with cancer. *J Pediatr Surg* 25:120–124, 1990.

19. Pegues D, Axelrod P, McClarren C, et al: Comparison of infections in Hickman and implanted port catheters in adult solid tumor patients. *J Surg Oncol* 49:156–162, 1992.

20. Brothers TE, Von Moll LK, Niederhuber JE, et al: Experience with subcutaneous infusion ports in three hundred patients. *Surg Gynecol Obstet* 166:295–301, 1988.

21. Hinke DH, Zandt-Stastny DA, Goodman LR, et al: Pinch-off syndrome: a complication of implantable subclavian venous access devices. *Radiology* 177:353–356, 1990.

22. Lafrenirre R: Indwelling subclavian catheters and a visit with the "pinch-off" syndrome. *J Surg Oncol* 47:261–264, 1991.

23. Denny DF, Dorfman GS, Greenwood LH, et al: Translumbar inferior vena cava Hickman catheter placement for total parenteral nutrition. *Am J Roentgenol* 148:621–622, 1987.

24. Denny DF, Greenwood LH, Morse SS, et al: Inferior vena cava: translumbar catheterization for central venous access. *Radiology* 170:1013–1014, 1989.

25. Kaufman JA, Greenfield AJ, Fitzpatrick GF: Transhepatic cannulation of the inferior vena cava. *J Vasc Interv Radiol* 2:331–334, 1991.

26. Robertson LJ, Jaques PF, Mauro MA, et al: Percutaneous inferior vena cava placement of tunnelled silastic catheters for prolonged vascular access in infants. *J Ped Surg* 25:596–598, 1990.

27. Lund GB, Lieberman RP, Haire WD, et al: Translumbar inferior vena cava catheters for long-term venous access. *Radiology* 174:31–35, 1990.

28. Azizkhan RG, Taylor LA, Jaques PF, et al: Percutaneous translumbar and transhepatic inferior vena caval catheters for prolonged vascular access in children. *J Ped Surg* 27:165–169, 1992.

29. Carasco CH, Richli WR, Chusilp C, et al: Technical note: repositioning misplaced central venous catheters. *Cardiovasc Intervent Radiol* 10:234–236, 1987.

30. Lois JF, Gomes AS, Pussey R: Non-surgical repositioning of central venous catheters. *Radiology* 165:329–333, 1987.

31. Olcott EW, Gordon RL, Ring EJ: The injection technique for repositioning central venous catheters: technical note. *Cardiovasc Intervent Radiol* 12:292–293, 1989.

32. Keohane PP, Attrill H, Northover J: Effect of catheter tunnelling and a nutrition nurse on catheter sepsis during parenteral nutrition. *Lancet* 17:1388–1390, 1983.

33. Kahn ML, Barboza RB, Kling GA, et al: Initial experience with percutaneous placement of the PAS PORT implantable venous access device. *J Vasc Interv Radiol* 3:459–461, 1992.

34. Hull JE, Hunter CS, Luiken GA: The Groshong catheter: initial experience and results of imaging-guided placement. *Radiology* 185:803–807, 1992.

35. Takasugi JK, O'Connell TX: Prevention of complications in permanent central venous catheters. *Surg Gynecol Obstet* 167:6–11, 1988.

36. Delmore JE, Horbelt DV, Jack BL, et al: Experience with the Groshong long-term central venous catheter. *Gynecol Oncol* 34:216–218, 1989.

37. Rubenstein RB, Alberty RE, Michels LG, et al: Hickman catheter separation. *J Parenter Enter Nutr* 9:754–757, 1985.

38. Haire WD, Lieberman RP, Lund GB, et al: Thrombotic complications of silicone rubber catheters during autologous marrow and peripheral stem cell transplantation: prospective comparison of Hickman and Groshong catheters. *Bone Marrow Transplant* 7:57–59, 1991.

39. Anderson AJ, Krasnow SH, Boyer MW, et al: Thrombosis: the major Hickman catheter complication in patients with solid tumor. *Chest* 95:71–75, 1989.

40. Bern MM, Lokich JJ, Wallach SR, et al: Very low doses of warfarin can prevent thrombosis in central venous catheters. *Ann Intern Med* 112:423–428, 1990.

41. Hoshal VL, Ause RG, Hoskins PA: Fibrin sleeve formation on indwelling subclavian central venous catheters. *Arch Surg* 102:353–358, 1971.

42. Moss JF, Wagman LD, Riihimaki DU, et al: Central venous thrombosis related to the silastic Hickman-Broviac catheters in an oncologic population. *J Parenter Enteral Nutr* 13:397–400, 1989.

43. Gray WJ, Bell WR: Fibrinolytic agents in the treatment of thrombotic disorder. *Semin Oncol* 17:228–237, 1990.

44. Clarke DE, Raffin TA: Infectious complications of indwelling long-term central venous access catheters. *Chest* 97:966–972, 1990.

45. Press OW, Ramsey PG, Larson EB, et al: Hickman catheter infections in patients with malignancies. *Medicine* 63:189–200, 1984.

46. Weightman NC, Simpson EM, Speller DCE, et al: Bacteremia related to indwelling central venous catheters: prevention, diagnosis, and treatment. *Eur J Clin Microbiol Infect Dis* 7:125–129, 1988.

CHAPTER 6

Intravascular Foreign Body Retrieval

J. Fritz Angle
Alan H. Matsumoto
Charles J. Tegtmeyer

The discovery of intravascular foreign bodies (FBs) predates the invention of modern catheters, wires, and filters. The earliest FBs were the product of war when bullet fragments entered the circulation, but venous catheters have become the most frequent source of intravascular FBs.[1,2]

In 1954, Turner reported a case in which embolization of a polyethylene catheter from the arm to the right atrium led to myocardial necrosis, mural thrombus, and death.[3] Since that report, the management of FBs has been a significant concern. A review by Wellman in 1968 identified 37 cases of catheter embolism.[4] Twenty-five of these patients had embolization to the heart and pulmonary arteries. At the time of the study, 13 of the 25 patients had died, with 6 of 13 deaths related to the catheter embolism. Findings at autopsy included perforation of the right atrium or ventricle, cardiac thrombus, pulmonary embolus, and bacterial and fungal endocarditis. Fisher reviewed 73 cases of untreated catheter embolization and found that 33% of the patients had life-threatening complications, while 38% died as a direct result of the embolization.[5] It is not surprising that embolized venous catheters are associated with a high morbidity, since 40% of indwelling catheters are contaminated with bacteria.[6] Foreign bodies on the left side of the heart or pulmonary veins are associated with systemic arterial embolization.[7]

Before the availability of percutaneous retrieval, most patients with cardiac FBs underwent thoracotomy to remove the FB because of the risk of thrombosis, endocarditis, or myocardial perforation.[1,5] Since the advent of percutaneous retrieval, extraction of FBs is now routine. In many cases FBs in the heart and great vessels have remained asymptomatic for prolonged periods of time, but most studies support an aggressive attempt to remove them.[1,4,5]

Percutaneous retrieval involves several steps: localizing the FB; choosing the appropriate retrieval device; capturing the FB; and removing it.

LOCALIZATION AND CAPTURE

In the thorax, frontal and lateral chest films and a good clinical history will localize most radiopaque FBs. If the retained object is known to be radiopaque, but is not visible at the expected locations, more extensive radiographic examinations are required to exclude peripheral embolization. Contrast venography is important when there is concern that the FB is partially or completely extravascular.

122

Fortunately, most catheters and surgical devices in use today are radiopaque. Rarely, radiolucent or minimally radiopaque FBs will enter the vascular system. These FBs can occasionally be localized with newer digital radiographs that use edge enhancement algorithms. Woo used ultrasound to localize and guide retrieval of a nonopaque venous catheter fragment from the inferior vena cava (IVC).[8] Morse used contrast venography to outline the filling defect caused by a large radiolucent cannula lost during cardiopulmonary bypass.[9]

Once the FB has been localized, an appropriate retrieval device can be selected. Regardless of the type of retrieval device used, it must be brought into contact with the FB. The most common reason for failure to retrieve a FB is the inability to engage the object. Capturing a FB can be challenging in a large cava, atrium, or ventricle. A rotating C-arm or biplane fluoroscopy is invaluable in positioning the retrieval device adjacent to the FB. Attempts at removing smaller objects in a peripheral pulmonary artery are complicated by the difficulty of advancing the retrieval device into the correct branch. Reference images made with digital subtraction angiography or roadmapping can facilitate superselective catheterization of the correct branch.

Foreign bodies may be oriented so that there is no free end to grasp. Use of a pigtail catheter, deflecting wire, forceps, or J-shaped wire to manipulate the end of the FB free from the vessel or heart wall will facilitate retrieval.[10,11] These instruments can be used simultaneously with the retrieval device using two access sites.[12] If the pigtail catheter has insufficient rigidity to pull the FB free, it may be possible to intertwine the two by rotating the pigtail catheter several times.[11] Once the pigtail catheter is braided around the FB, more force can be exerted.

Recently embolized FBs are easily freed from the vessel wall, whereas chronic lines, such as pacer wires, are adherent due to endothelialization of their tines to the vessel or heart wall. Chronically retained FBs may also be encased in organized thrombus or become incorporated into the vessel wall by a fibrin sheath. Catheters may even be inadvertently sutured to the vessel wall (Figure 6.1). In these circumstances, a sheath advanced to the site of catheter fixation provides countertraction that minimizes shearing forces on the vessel wall during FB extraction.[13]

RETRIEVAL DEVICES

Forceps

The first percutaneous FB retrieval was performed from a femoral approach using bronchoscopic forceps.[14] This technique is limited by the rigid shaft of the instrument. The right internal jugular vein is the best approach for retrievals from the superior vena cava (SVC) or right heart when the retrieval device is rigid.[15] Bronchoscopic and urologic forceps provide excellent control, but the risk of vessel perforation is fairly high with these rigid devices. Smaller profile forceps with a flexible shaft (Cook Urologic, Spencer, IN) have been successfully employed (Figure 6.2).[16] The limited control with the flexible shaft forceps can be partially overcome by using a preshaped, torqueable guiding catheter. Some of the flexible shaft forceps have a shapeable shaft that allows greater directional control. Endomyocardial and gastrointestinal biopsy forceps are also flexible and provide good grasping force, but the small grasping surface makes them difficult to use (Figure 6.2). Extra care must be taken with biopsy forceps so as not to cut through a retained catheter. One of the major advantages of forceps is that they make it possible to capture a FB even though there is no free end to grasp.

Loop Snare

Loop snare retrieval, the most widely used method of FB retrieval, was first performed in 1967.[17] A small-caliber guidewire was folded over and introduced through a large,

Text continues on page 128

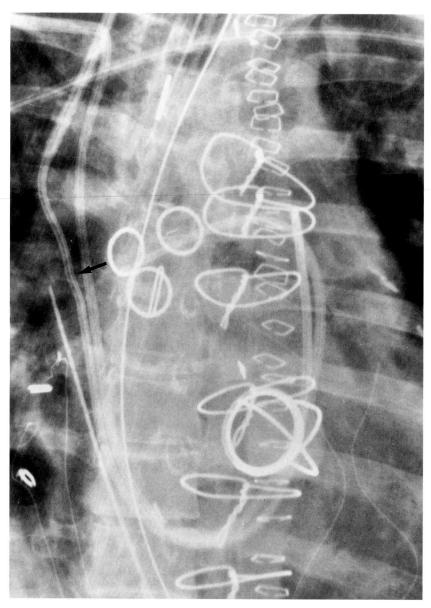

A

Figure 6.1 A. Right internal jugular (IJ) Swan-Ganz catheter was inadvertently sewn to the SVC during a valve replacement procedure. There is a second central line entering through the right subclavian vein. B, C, D, and E. Following pages.

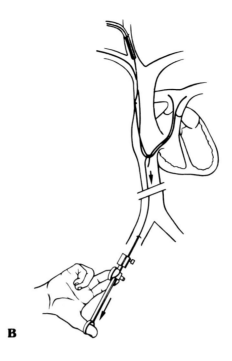

B

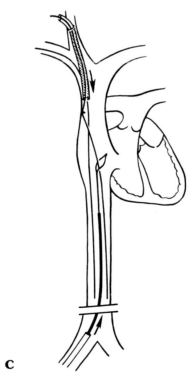

C

Figure 6.1 B. Tip-deflecting wire was used to pull the central lines into the IVC. C. A sheath was advanced over the IJ catheter to the site of the suture. A loop snare was advanced from a femoral vein approach over the tip of the catheter to the site of the suture. D and E. Following page.

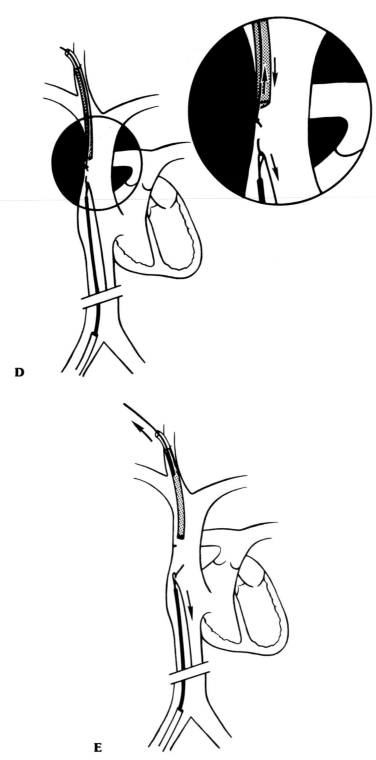

D

E

Figure 6.1 D. Traction was then applied to both ends of the catheter while counterpressure was kept on the sheath against the suture. The catheter fractured at the suture site. E. The two fragments were removed through the jugular and femoral sheaths. (Reprinted with permission from Matzko et al.[13])

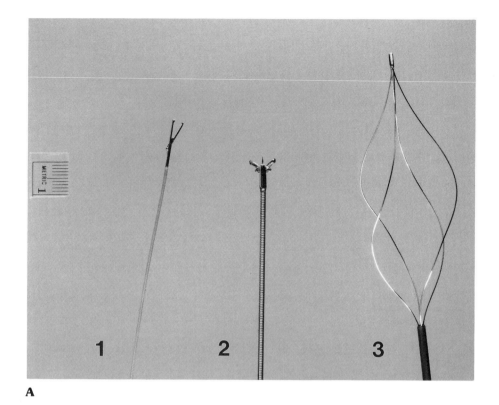

A

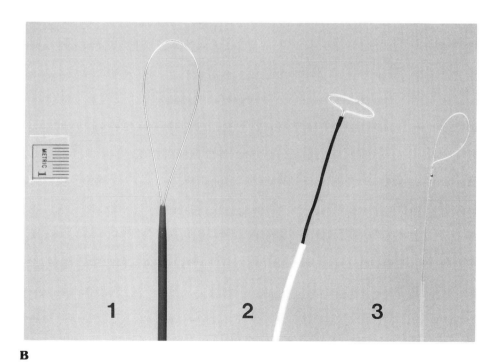

B

Figure 6.2 A. (1) Cook flexible alligator forceps, (2) endoscopic biopsy forceps (Olympus, Columbia, MD), and (3) Dotter intravascular retrieval basket. B. (1) Curry loop snare, (2) Nitinol gooseneck loop snare, and (3) Tracker loop snare.

nontapered catheter.[5] Commercially available kits include the Curry Loop Snare Retrieval Set (Cook, Bloomington, IN) which uses a 300-cm length of 0.021-inch wire doubled over to form a loop in an 8-Fr guiding catheter (Figure 6.2).[18]

The retrieval technique is similar for all types of loop snares. A guiding catheter is positioned at the site of the FB. The wire loop is advanced to the tip of the guiding catheter and the catheter is then withdrawn to expose the loop. The loop is placed orthogonal to the object to facilitate engagement of the FB. The wire loop is manipulated to "lasso" the object. The guiding catheter is advanced over the wire loop to entrap the FB. If the operator pulls on the loop instead of advancing the guiding catheter, the object may disengage from the loop. The loop snare should be secure enough to allow removal of the FB. Overtightening of the loop snare may shear or fragment a plastic FB. Different shapes of guiding catheters can facilitate steering and positioning the loop snare.

Since most FBs are oriented parallel to the vessel wall, it may be preferable to place a right angle bend on the wires so that the loop exits the catheter perpendicular to the vessel.[19] In 1991, Microvena (Vadnais Heights, MN) introduced the preshaped Amplatz Gooseneck nickel-titanium (nitinol) loop snare with an angled, guiding catheter containing a radiopaque tip (Figure 6.2). This device is unique because the flexible, nonkinking, nitinol wire quickly regains its original shape. The formed loop exits the catheter tip oriented perpendicular to the catheter shaft, making it easier to engage most intravascular FBs. The kits are available in loop sizes of 5, 10, 15, 25, and 35 mm.[20] This device has proved to be very useful in the clinical arena.[21]

A loop snare on a microcatheter (Target Therapeutics, Fremont, CA) can be used to enter smaller vessels. The 3-Fr catheter contains a preloaded loop, and the unit can be advanced coaxially through a 6-Fr (internal diameter) guiding catheter (Figure 6.2).

Balloons

The Fogarty balloon (Baxter Health Care Co., Santa Ana, CA) has limited use in percutaneous FB retrievals. It has been used in the removal of peripheral venous FBs, but extraction is difficult because the balloon affords no control over the FB and a surgical venotomy is usually required to remove the foreign body. Balloon retrievals in the heart and great vessels have been described,[22] but are best limited to smaller vessels due to size constraints of the balloon and the effect of large vessel flow on the balloon.

Baskets

The Dotter Intravascular Basket Retrieval Set (Cook, Bloomington, IN) consists of a large helical wire basket and an 8-Fr guiding catheter (Figure 6.2).[15] A variety of baskets has been used for vascular retrieval, and results have been excellent. A guiding catheter is advanced over a standard guidewire to the site of the FB. The basket is advanced through the catheter, which is then withdrawn to uncover the basket in proximity to the FB. The basket is carefully manipulated to grasp an end of the FB, and the guiding catheter is advanced over the basket to firmly entrap the object. The catheter and basket are withdrawn as a unit through the vascular access sheath. Extreme care must be taken not to entrap right ventricular trabeculae or valve structures when working in or through the heart.

REMOVAL

An introducer sheath should be inserted prior to engaging a FB. Captured catheters and wires will often become folded over. Therefore, the sheath at the exit site must be sized accordingly. Once the FB is grasped, it can be withdrawn into the sheath at the puncture site. It may not be possible to pull the FB through the sheath, but the sheath and FB can be removed as a unit. Needles and other rigid objects that can easily penetrate the heart or vessel wall must be carefully manipulated. More than one loop snare may be required to remove sharp FBs. It may be impossible to extract a large FB through a percutaneous access, but moving it into the common femoral or internal jugular vein makes removal by surgical cutdown easier.

SPECIFIC FOREIGN BODIES

Techniques that greatly facilitate removal of FBs and methods of managing several common FBs are presented below.

Central Venous Lines and Guidewires

The most common intravascular FBs are central line fragments and guidewires. Where the catheter fragment or guidewire lodges depends on the length and stiffness of the FB. Longer, stiffer fragments may remain in the SVC or IVC, while shorter, softer FBs embolize to the right ventricle or pulmonary artery. Most intravascular retrievals are performed very shortly after the catheter fragment has embolized, but successful removal of a right heart FB 13 months after the initial embolization has been reported.[23]

Bullet Fragments

Bullets, shrapnel, and other penetrating objects can migrate intravascularly. In the venous system, bullets can migrate to the heart and pulmonary arteries. Bullets in the pulmonary veins have been found to migrate to the arterial system.[7]

In the pulmonary artery, bullet fragments can cause symptoms of pulmonary embolism and can lead to pulmonary infarction, secondary thrombosis, infection, hemorrhage, vessel erosion, and extravascular migration. These risks lead most authors to recommend removal of all bullet fragments that migrate to the pulmonary arteries.[24] Others believe that small bullet emboli can be safely left in place.[25] Percutaneous removal is possible, but a large sheath or surgical cutdown is required to remove most intact bullets or large bullet fragments.[24,26]

Inferior Vena Cava Filters

Although most IVC filters migrate to or are inadvertently deployed in the heart during filter placement, there are several reports of delayed, spontaneous, migration to the right atrium, right ventricle, or pulmonary arteries.[27,28] Filters have also been displaced into the right atrium or SVC/innominate vein when the guidewire used to insert or change a central venous line becomes entangled with the filter.[29,30]

Filters in the right atrium or right ventricle are associated with a high risk of arrhythmias and/or myocardial injury and, whenever possible, should be removed or repositioned percutaneously. Filters have been successfully retrieved or repositioned from the heart to the IVC (Figure 6.3).[28,31,32] Dondelinger et al. used urologic forceps and the Gunther filter retrieval set (Cook Europe, Bjaevershov, Denmark) to rotate a Gunther filter in the right atrium and withdraw it into the IVC from a combined right axillary and right femoral approach.[2] Similarly, a Bird's Nest filter (Cook, Bloomington, IN) and a Greenfield filter (Medi-Tech, Watertown, MA) have been repositioned from the right atrium to the suprarenal IVC by means of a tip-deflecting wire and Curry loop snare.[28] Greenfield has also described using a filter retrieval device to capture a filter in the right atrium and then redeploy it in the IVC.[33]

Not all filters that migrate need to be retrieved. LaPlante reported a Nitinol filter (Nitinol Medical Technologies, Woburn, MA) that migrated to the pulmonary artery

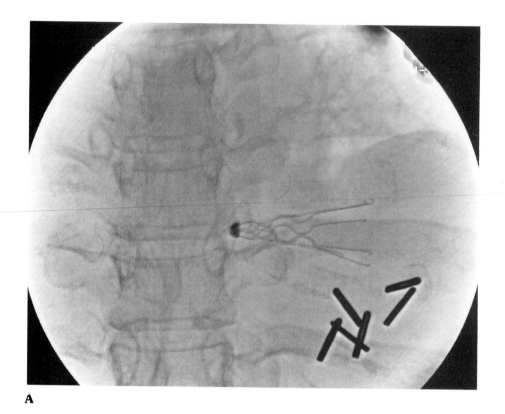

A

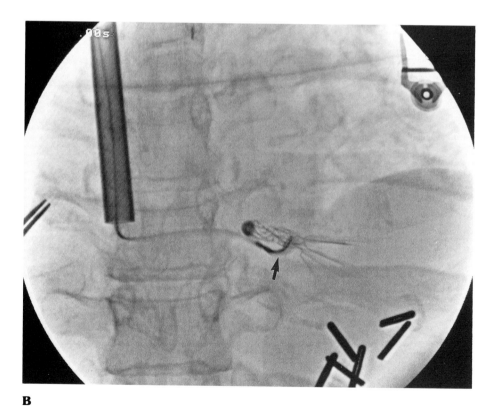

B

Figure 6.3 A. Greenfield filter lost in the right ventricle during operative placement. B. A 28-Fr sheath was placed into the right IJ vein and a loop snare was advanced over the filter (arrow). C and D. Following page.

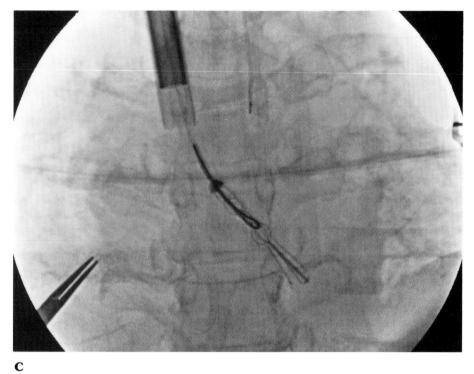

C

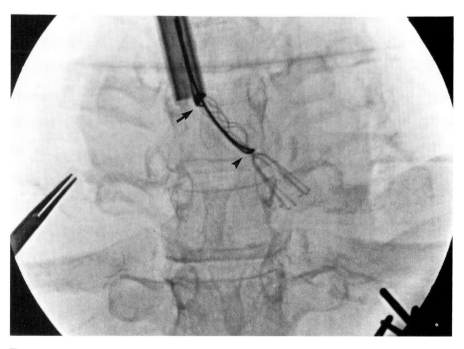

D

Figure 6.3 C. The filter could be only partially withdrawn. D. A second loop snare (arrow) was advanced over the first (arrowhead) to further reduce the profile of the filter and help guide it into the sheath.

immediately after deployment. The patient was symptom-free and the filter was not removed, but no follow-up was reported.[27] Filters that have migrated to the right heart, but could not be removed percutaneously, have been observed for as long as 88 months without significant symptoms.[34]

Interventional Devices

Spontaneous migration of metal stents placed in the central veins has been reported.[35] Arterial stents have also been misplaced or dislodged, or have migrated.[36] Vascular stent retrievals usually occur during the initial attempt to place a stent. Misplaced or partially deployed balloon-expanded stents are easier to retrieve if wire access is maintained through the stent. In this situation, a loop snare can be inserted through the introducer sheath with the loop placed over the end of the guidewire.[36] Once the loop is advanced to the level of the stent, it is much easier to advance the loop snare coaxially over the guidewire and the stent. The loop snare is used to compress and withdraw the stent. If needed, a balloon can be advanced into the stent over the existing guidewire and gently inflated. Once affixed to the inflated balloon, the stent can be redeployed in another vessel, such as the iliac vein. Alternatively, a loop snare can then be advanced over the stent.[37] In certain cases, alligator forceps or a tip-deflecting wire can be used to grasp the stent (Figure 6.4), and a loop snare can then be used to compress the stent.[38]

Coils placed in venous lesions or other abnormalities with arteriovenous shunting can migrate to the heart or pulmonary circulation. Percutaneous retrieval of coils has been performed with baskets, forceps, and loop snares.[2,39,40] Successful retrieval depends largely on the size of the vessel. Coils that have a tail extending into a larger vessel are more easily grasped than coils in smaller vessels. Once captured, coils are pliable and can be easily removed through an introducer sheath. Not all misplaced coils need to be removed; patients with coils that embolize to the pulmonary artery have been free of symptoms of pulmonary embolism. Misplaced peripheral arterial coils should be retrieved because of the risk of arterial thrombosis or distal thromboemboli.

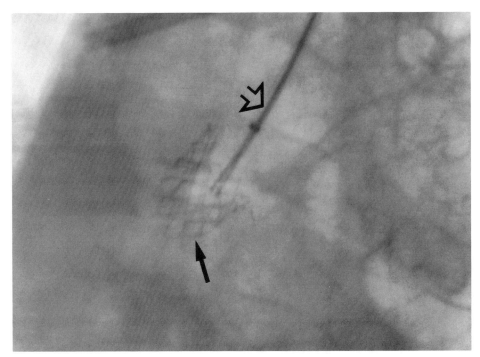

Figure 6.4 Palmaz stent (Johnson and Johnson Interventional Systems Co., Warren, NJ) (arrow) is being grasped with rat tooth forceps (open arrow) for subsequent removal.

In rare instances, angioplasty balloons can separate from the balloon catheter and embolize. These fragments are unfortunately radiolucent, but have been retrieved with forceps and loop snares.[21,41]

Balloon fragments, guidewire fragments, and laser catheter tips have all been left in previously occluded arterial segments without significant sequelae.[42] Conversely, fractured segments of guidewires left in the coronary circulation after an otherwise successful coronary artery angioplasty have led to vessel narrowing on follow-up.[43] Guidewire fragments in a coronary artery can be retrieved from the vessel with an angioplasty balloon or a loop snare, or by creating a braid around the wire fragment with two additional coronary guidewires.[42]

Pacemaker Wires

Permanent intravenous pacemakers are widely used. Fractured leads, leads that break free of the pacer unit, and leads that are no longer in use but are sewn to the subcutaneous tissues at the vessel entry site can all embolize. The most common indications for removal of pacer leads are septicemia, pocket infection, and the need for lead replacement.[44] Noninfected leads that are not in use may often be left in place since the risk of embolization and venous thrombosis may be less than the risk of percutaneous retrieval.[45]

Fearnot described a series of 228 pacer lead extractions.[46] The leads were in place for an average of 55 months. Extraction was successful in 85% of cases. An additional 8% of leads were partially extracted. One patient required thoracotomy for atrial wall repair. Two other patients developed a significant hemothorax. Before lead removal was attempted, appropriate pacer backup was established. The retrievals were performed through a cutdown on the original vessel of entry. A Cook pacemaker lead removal kit (Cook Pacemaker, Leechburg, PA) (Figure 6.5) was used in the most cases. The kit provides a core wire to stiffen and lengthen the pacer lead. This core wire is advanced to the tip of the hollow pacer lead where rotation of the wire locks the threaded end of the core wire into the pacer lead. Traction on a pacer lead without the core wire can easily cause the lead to fracture. A series of dilators are then advanced over the pacer lead. A sheath is eventually advanced over the lead to its tip in the ventricle or atrium. The sheath helps to free the pacer lead from any fibrin sheath along its course in the vessel and provides countertraction against the myocardium when the pacer lead is pulled (Figure 6.6). This technique greatly reduces the risk of cardiac wall avulsion or perfora-

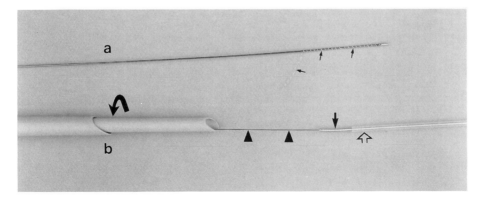

Figure 6.5 Cook pacemaker lead retrieval kit: **A.** Core wire: a fine wire (small arrows) is welded to and loosely wound around the end of the mandril of the core wire. This fine wire is designed to lock the core wire to the end of the pacer lead. **B.** The core wire (arrowheads) is shown inserted into the central lumen of the pacer lead (straight arrow). The pacer lead has an outer polymer sleeve (open arrow). Once the core wire has been advanced to the tip of the lead, the core wire is rotated to engage the locking mechanism. A coaxial dilator/sheath system (curved arrow) is shown partially advanced over the core wire.

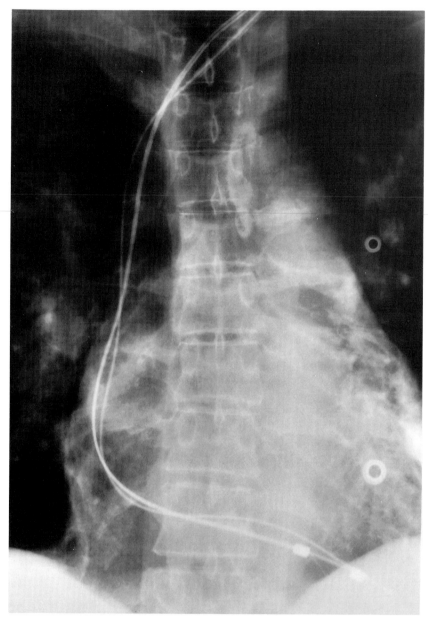

A

Figure 6.6 A. A failed pacer lead was present in the left jugular vein. The tip was firmly implanted in the wall of the right ventricle. A temporary pacer has been placed through the left subclavian vein. **B.** Following page.

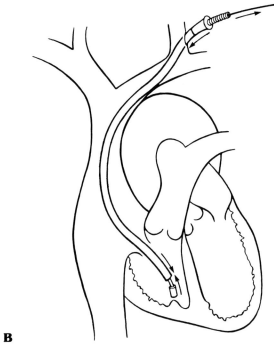

B

Figure 6.6 B. A Cook pacemaker lead removal kit core wire (open arrow) is used to stiffen and lengthen the pacer lead. A sheath (curved arrows) is advanced over the wire to near the distal tip. With the sheath being used for countertraction, the wire is pulled free from the ventricular wall.

tion. A femoral approach may be required when there is lead retraction or fracture or an inability to advance dilators over the pacer lead from the upper extremity site. In this situation, a combination of retrieval devices may be required.

RESULTS

Percutaneous FB retrieval is successful in 90–95% of patients.[2,21] Failure is most likely to occur with attempts at retrieving very small objects that have embolized to a peripheral pulmonary artery or into right heart pectinate muscles, objects that have already been incorporated into the vascular wall, very firmly incorporated pacemaker leads, or large, rigid, metallic FBs.

RISKS

The risk of retrieving a FB must always be weighed against the long-term risk of leaving the FB in the patient. Because risks have been reduced by refinements in percutaneous techniques, retrieval of most intravascular FBs should be attempted. Overall, the risk of a complication during a percutaneous retrieval is minimal.[2,15] Embolization of thrombus associated with a FB retrieval is a potential complication, especially with FBs that have been present for several days to weeks. A venogram or arteriogram before manipulation of the retained object may help to identify cases at high risk.

Any FB in the venous system may embolize to the pulmonary circulation during manipulation and attempted removal. Catheter fragments that have been in place for a long time can be brittle, and manipulation can lead to further fragmentation of the retained fragments. Fragmented intra-arterial FBs can embolize to the cerebral, coronary, or peripheral arteries.

Great care must be taken to avoid air emboli during venous retrieval procedures. Sheaths with hemostatic valves and catheters with rotating hemostatic valves are recommended. Some type of valve is also needed for intra-arterial retrievals to prevent excessive blood loss.[47]

Cardiac arrhythmias frequently occur during percutaneous removal of FBs from the heart or pulmonary circulation.[5] Although most are asymptomatic, life-threatening arrhythmias may arise from prolonged catheter manipulation in the heart. Other potential cardiac complications include myocardial contusion or perforation or disruption of a chorda tendinea. Such complications are of greater concern with the use of forceps and baskets. Pacemaker lead extraction and removal of IVC filters that have migrated to the heart are associated with the greatest risk of myocardial perforation or valve injury.

CONCLUSION

Central lines account for most intravascular FBs. Failure to remove them is associated with a very high morbidity and mortality. This, in combination with the very high success rate of percutaneous FB retrieval and a low complication rate, suggests that an aggressive approach to FB retrieval should generally be maintained. Asymptomatic patients with small, sterile, blunt FBs in the peripheral pulmonary circulation may be an exception. This type of FB is associated with a relatively low morbidity and is also relatively difficult to retrieve. Large, stiff FBs may be very difficult to retrieve percutaneously. Some of these FBs, such as IVC filters in the pulmonary artery, have been left in place without symptomatic complications at several years of follow-up.

REFERENCES

1. Decker R: Foreign bodies in the heart and pericardium—should they be removed? *J Thorac Surg* 9:62–67, 1940.
2. Dondelinger RF, Lepoutre B, Kurdziel JC: Percutaneous vascular foreign body retrieval: experience of an 11-year period. *Eur J Radiol* 12:4–10, 1991.
3. Turner DD, Sommers SC: Accidental passage of a polyethylene catheter from cubital vein to right atrium. *N Engl J Med* 251:744–745, 1954.
4. Wellman KF, Reinhard A, Salazar EP: Polyethylene catheter embolism: review of the literature and report of a case with associated fatal tricuspid and systemic candidiasis. *Circulation* 37:380–392, 1968.
5. Fisher RG, Ferreyro R: Evaluation of current techniques for nonsurgical removal of intravascular iatrogenic foreign bodies. *Am J Roentgenol* 130:541–548, 1978.
6. Druskin MS, Siegel PD: Bacterial contamination of indwelling intravenous polyethylene catheters. *JAMA* 185:966–968, 1963.
7. Kerr A, Louie W: Bullet embolus from a pulmonary vein to the right axillary artery. *Cardiovasc Intervent Radiol* 16:178–179, 1993.
8. Woo VL, Gerber M, Scheible W, et al: Real-time ultrasound guidance for percutaneous transluminal retrieval of nonopaque intravascular catheter fragment. *Am J Roentgenol* 133:760–761, 1979.
9. Morse SS, Strauss EB, Hashim SW, et al: Percutaneous retrieval of an unusually large, nonopaque intravascular foreign body. *Am J Roentgenol* 146:863–864, 1986.
10. McSweeney WJ, Schwartz DC: Retrieval of a catheter foreign body from the right heart using a guidewire deflector system. *Radiology* 100:61–62, 1971.
11. Ferrel H, Kimura Y, Amplatz K: Retrieval of an entrapped guide wire with a braiding maneuver. *J Vasc Interv Radiol* 5:649–651, 1994.

12. Khaja F, Lakier J: Foreign body retrieval from the heart by two catheter technique. *Cathet Cardiovasc Diagn* 5:263–268, 1979.

13. Matzko J, Matsumoto AH, Tegtmeyer C, et al: Percutaneous removal of a Swan-Ganz catheter sutured to the superior vena cava. *J Vasc Interv Radiol* 5:653–656, 1994.

14. Thomas J, Sinclair-Smith B, Bloomfield D, Davachi A: Non-surgical retrieval of a broken segment of steel spring guide from the right atrium and inferior vena cava. *Circulation* 30:106–108, 1964.

15. Dotter CT, Rosch J, Bibao MK: Transluminal extraction of catheter and guide fragments from the heart and great vessels; 29 collected cases. *Am J Roentgenol* 111:467–472, 1971.

16. Selby JB, Tegtmeyer CJ, Bittner GM: Experience with new retrieval forceps for foreign body removal in the vascular, urinary, and biliary systems. *Radiology* 176:535–538, 1990.

17. Massumi RA, Ross AM: Atraumatic, nonsurgical technique for removal of broken catheters from the cardiac cavities. *N Engl J Med* 277:195, 1967.

18. Curry JL: Recovery of detached intravascular catheter or guide wire fragments. *Am J Roentgenol* 105:894, 1969.

19. Hubert JW, Krone RJ, Shatz BA, et al: An improved snare system for the nonsurgical retrieval of intravascular foreign bodies. *Cathet Cardiovasc Diagn* 6:405–411, 1980.

20. Yedlicka JW Jr, Carlson JE, Hunter DW, et al: Nitinol gooseneck snare for removal of foreign bodies; experimental study and clinical evaluation. *Radiology* 178:691–693, 1991.

21. Cekirge S, Weiss JP, Foster RG, et al: Percutaneous retrieval of foreign bodies: experience with the nitinol gooseneck snare. *J Vasc Interv Radiol* 4:805–810, 1993.

22. Swersky RB, Reddy K, Hamby RI: Balloon catheter technique for removing foreign bodies from heart and great vessels. *N Y State J Med* 75:1077–1079, 1975.

23. Whitaker JA, Faruqui AM: Successful percutaneous removal of cardiac foreign body after 13 months in situ. *South Med J* 74:645–646, 1981.

24. Bernini CO, Junqueira AR Jr, Horita LT, et al: Pulmonary embolism from gunshot missiles. *Surg Gynecol Obstet* 156:615–619, 1983.

25. Unkle D, Shaikh KA: Iliac vein to pulmonary artery missile embolus: case report and review of the literature. *Heart Lung* 17:363–364, 1988.

26. Gaylord GM, Johnstrude IS: Split 24-Fr Amplatz dilator for percutaneous extraction of an intravascular bullet: case report and technical note. *Radiology* 170:888–889, 1989.

27. LaPlante JS, Contractor FM, Kiproff PM, et al: Migration of the Simon nitinol vena cava filter to the chest. *Am J Roentgenol* 160:385–386, 1993.

28. Ferris EJ, McCowan TC, Carver DK, et al: Percutaneous inferior vena caval filters: follow-up of seven designs in 320 patients. *Radiology* 188:851–856, 1993.

29. Marelich GP, Tharratt RS: Greenfield inferior vena cava filter dislodged during central venous catheter placement. *Chest* 106:957–959, 1994.

30. Urbaneja A, Fontaine AB, Bruckner M, et al: Evulsion of a vena tech filter during insertion of a central venous catheter. *J Vasc Interv Radiol* 5:783–785, 1994.

31. Siegel EL, Robertson EF: Percutaneous transfemoral retrieval of a free-floating titanium Greenfield filter with an Amplatz gooseneck snare. *J Vasc Interv Radiol* 4:565–568, 1993.

32. Tsai FY, Myers TV, Ashraf A, et al: Aberrant placement of a Kimray-Greenfield filter in the right atrium: percutaneous retrieval. *Radiology* 167:423–424, 1988.

33. Greenfield LJ, Crute SL: Retrieval of the Greenfield vena caval filter. *Surgery* 80:719–722, 1980.

34. Rodriguez LF, Saltiel FS: Long-term follow-up of ectopic intracardiac Greenfield filter. *Chest* 104:611–612, 1993.

35. Carrasco CH, Charnsangavej C, Wright KC, et al: Use of the Gianturco self-expanding stent in stenoses of the superior and inferior venae cavae. *J Vasc Interv Radiol* 3:409–419, 1992.

36. Pan M, Medina A, Romero M, et al: Peripheral stent recovery after failed intracoronary delivery. *Cathet Cardiovasc Diagn* 27:230–233, 1992.

37. Cekirge S, Foster RG, Weiss JP, et al: Percutaneous removal of an embolized Wallstent during a transjugular intrahepatic portosystemic shunt procedure. *J Vasc Interv Radiol* 4:559–560, 1993.

38. Eeckhout E, Sauffer JC, Goy JJ: Retrieval of a migrated coronary stent by means of an alligator forceps catheter. *Cathet Cardiovasc Diagn* 30:166–168, 1993.

39. Weber J: A complication with the Gianturco coil and its non-surgical management. *Cardiovasc Intervent Radiol* 3:156–158, 1980.

40. Kim MS, Horton JA: Intra-arterial foreign body retrieved using endoscopic biopsy forceps. *Radiology* 149:597, 1983.

41. Selby JB Jr, Oliva VL, Tegtmeyer CJ: Circumferential rupture of an angioplasty balloon with detachment from the shaft: case report. *Cardiovasc Intervent Radiol* 15:113–116, 1992.

42. Gurley JC, Booth DC, Hixson C, et al: Removal of retained intracoronary percutaneous transluminal coronary angioplasty equipment by a percutaneous twin guidewire method. *Cathet Cardiovasc Diagn* 19:251–256, 1990.

43. Doorey AJ, Stillabower M: Fractured and retained guide-wire fragment during coronary angioplasty—unforeseen late sequelae. *Cathet Cardiovasc Diagn* 20:238–240, 1990.

44. Byrd CL, Schwartz SJ, Hedin N: Intravascular techniques for extraction of permanent pacemaker leads. *J Thorac Cardiovasc Surg* 101:989–997, 1991.

45. Choo MH, Holmes DR, Gersh BJ, et al: Permanent pacemaker infections: characterization and management. *Am J Cardiol* 48:559–564, 1981.

46. Fearnot NE, Smith HJ, Goode LB, et al: Intravascular lead extraction using locking stylets, sheaths, and other techniques. *PACE* 13:1864–1870, 1990.

47. Smith PL: An improved method for intra-arterial foreign body retrieval. *Radiology* 145:539, 1982.

C H A P T E R
7

Percutaneous Transluminal Angioplasty of Brachiocephalic Arteries

J. Bayne Selby, Jr
Alan H. Matsumoto
John F. Angle
Charles J. Tegtmeyer

Since the original report by Dotter and Judkins in 1964,[1] percutaneous transluminal angioplasty (PTA) has been used in almost every portion of the vascular system. Bachman and Kim first described PTA in the brachiocephalic circulation in 1980.[2] Advances in technique and equipment have further refined the safety and efficacy of this intervention since then. With careful patient selection and meticulous technique, experienced operators can expect gratifying long-term results for their patients.[3–5]

ANATOMY

To avoid confusion, we will use *brachiocephalic arteries* as a general term to describe the arteries originating off the aortic arch. The first major vessel arising from the thoracic aorta is the innominate artery. The left common carotid artery is the second and the left subclavian artery the third. There are numerous variants to this anatomy and all have implications for PTA.

The most common normal variant is the innominate and left common carotid arteries arising from the aorta as a common (bovine) trunk. If a stenosis occurs in a bovine trunk, the relative risk of PTA is greatly increased since the entire anterior cerebral circulation is dependent on this common trunk. The incidence of significant occlusive disease in this setting is unknown.

The left vertebral artery can arise directly from the aortic arch. In this setting, left subclavian artery PTA can be performed without putting any of the cerebral circulation at risk. A third variant that can be encountered is an aberrant right subclavian artery. Although the presence of this anatomic variant is uncommon, an aberrant right subclavian artery may be prone to the development of occlusive or aneurysmal disease when compared to a nonaberrant right subclavian artery.[3,6] The angle of takeoff and the more distal origin of an aberrant right subclavian artery from the aortic arch also simplifies the technical aspects of PTA from a femoral approach, and makes the procedure safer because the balloon catheter does not traverse the carotid arteries.

139

ETIOLOGIES

The majority of brachiocephalic arterial stenoses are due to atherosclerosis. The sites affected by atherosclerosis are fairly predictable: the origins of the great vessels, the bifurcation of the innominate artery into the right subclavian and right common carotid arteries, and the left subclavian artery trunk (Figure 7.1). The left subclavian artery is the most common site of a hemodynamically significant narrowing in the proximal brachiocephalic vessels.[3,4]

Involvement of the brachiocephalic arteries with diffuse long segments of disease, especially in more than one vessel, should raise the question of an arteritis[7,8] (Figure 7.2). Takayasu's is the most common arteritis to affect the arteries of the aortic arch.[8–10] The "activity" of the arteritis is approximated by the degree of elevation in the erythrocyte sedimentation rate (ESR): the higher the ESR, the more active the disease process. The surgical literature has shown that a graft placed into a vessel with ongoing, active arteritis is likely to fail.[11] Angioplasty may be affected by the same limitation. In fact, there has been some suggestion that PTA in an area of active arteritis intensifies the inflammatory process.[9] Despite the concern for performing PTA in the setting of an elevated ESR, all six patients in one series with focal lesions (<3 cm) and persistently elevated ESRs demonstrated sustained patency following PTA.[10] In contrast, long-segment disease or complete occlusions in patients with nonspecific aortoarteritis seem to respond poorly to PTA, regardless of the ESR.[9,10] Giant cell arteritis is also known to affect the braciocephalic arteries and can be treated with PTA (Figure 7.3).

Radiation can also induce segmental or diffuse vessel narrowing in the brachiocephalic vessels.[12,13] Arterial stenosis can arise secondary to irradiation in three ways:

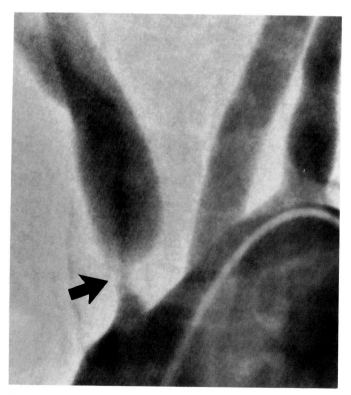

A

Figure 7.1 Characteristic location of atherosclerotic lesions involving the brachiocephalic arteries: **A.** origin of the innominate artery (arrow); **B** and **C.** Following page.

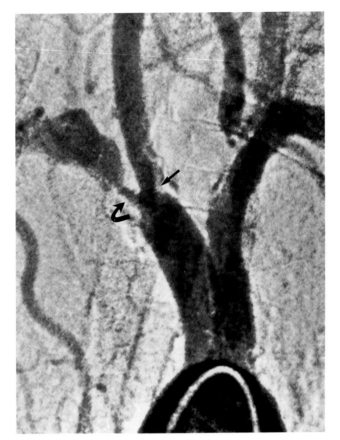

B

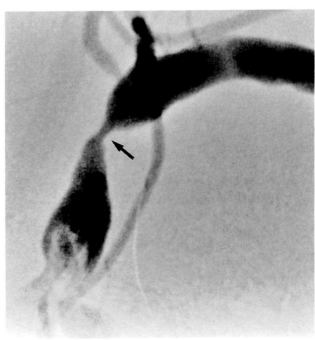

C

Figure 7.1 B. The bifurcation of the innominate artery into the right subclavian (curved arrow) and right common carotid (straight arrow) arteries; and C. the trunk of the left subclavian artery (arrow).

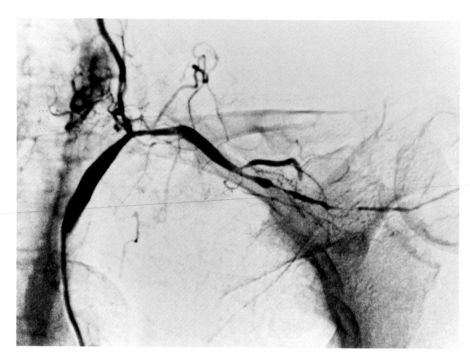

Figure 7.2 Selective catheterization and injection of the left subclavian artery demonstrates long irregular stenotic disease involving the subclavian and axillary arteries characteristic of a nonatherosclerotic etiology to the vascular disease. This patient was a 75-yr-old woman with giant cell arteritis.

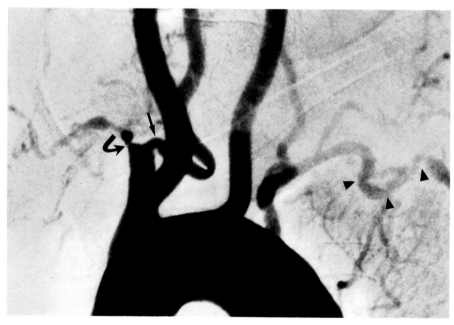

A

Figure 7.3 A 74-yr-old woman with a known history of giant cell arteritis presents with the subacute onset of right arm claudication several months after a right common carotid to right axillary artery bypass graft. **A.** An arch aortogram shows severe narrowing of the right subclavian artery (curved arrow) just beyond the origin of the vertebral artery (straight arrow). There is also diffuse narrowing of the left subclavian artery (arrowheads). The right common carotid to right axillary artery bypass graft is occluded. **B** and **C.** Following page.

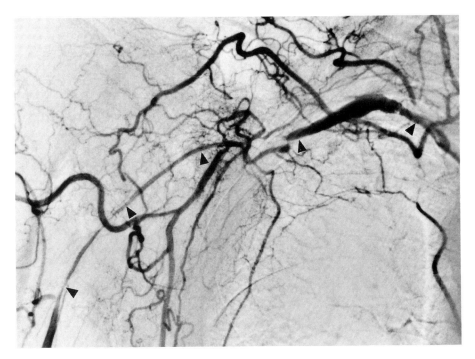

B

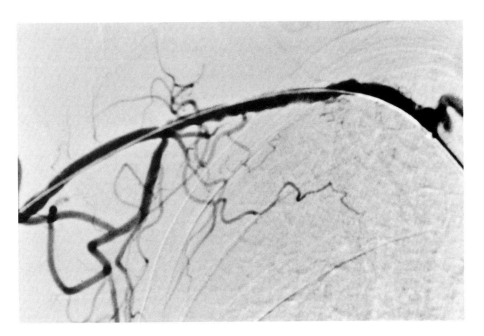

C

Figure 7.3 B. Selective right subclavian arteriogram reveals diffuse narrowing of the subclavian, axillary, and proximal brachial arteries (arrowheads) **C** and **D** (following page). Following dilatation of the entire diseased segment with an angioplasty balloon 4 mm in diameter by 10 cm in length, the caliber of the arteries is significantly improved. The radial artery pulse at the wrist, which was not palpable prior to the procedure, was now easily palpable. The patient remained asymptomatic until she expired 6 months later.

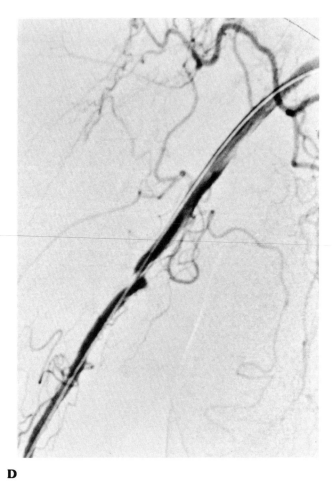

D

Figure 7.3 (*Continued.*)

(1) dense periarterial fibrosis, (2) arterial wall fibrosis with secondary damage to the vasa vasorum, and (3) acceleration of the atherosclerotic process.[13,14] A common scenario is a patient with lymphoma who undergoes successful radiation treatment, but returns later in life with a symptomatic stenosis in the radiation field. Although data are limited, radiation-induced lesions have responded to balloon PTA.[15,16]

Although fibromuscular dysplasia has been reported in the extracranial carotid and vertebral arteries, it is extremely rare in the chest.[17,18]

PATIENT SELECTION

As in other areas of the body, PTA should only be performed in those patients who have both a hemodynamically significant lesion and corresponding clinical symptoms.[19-21] Because of the central location of the brachiocephalic vessels, clinical symptoms can be variable. Indications for treatment can be categorized on the basis of the clinical presentation of the patient: (1) upper extremity ischemia; (2) cerebral ischemia; and (3) angina in patients with an internal mammary to coronary artery bypass graft or lower extremity ischemia in patients with an axillobifemoral bypass graft. Although the prevalence of ischemia is less in the upper than in the lower extremity, if the dominant arm is affected, symptoms can be quite disabling. The clinical symptoms are analogous to those that occur in the legs: claudication or fatigue, rest pain, and nonhealing ulcers (Figure 7.4).

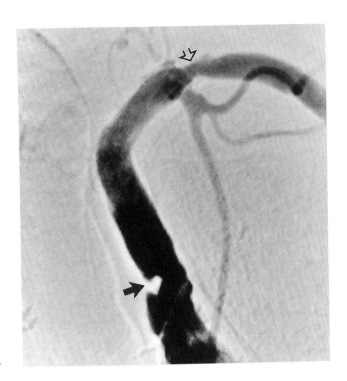

A

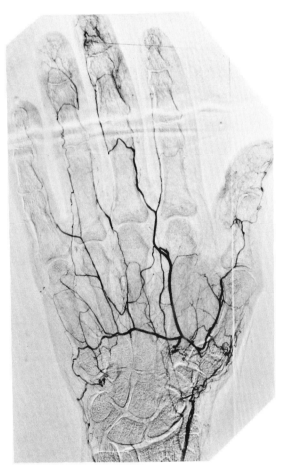

B

Figure 7.4 A 65-yr-old woman with severe peripheral vascular disease presents with non-healing ulcers of the thumb and fourth finger of the left hand with a diminished left brachial pulse. **A.** A selective left subclavian arteriogram demonstrates an asymmetric plaque involving the proximal left subclavian artery (closed arrow) and a more concentric stenosis (open arrow) involving the left subclavian artery just beyond the left internal mammary artery. **B.** Arteriogram of the left hand reveals proximal radial and ulnar artery occlusions with diffuse disease of the common palmar and proper digital arteries. **C.** Following page.

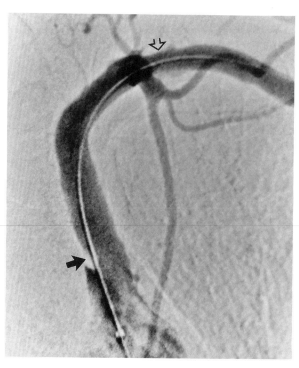

C

Figure 7.4 C. Following dilatation of the proximal subclavian artery lesion with a 10-mm balloon and the midsubclavian lesion with a 7-mm balloon, the control arteriogram demonstrates a satisfactory angiographic appearance to both lesions (arrows). There was equalization of the blood pressure in both upper extremities and the patient's ischemic left hand rest pain resolved.

Cerebral ischemia can be subdivided into the carotid (anterior) and vertebral (posterior) circulations. Since the left subclavian artery is the most common proximal brachiocephalic vessel affected, "subclavian steal" with symptoms of vertebrobasilar insufficiency is a common manifestation of cerebrovascular insufficiency. Similar symptoms can also occur with right subclavian artery stenosis. It is important to carefully evaluate the bifurcation of both common carotid arteries in this situation since most patients with vertebrobasilar symptoms and subclavian artery disease usually have associated narrowings of the anterior circulation.[22] A patient with a lesion in the innominate artery or either proximal common carotid arteries can present with amaurosis fugax, transient ischemia attacks, and/or a stroke (Figure 7.5).

A more recent indication for left subclavian artery PTA has been the need to improve inflow to a coronary artery graft bypass.[3,23–29] Use of the left internal mammary artery (LIMA) as a conduit to bypass coronary artery disease is associated with improved long-term results for coronary revascularization because of a low incidence of atherosclerosis in this vessel.[28–30] However, the internal mammary artery arises distal to a common site of significant atherosclerosis, the proximal left subclavian artery. Therefore, PTA of the left subclavian proximal to a LIMA to coronary artery graft will probably become more commonplace in the near future (Figure 7.6).

TECHNIQUE

The technique of PTA of the brachiocephalic arteries is similar to previously described techniques for peripheral artery PTA, although the risk associated with a bad outcome is fairly significant. Therefore, proper patient selection, meticulous technique, and close monitoring of the patient are requisite.

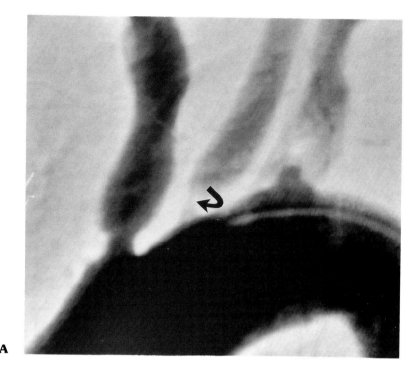

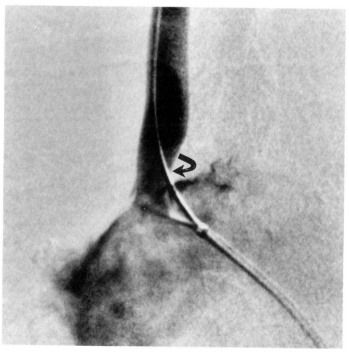

Figure 7.5 A. An arch aortogram in the right posterior oblique (RPO) projection in a 63-yr-old woman with left hemispheric transient ischemic attacks demonstrates a 90% stenosis at the origin of the left common carotid artery (curved arrow). The left internal carotid artery was widely patent. There is also a 50% stenosis at the origin at the innominate artery. **B.** Following dilatation with an 8-mm-diameter balloon, the control arteriogram shows a widely patent origin to the left common carotid artery (curved arrow). The patient's symptoms resolved.

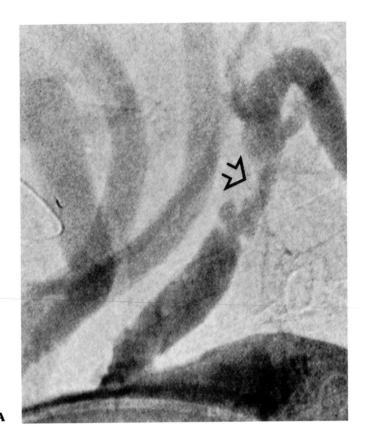

Figure 7.6 A 76-yr-old man with a known abdominal aortic aneurysm presents with unstable angina. The patient had a prior LIMA to coronary artery bypass graft and now has a diminished blood pressure in the left upper extremity. **A.** An arch aortogram in the RPO projection reveals an irregular stenosis involving the left subclavian artery (open arrow) proximal to the origin of the left vertebral artery. **B.** Following dilatation with a 9-mm-diameter balloon, the control arteriogram demonstrates a widely patent left subclavian artery (arrows). The patient's angina resolved and his blood pressure in both arms equalized.

Possibly the most important aspect of the procedure is the diagnostic angiogram. High-quality cut-film thoracic angiography supplemented with digital subtraction arteriography (DSA) is highly recommended. Selective injections should be made when necessary. The location and extent of the lesion should be completely defined before the interventional portion of the procedure begins (Figure 7.7). The status of the vascular bed distal to the stenosis, whether in the arm or the head, should also be studied angiographically prior to the PTA procedure. As much anatomy as possible should be visualized prior to the PTA so that there are no surprises during the procedure.

Rupture of one of the brachiocephalic vessels is potentially fatal, so great care should be exercised in choosing the appropriate balloon size. Although some methods have been developed for measuring blood vessels by DSA techniques, we still feel that an anteroposterior (AP) cut-film angiogram provides the safest, most consistent measurement of vessel size. The balloon diameter is chosen according to the size of the artery on the AP cut-film arteriogram; no allowance is made for magnification. This results in a slight, but consistent (20% at our institution) overdilation of the artery. If there is a question about balloon size, it is prudent to use the smaller balloon. The right posterior oblique view of the aortic arch is used to better delineate the vessel origins.

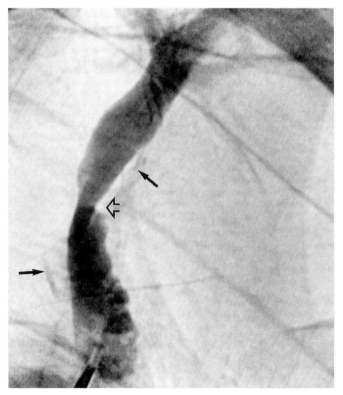

A

Figure 7.7 A 63-yr-old man, 2 yr after a LIMA to coronary artery bypass graft, had unstable angina despite intravenous heparin and nitroglycerin therapy. A cardiac catheterization done 1 wk earlier from a left brachial artery approach showed a significant left subclavian artery stenosis. Injection of the LIMA at the time of cardiac catheterization revealed a stenosis in the coronary circulation not amenable to percutaneous transluminal coronary angioplasty. **A.** A selective left subclavian arteriogram demonstrates the spiraling stenosis of the proximal left subclavian artery (open arrow) with evidence for intramural contrast (straight arrows), suggesting a dissection of the left subclavian artery. **B** and **C.** Following page.

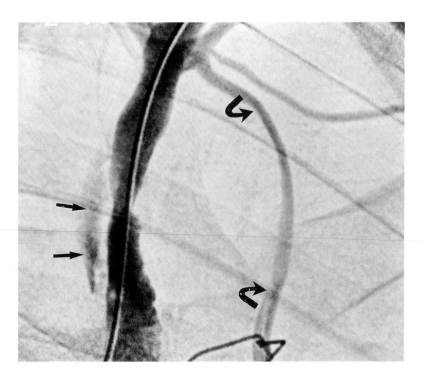

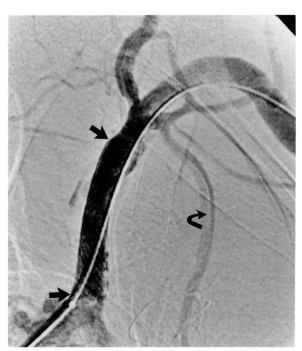

Figure 7.7 B. The irregular stenosis of the left subclavian artery was carefully traversed with a guidewire. Following dilatation with a balloon 8 mm in diameter, there was still a significant residual stenosis with intramural collection of contrast (straight arrows). The LIMA was also better visualized and showed evidence of dissection (curved arrows). C. Because of a residual 10 mm Hg gradient, a Wallstent 8 mm in diameter and 20 mm in length was deployed in the left subclavian artery (straight arrows). The gradient after stent deployment was zero. The control arteriogram revealed rapid flow through the left subclavain artery with better opacification of the LIMA. The dissection flap within the LIMA was also more clearly defined (curved arrow). The patient did well following the procedure.

The lesion is crossed with a guidewire from the easiest approach. The femoral artery is associated with lower puncture site complications, while the ipsilateral high brachial artery provides a more direct access for subclavian lesions.[31] If crossing the lesion is not possible or seems excessively risky from one direction, an alternative approach is used. Occasionally, both a femoral and brachial artery approach may be necessary. An introducer sheath may be used, depending on operator preference.

A floppy-tipped guidewire (0.035-inch Bentson; Cook, Inc., Bloomington, IN) is initially used to cross the lesion. Occasionally, a steerable 0.035-inch Terumo wire (Medi-Tech/Boston Scientific, Natick, MA) facilitates lesion traversal. A 5-Fr diagnostic catheter is advanced over the wire beyond the lesion, and contrast material is injected to confirm an intraluminal location. We routinely give 2,000–3,000 units of heparin, but no antispasmodic agents. An exchange length wire is used to advance a balloon catheter of appropriate diameter to the lesion. A long shaft on the balloon catheter (e.g., 100–120 cm) may be required to reach a brachiocephalic lesion from a femoral artery approach.

The balloon is prepared *ex vivo* to eliminate the air from the balloon and inflation device in order to minimize the chance for an air embolism to the brain should the balloon rupture during its inflation. The balloon is initially inflated for approximately 10–30 sec to a pressure sufficient to eliminate any "waist" on the balloon. The patient may experience some pain during balloon inflation, but the pain should rapidly abate with balloon deflation. If the pain does not decrease following balloon deflation, a control arteriogram should be done immediately to exclude vessel rupture. If the patient experiences severe pain during balloon inflation, a smaller balloon should be used.

For procedures that directly affect the carotid circulation (Figures 7.5 and 7.8), the patient is asked to count continuously during balloon inflation. Counting provides a

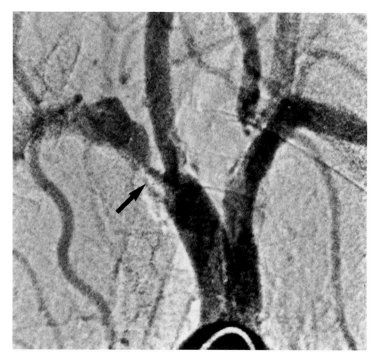

A

Figure 7.8 A 56-yr-old man was referred for evaluation of recurrent syncope following the use of his right arm. **A.** An arch aortogram in the left posterior oblique (LPO) projection demonstrated a 90% stenosis involving the origin of the right subclavian artery (arrow). The plaque appeared calcified and partially engulfed the origin of the right carotid artery. **B, C,** and **D.** Following pages.

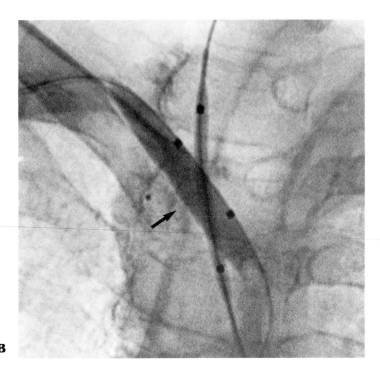

B

C

Figure 7.8 B. From the right high brachial artery approach, a balloon 9 mm in diameter was advanced across the subclavian artery stenosis and using the "kissing balloon" technique with a 4-mm balloon in the right common carotid artery, the right subclavian artery was dilated. Digital spot film revealed the calcified nature of the lesion (arrow). C. Control arteriogram showed a residual stenosis of 30% (arrow), but the blood pressure in the left and right arm were now equal. The patient's clinical symptoms resolved. **D.** Following page.

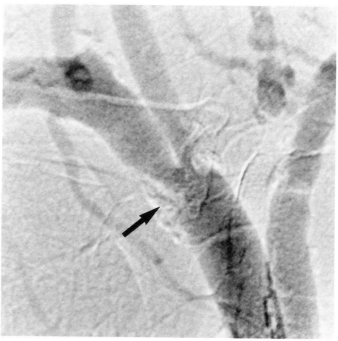

D

Figure 7.8 D. A follow-up arteriogram 28 months following the balloon angioplasty demonstrates the large calcified plaque engulfing the origins of the right subclavian and common carotid arteries. The stenosis has not significantly progressed and the patient remains asymptomatic relative to the right subclavian artery.

means to monitor the adequacy of cerebral perfusion during the procedure. If the patient loses the ability to count, the balloon should be immediately deflated, and the neurologic status of the patient should be reassessed. In this situation, a few rapid balloon inflations and deflations in the lesion may be all that is tolerated. In addition, more aggressive anticoagulation (i.e., bolus of 5,000 units of heparin) is used to minimize any chance for thrombus formation during the procedure.

Following the angioplasty, the result should be checked immediately. If the lesion is dilated from a femoral artery approach, a 0.018-inch guidewire is placed through the balloon catheter by using a side-arm adapter. The tip of the small wire is left across the lesion and the balloon catheter is withdrawn proximal to the area of dilatation. A control arteriogram can then be performed. Alternatively, the balloon catheter can be removed and a 6-Fr nontapered catheter with an 0.061-inch internal diameter (ID) and a radiopaque marker at its tip (Microvena Corp, Vadnais, MN) can be fitted with a side-arm adapter and advanced over the 0.035-inch exchange wire proximal to the area dilated (Figure 7.9). Although this method requires the use of a sheath, we have found that control arteriograms are of better quality than those obtained with the 0.018-inch wire system described above.

If the lesion was dilated from a high brachial artery approach and a diagnostic catheter was placed from a femoral artery approach, the diagnostic catheter can be used to check the PTA result. When a high brachial artery approach is used alone, the balloon catheter is advanced central to the lesion. The wire is removed, and a control arteriogram is obtained.

Additional dilatations are performed for residual stenoses greater than 30%, residual gradients greater than 5–10 mm Hg, or persistent subclavian "steal". Standard checks of neurologic status are done before and after all procedures.

After the procedure, the patient is treated with 2,000 units of heparin subcutaneously every 6 hr while in the hospital. Patients are instructed to take 325 mg acetyl-

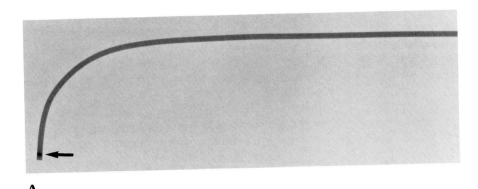

A

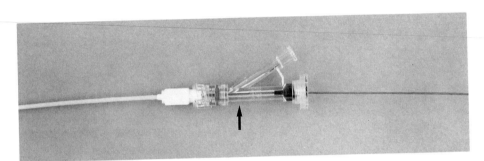

B

Figure 7.9 A. A 6-Fr nontapered catheter (Microvena Corp.) with a 0.061-inch internal diameter (ID) and a radiopaque marker at its tip (arrow) is shown. It is available in lengths of 75 and 100 cm. B. The catheter, which costs about $33, can be fitted with a side-arm adapter (arrow) and advanced over a 0.035-inch guidewire. Figures 8.4C, 8.5B, 8.6B, and 8.7C are examples of control arteriograms performed using this 6-Fr nontapered catheter system. The radiopaque tip of the catheter is seen on the control arteriograms.

salicylic acid daily for life. Dipyridamole, 75 mg two times a day for 6 months, can also be added to the postprocedural medication regimen. Patients are asked to quit smoking if they are smokers and to perform daily exercises with the affected arm (if the dilated vessel serves an extremity). Follow-up pulse volume recordings and segmental Doppler pressures of the upper extremities are also obtained in patients treated for subclavian artery stenosis.

RESULTS

The immediate technical and the long-term clinical results should be considered when evaluating the efficacy of PTA. It is also necessary to distinguish between the treatment of stenoses and occlusions when comparing the results of PTA with surgical alternatives. Kachel et al. reviewed results of PTA of 774 supra-aortic artery occlusions and stenoses and found an overall technical success rate of 95.3%.[4] Although the compilation included lesions involving the internal carotid artery, subclavian artery dilatations were the largest subset of procedures (N = 436). Hebrang et al. were technically successful with PTA in 40 of 43 (93%) patients with stenoses of the subclavian artery.[5] In our series of 32 stenoses in 29 patients, the technical success rate was 100%.[3] Reviewing the published results and taking into account refinements in technique and improvements in equipment, the technical success rate for PTA of brachiocephalic arterial stenoses should approach 95%[3–5,31–39] (Table 7.1).

TABLE 7.1 Summary of Largest Series of PTA of Brachiocephalic Arterial Stenoses

Authors	No. of Lesions	Technical Success	Long-term Primary Clinical Success	Complications Neurologic	Complications Other	Months Follow-up (mean)
Selby et al.[3]	32	32/32 (100%)	31/32 (97%)	0	2	4–88 (36)
Kachel et al.[4]	47	47/47 (100%)	45/47 (96%)	0	2	3–109 (58)
Hebrang et al.[5]	43	40/43 (93%)	34/43 (79%)	0	0	6–48 (29)
Dorros et al.[31]	22	22/22 (100%)	21/22 (95%)	0	2	2–73 (28)
Motarjeme et al.[32]	16	16/16 (100%)	16/16 (100%)	0	0	8/60 (27)
Vitek et al.[33]	35	35/35 (100%)	—	0	0	—
Burke et al.[34]	29	26/29 (90%)	—	1	1	(37)
Insall et al.[35]	34	34/34 (100%)	30/34 (89%)	1	2	2–90 (26)
Romanowski et al.[36]	25	23/25 (92%)	17/25 (68%)	0	0	8–111 (50)
Erbstein et al.[37]	21	18/21 (86%)	17/21 (81%)	—	—	18–26
Millaire et al.[38]	46	45/46 (98%)	37/44 (84%)	1	4	9–101 (41)
Wilms et al.[39]	23	21/23 (91%)	18/21 (86%)	1	2	6–60 (25)
Farina et al.[53]	23	21/23 (91%)	(54%)	—	1	5-yr actuarial (30)
Overall	396	380/396 (96%)	239/305 (78%)*	4	16	—

*Ten of the 13 series (unable to determine for references 33, 34, and 52).

155

TABLE 7.2 Summary of Largest Series of PTA of Brachiocephalic Arterial Occlusions

Authors	No. of Occlusions	Technical Success	Long-term Primary Clinical Success	Complications Neurologic	Complications Other	Months Follow-up (mean)	No. of Patients Receiving Stents
Kachel et al.[4]	7	1/7 (15%)	—	—	—	—	0
Hebrang et al.[5]	9	5/9 (56%)	—	—	—	—	0
Dorros et al.[31]	11	11/11 (100%)	—	0	3	(28)	
Motarjeme et al.[32]	7	1/7 (15%)	1/1 (100%)	0	0	—	0
Mathias et al.[40]	46	38/46 (83%)	32/38 (84%)	0	0	(33)	7
Duber et al.[41]	8	7/8 (88%)	3/7 (43%)	0	2	8–37	7
Bates et al.[42]	5	5/5 (100%)	—	0	—	—	5
Totals	93	68/93 (73%)	36/46 (78%)	—	—	—	19

It is more difficult to estimate the likelihood of a technical success of PTA in a complete occlusion, but it appears to be lower than for stenoses[4,5,31,32,40–42] (Table 7.2). In the review by Kachel et al., there were seven technical failures of subclavian artery PTA; six occurred in total occlusions and the seventh failure was not specified.[4] Hebrang et al. were technically successful in only 5 of 9 (55%) patients with subclavian artery occlusions.[5] Mathias et al. treated 46 patients with subclavian artery occlusions and were successful in 38 (83%).[40] The authors did note that traversing the obstructed subclavian artery was very difficult in 29 of the 38 (76%) successful cases. Seven of the patients also required implantation of a vascular stent. Duber et al. treated eight patients with proximal left subclavian artery occlusions.[41] Technical success was achieved in 7 of 8 (87.5%) patients.

The long-term clinical success rate for PTA of brachiocephalic arterial stenoses appears to be high (Table 7.1). Kachel et al. reported that 42 of 44 (95%) patients in their series who underwent subclavian artery PTA remained symptom-free at a follow-up of 3 to 109 months (mean = 58 months).[4] On the basis of life-table analysis, Hebrang et al. projected a 4-yr patency rate of 78.8% for subclavian artery PTA.[5] Life-table analysis in our series of 29 patients projected a 7.5-yr cumulative primary patency rate of 96.6%, with a standard error of 4.3%. Follow-up ranged from 4 to 88 months (mean = 36 months). The one clinical failure in our series occurred 8 months after the initial PTA and the recurrent stenosis was successfully redilated. The patient remained asymptomatic until she died of lymphoma 19 months later. The patient was receiving upper thoracic and mediastinal radiation therapy which is known to accelerate occlusive vascular disease.

The excellent long-term clinical success rate found with PTA of brachiocephalic arterial stenoses can be explained by a number of factors. Brachiocephalic arteries are large vessels with high flow. The best results with PTA of the lower extremities are achieved in the aortoiliac vessels, which are similar in size to the brachiocephalic arteries.[43] In addition, "poor run-off" and multiple tandem lesions in brachiocephalic arteries are uncommon. Therefore, patients are unlikely to develop recurrent symptoms because of progression of more distal disease.

The long-term clinical success for PTA of brachiocephalic artery occlusions is less clear because of the absence of good follow-up data (Table 7.2). In the series of Mathias et al, 6 of 38 (16%) patients developed recurrent disease at the site of prior recanalization at a mean follow-up of 33 months.[40] Duber et al. reported a recurrence rate of 57% (4 of 7 patients) within 16 months.[41] In general, we refer patients with complete occlusions of brachiocephalic arteries for surgical bypass because of the relatively low technical success rates and the absence of good long-term follow-up data from PTA. Kachel et al. have made a similar recommendation.[4]

SURGICAL ALTERNATIVES

Surgical intervention for the treatment of supra-aortic occlusive disease has continued to evolve. Direct endarterectomy and aortobrachiocephalic bypass grafting have been largely replaced by extrathoracic surgical procedures.[44,45] The current initial surgical approach to proximal brachiocephalic arterial disease includes common carotid–subclavian bypass grafting, extra-anatomic bypass grafts, and subclavian–carotid transposition. These surgical procedures are associated with relatively low morbidity (<5%) and mortality (<2%) rates and good long-term patency rates (70–100%).[44–51]

Because the ipsilateral internal carotid artery can be diseased, concomitant carotid endarterectomy may be necessary in as many as 23% of patients undergoing a common carotid to subclavian bypass for subclavian artery disease, exposing these patients to additional risks.[46,52] In patients in whom the ipsilateral common carotid artery is a poor donor inflow vessel, a contralateral common carotid to subclavian or axillary to axillary bypass graft can be used. Long-term patency rates with these extra-anatomic bypass grafts approach 95%, but tracheal or skin erosion, graft infections, and adjacent nerve injury remain somewhat problematic.[48,51]

There are no randomized trials comparing surgery to PTA in the treatment of brachiocephalic arterial disease. A retrospective, nonrandomized study from a single institution compared the two therapeutic modalities.[53] There were 36 patients treated, 21 with PTA and 16 with surgery. The technical success rate was 91% (19 of 21) for PTA and 86% (13 of 15) surgery. Significant complications occurred in 1 PTA patient and 2 surgical patients. Actuarial patency rates at 3 and 5 yr for PTA were 86% and 54%, respectively, versus 86% and 87%, respectively for surgery.

COMPLICATIONS OF PTA

The complication rates reported with PTA of the brachiocephalic arteries are low. In the review by Kachel et al., of 774 supraaortic lesions treated with PTA, major complications occurred in 0.5% and minor complications in 3.5%.[4] In the report by Mathias et al., no significant embolic complications occurred in the 38 patients with total occlusions who underwent successful percutaneous revascularization.[40] Two of the 29 (6.6%) patients in our series had complications, both related to the puncture site.[3] These occurred early in our experience when relatively large catheters were used for both the diagnostic and interventional portions of the study. We have now treated 58 patients with stenoses of the brachiocephalic arteries and have had no clinically significant complication in our last 40 patients.

Neurologic complications related to PTA of the brachiocephalic arteries have been rare. For subclavian artery PTA, there may be an intrinsic mechanism to protect the patient from having emboli to the central nervous system during the procedure. Investigators have shown that, when subclavian steal is related to a proximal subclavian artery lesion, reversal of retrograde to antegrade flow in the vertebral artery does not occur for at least 20 sec after reestablishment of normal antegrade flow in the subclavian artery.[54] Therefore, if any embolization occurred during the PTA procedure, at least initially, the emboli would probably travel to the arm. Other investigators have confirmed an extremely low clinical incidence of complications involving the vertebral artery circulation, even when PTA of the subclavian artery involved the origin of the vertebral artery.[55] Although some angiographers attempt to maximize flow in the extremity ipsilateral to a subclavian artery lesion by using vasodilators so that an embolus would be more likely to flow down the arm, we do not believe that this maneuver is necessary.

When PTA is performed on the innominate or left common carotid artery origin, the anterior circulation to the brain is placed at risk. Although the literature reflects that neurologic complications in this setting are very rare, when they do occur, they can be catastrophic.[56]

ARTERIAL STENTS

Although the long-term success associated with PTA of the brachiocephalic arteries is high, metal stents hold promise for improving the outcome in technical and early clinical failures and in the treatment of complete arterial occlusions.[40] Data related to the use of stents in the brachiocephalic arteries are currently limited. Mathias has recently presented his experience with the Wallstent (Schneider USA, Inc., Minneapolis, MN) in 23 patients.[57] In this series, stents were only placed following a suboptimal result with PTA. Stent placement was successful in 22 of 23 (96%) cases, and all have remained patent at 22 months of follow-up.

It is reasonable to expect that the experience with stents in the brachiocephalic arteries will be comparable to that in the iliac arteries, since the brachiocephalic and iliac arteries are both large vessels with high flow.[58] Indeed, there is a group that advocates primary stenting for subclavian artery stenosis.[42] In contrast to these authors, we reserve the use of stents for cases in which we have had a suboptimal PTA result ($\geq$ 30% residual stenosis, residual gradient $\geq$ 5–10 mm Hg, or flow-obstructing intimal flap) (Figure 7.10). We have also found it to be very difficult to predict which brachiocephalic stenoses will be responsive to PTA alone (Figure 7.11) and which will require the supplemental use of a stent (Figure 7.12). Stents are not approved by the FDA for use in the brachiocephalic vessels. They are also expensive. Moreover, data about long-term patency rates with the use of stents in this vascular bed are lacking. Therefore, we do not recommend primary stenting of brachiocephalic stenoses, although we suspect that stents will assume a more prominent role in the treatment of lesions that respond poorly to PTA.

We have placed stents in the left subclavian artery in four patients. In each case, elastic recoil or a dissection flap resulted in a suboptimal PTA. Placement of the stent resulted in immediate improvement and reduction of the gradient across the lesion to less than 5 mm Hg. No long-term anticoagulation was needed although our patients have been maintained on antiplatelet agents.

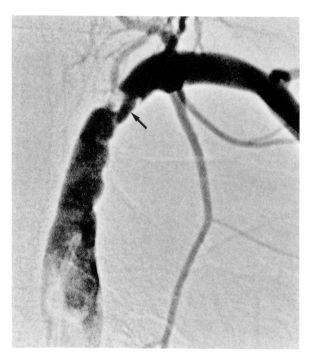

A

Figure 7.10 A 60-yr-old man with painful, ischemic, blue digits of the left hand presents for evaluation. **A.** Selective left subclavian arteriogram reveals an asymmetric plaque of the left subclavian artery (arrow) in close proximity to the left vertebral artery, but proximal to the LIMA. **B** and **C.** Following page.

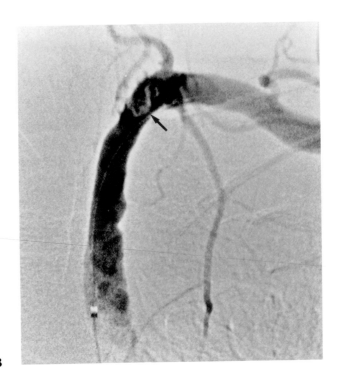

B

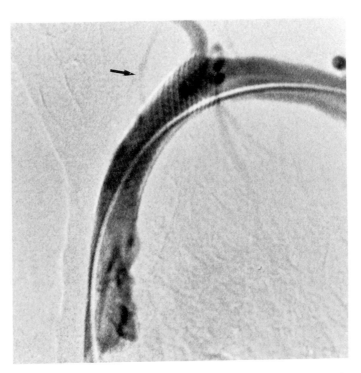

C

Figure 7.10 B. Following dilatation with an 8-mm balloon, residual narrowing of the vessel by the asymmetric plaque is still identified (arrow). C. Following deployment of a Wallstent 8 mm in diameter and 20 mm in length, the appearance of the left subclavian artery is markedly improved. There is still some antegrade flow through the diminutive left vertebral artery (arrow). Of note, the right vertebral artery was the dominant vertebral vessel. The patient had resolution of his symptoms.

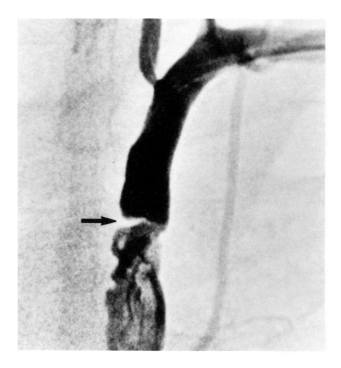

A

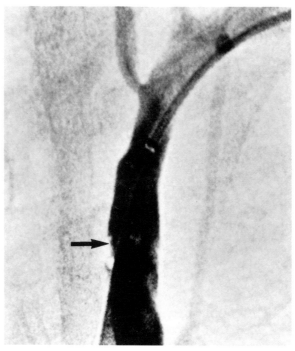

B

Figure 7.11 A 67-yr-old man with a prior left axillobifemoral bypass graft presented with the acute onset of left lower extremity numbness and right lower extremity claudication. **A.** A selective left subclavian arteriogram shows an asymmetric, irregular stenosis involving the proximal left subclavian artery (arrow). The gradient across the lesion measured 40 mm Hg. The left axillobifemoral bypass graft was also occluded. **B.** Following balloon dilatation of the left subclavian artery stenosis from a left high brachial artery approach, the pressure gradient was eliminated. The control arteriogram demonstrates an excellent result (arrow). The axillobifemoral bypass graft was subsequently thrombolysed and underlying lesions of the distal graft anastomosis on the left and the native right superficial femoral artery were balloon dilated. The patient was discharged with resolution of his symptoms and palpable pedal pulses.

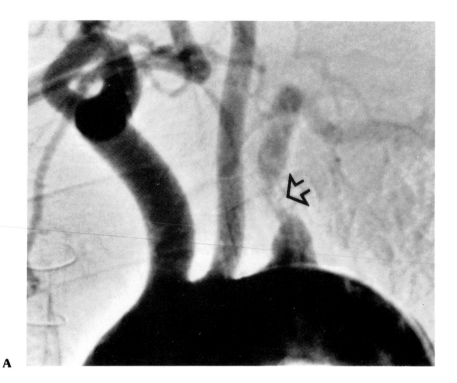

A

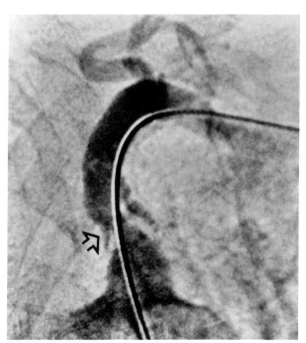

B

Figure 7.12 A 69-yr-old woman with a prior history of a myocardial infarction and LIMA bypass graft to the left anterior descending coronary artery presented with unstable angina and a blood pressure in the left arm 60 mm Hg less than in the right arm. A. An RPO arch aortogram demonstrates a symmetric stenosis involving the left subclavian artery (open arrow). B. Following dilatation with balloons 7 and 8 mm in diameter, there was a dissection flap (open arrow) and a residual 12 mm Hg gradient. C. Following page.

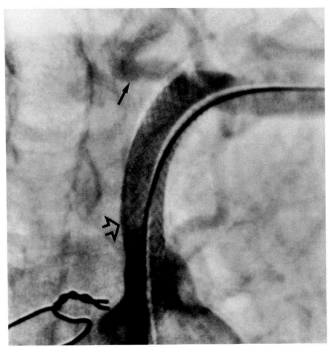

C

Figure 7.12 C. A Wallstent 8 mm in diameter and 20 mm in length was deployed, but did not cover the lesion completely. A second similar-sized Wallstent was placed across the lesion (open arrow) and the trans-stenotic gradient was eliminated. Although one of the stents covers the origin of the vertebral artery, antegrade flow in the vertebral artery (closed arrow) is seen. Following the procedure, this patient's angina resolved.

INFLOW TO INTERNAL MAMMARY GRAFTS

Patients who have undergone or will undergo coronary artery bypass grafting using the LIMA will need treatment if a left subclavian artery stenosis is present or develops after the bypass surgery. Since 1991, there have been a number of case reports detailing the success of PTA in this clinical situation.[24–29] More recently, a small series of eight patients with left subclavian artery stenosis and either a LIMA to coronary bypass graft (n = 4) or plans for a LIMA graft (n = 4) were successfully treated with subclavian artery PTA.[23] All four patients who developed coronary ischemia after a LIMA graft have remained asymptomatic following the subclavian PTA for a mean follow-up period of 31 months. Three of the four patients treated with subclavian PTA prior to the LIMA graft have remained free of angina for a mean period of 14 months. We have successfully dilated or stented eight subclavian arteries to improve inflow to an existing LIMA graft or in preparation for coronary bypass surgery (Figures 7.6, 7,7, and 7.12).

Directional atherectomy has been successfully used for treatment of subclavian artery stenoses in three patients with coronary–subclavian steal syndrome.[59] One of these three patients had recurrence of the subclavian lesion at 9 months and underwent repeat atherectomy. Although atherectomy can be used for treatment of a proximal subclavian stenosis, it does not appear to offer any advantage over balloon angioplasty.

DISCUSSION

Although PTA has been demonstrated to be a safe and effective method for treating occlusive vascular disease of the brachiocephalic arteries, the indications for intervention must be considered carefully. When stenotic lesions are identified angiographically, they should be correlated with the patient's clinical symptoms.[21] It has been well established that an isolated subclavian artery stenosis, even in the presence of vertebral artery "steal," is well tolerated and rarely progressive to stroke.[19,20,22] Indeed, in one study, spontaneous remission of blurred vision and vertigo occurred in 50% of patients who had proximal subclavian artery disease and subclavian steal syndrome.[60] However, when intervention is indicated, PTA should be considered as a first line of therapy.

Although the complication rate is low with brachiocephalic artery PTA, the potentially serious nature of complication should limit this procedure to well-trained, experienced angiographers who have access to good angiographic equipment. If meticulous attention is paid to patient selection, procedural technique, and follow-up, not only will the results be gratifying, but also endovascular interventions in this vascular bed will become better recognized as a minimally invasive therapeutic alternative.

REFERENCES

1. Dotter CT, Judkins MP: Transluminal treatment of arteriosclerotic obstruction: description of a new technique and preliminary report of its application. *Circulation* 30:654–670, 1964.
2. Bachman DM, Kim RM: Transluminal dilatation for subclavian steal syndrome. *Am J Roentgenol* 135:983–988, 1980.
3. Selby JB, Matsumoto AH, Tegtmeyer CJ, et al: Balloon angioplasty above the aortic arch: immediate and long-term results. *Am J Roentgenol* 160:631–635, 1993.
4. Kachel R, St Basche, Heerklotz I, et al: Percutaneous transluminal angioplasty (PTA) of supra-aortic arteries: especially the internal carotid artery. *Neuroradiology* 33:191–194, 1991.
5. Hebrang A, Maskovic J, Tomac B: Percutaneous transluminal angioplasty of the subclavian arteries: long-term results in 52 patients. *Am J Roentgenol* 156:1091–1094, 1991.
6. Kieffer E, Bahnini A, Koskas F: Aberrant subclavian artery: surgical treatment in thirty-three adult patients. *J Vasc Surg* 19:100–111, 1994.
7. Park J, Han M, Kim S, et al: Takayasu arteritis: angiographic findings and results of angioplasty. *Am J Roentgenol* 153:1069–1074, 1989.
8. Staller BJ, Maleki M: Percutaneous transluminal angioplasty for innominate artery stenosis and total occlusion of subclavian artery in Takaysu's-type arteritis. *Cathet Cardiovasc Diagn* 16:91–94, 1989.
9. Tanimoto A, Hiramatsu K: Percutaneous transluminal angioplasty for Takayasu's arteritis. *Semin Intervent Radiol* 10:1–7, 1993.
10. Joseph S, Mandalam KR, Rao VR, et al: Percutaneous transluminal angioplasty of the subclavian artery in nonspecific aortoarteritis: results of long-term follow-up. *J Vasc Interv Radiol* 5:573–580, 1994.
11. Weaver FA, Yellin AE, Campen DH, et al: Surgical procedures in the management of Takayasu's arteritis. *J Vasc Surg* 12:429–439, 1990.
12. Staab GE, Tegtmeyer CJ, Constable WC: Radiation-induced renovascular hypertension. *Am J Roentgenol* 126:634–637, 1976.
13. Kretschmer G, Niederle B, Polterauer P, et al: Irradiation-induced changes in the subclavian and axillary arteries after radiotherapy for carcinoma of the breast. *Surgery* 99:658–663, 1986.
14. Johnson AG, Lane B, Harding-Rains AJ, et al: Large artery damage after x-radiation. *Br J Radiol* 42:937–939, 1969.
15. McBride KD, Beard JD, Gaines PA: Percutaneous intervention for radiation damage to axillary arteries. *Clin Radiol* 49:630–633, 1994.
16. Guthaner DF, Schmitz L: Percutaneous transluminal angioplasty of radiation-induced arterial stenosis. *Radiology* 144:77–78, 1982.

17. Phadke RV, Taori KB, Divek VK, et al: Fibromuscular dysplasia of common carotid artery: a case report. *Austr Radiol* 34:350–352, 1990.

18. Heiserman JE, Drayer BP, Fram EK, et al: MR angiography of cervical fibromuscular dysplasia. *AJNR* 13:1454–1457, 1992.

19. Bornstein NM, Norris JW: Subclavian steal: a harmless hemodynamic phenomenon? *Lancet* 2:303–305, 1986.

20. Hennerici M, Klemm C, Routenberg W: The subclavian steal phenomenon: a common vascular disorder with rare neurologic deficits. *Neurology* 38:669–673, 1988.

21. Ueda K, Toole JF, McHenry LC Jr: Carotid and vertebrobasilar transient ischemic attacks: clinical and angiographic correlation. *Neurology* 29:1094–1101, 1979.

22. Fields WS, Lemak NA: Joint study of extracranial arterial occlusion. *JAMA* 222:1139–1143, 1972.

23. Hallisey MJ, Rees JH, Meranze SG, et al: Use of angioplasty in the prevention and treatment of coronary subclavian steal syndrome. *J Vasc Interv Radiol* 6:125–129, 1995.

24. Levitt RG, Wholey MH, Jamolowski CR: Subclavian artery angioplasty for treatment of coronary artery steal syndrome. *J Vasc Interv Radiol* 3:73–76, 1992.

25. Soulen MC, Sullivan KL: Subclavian artery angioplasty proximal to a left internal mammary-coronary artery bypass graft: case report. *Cardiovasc Intervent Radiol* 14:355–357, 1991.

26. Belz M, Marshall JJ, Cowley MJ: Subclavian balloon angioplasty in the management of coronary-subclavian steal syndrome. *Cathet Cardiovasc Diagn* 25:161–163, 1992.

27. Georges NP, Ferretti JA: Percutaneous transluminal angioplasty of subclavian artery occlusion for treatment of coronary-subclavian steal. *Am J Roentgenol* 161:399–400, 1993.

28. Laub GW, Muralidharan S, Naidech H, et al: Percutaneous transluminal subclavian angioplasty in a patient with postoperative angina. *Ann Thorac Surg* 52:850–851, 1991.

29. Levitt RG, Wholey MH, Jamolowski CR: Subclavian artery angioplasty for treatment of coronary artery steal syndrome. *J Vasc Interv Radiol* 3:73–76, 1992.

30. Siegal W, Loop FD: Comparison of internal mammary artery and saphenous vein bypass grafts for myocardial revascularization circulation. *Circulation* 3(Suppl 34):1–3, 1976.

31. Dorros G, Lewin RF, Jamnadas P, et al: Peripheral transluminal angioplasty of the subclavian and innominate arteries utilizing the brachial approach: acute outcome and follow-up. *Cathet Cardiovasc Diagn* 19:71–76, 1990.

32. Motarjeme A, Keifer JW, Zuska AJ, et al: Percutaneous transluminal angioplasty for treatment of subclavian steal. *Radiology* 155:611–613, 1985.

33. Vitek JJ, Keller FS, Duvall ER, et al: Brachiocephalic artery dilation by percutaneous transluminal angioplasty. *Radiology* 158:779–785, 1986.

34. Burke DR, Gordon RL, Mishkin JD, et al: Percutaneous transluminal angioplasty of subclavian arteries. *Radiology* 164:699–704, 1987.

35. Insall RL, Lambert D, Chamberlain J, et al: Percutaneous transluminal angioplasty of the innominate, subclavian, and axillary arteries. *Eur J Vasc Surg* 4:591–595, 1990.

36. Romanowski CAJ, Fairlie NC, Procter AE, et al: Percutaneous transluminal angioplasty of the subclavian and axillary arteries: initial results and long term follow-up. *Clin Radiol* 46:104–107, 1992.

37. Erbstein RA, Wholey MA, Smoot S: Subclavian artery steal syndrome: treatment by percutaneous transluminal angioplasty. *Am J Roentgenol* 151:291–294, 1988.

38. Millaire A, Trinca M, Marache P, et al: Subclavian angioplasty: immediate and late results in 50 patients. *Cathet Cardiovasc Diagn* 29:8–17, 1993.

39. Wilms G, Baert A, Dewaele D, et al: Percutaneous transluminal angioplasty of the subclavian artery: early and late results. *Cardiovasc Intervent Radiol* 10:123–128, 1987.

40. Mathias KD, Luth I, Haarmann P: Percutaneous transluminal angioplasty of proximal subclavian artery occlusions. *Cardiovasc Intervent Radiol* 16:214–218, 1993.

41. Duber C, Klose KJ, Kopp H, et al: Percutaneous transluminal angioplasty for occlusion of the subclavian artery: short- and long-term results. *Cardiovasc Intervent Radiol* 15:205–210, 1992.

42. Bates MC, Dorros G, Kumar K, et al: Primary Palmaz stent implantation in patients with subclavian artery stenosis (abstract). *Cardiovasc Intervent Radiol* 16:56, 1993.

43. Tegtmeyer CJ, Hartwell GD, Selby JB, et al: Results and complications of angioplasty in aortoiliac disease. *Circulation* 83(Suppl I):I-53–I-60, 1991.

44. Vogt DP, Mertzer NR, O'Hara, et al: Brachiocephalic arterial reconstruction. *Ann Surg* 196:541–542, 1982.

45. Shumaker HB Jr, Isch JH, Jolly WW, et al: The management of stenotic and obstructive lesions of the aortic arch branches. *Am J Surg* 133:351–360, 1977.

46. Sandmann W, Kniemeyer HW, Jaeschock R, et al: The role of subclavian-carotid transposition in surgery for supra-aortic occlusive disease. *Vasc Surg* 5:53–58, 1987.

47. Fry WR, Martin JD, Clagett GP, et al: Extrathoracic carotid reconstruction: the subclavian-carotid artery bypass. *J Vasc Surg* 18:83–89, 1992.

48. Cherry KJ Jr: Carotid-subclavian bypass and other extra-anatomic revascularizations for proximal subclavian artery stenosis causing cerebral steal syndrome. In Ernst CB, Stanley JC (eds): *Current Therapy in Vascular Surgery*, ed 2. St Louis, MO, Mosby Year Book Inc, 1991, pp 125–128.

49. Zelenock GB, Podrazik RM: Surgical treatment of innominate artery atherosclerosis. In Ernst CB, Stanley JC (eds): *Current Therapy in Vascular Surgery*, ed 2. St Louis, MO, Mosby Year Book Inc, 1991, pp 128–133.

50. Williams SJ: Chronic upper extremity ischemia: current concepts in management. *Surg Clin North Am* 66:355–375, 1986.

51. Owens LV, Tinsley EA Jr, Criado E, et al: Extrathoracic reconstruction of arterial occlusive disease involving the supraaortic trunks. *J Vasc Surg* 22:217–222, 1995.

52. Musser DJ, Nicholas GG, Reed JF: Death and adverse cardiac events after carotid endarterectomy. *J Vasc Surg* 19:615–627, 1994.

53. Farina C, Mingoli A, Schultz RD, et al: Percutaneous transluminal angioplasty versus surgery for subclavian artery occlusive disease. *Am J Surg* 158:511–514, 1989.

54. Ringelstein B, Zeumer H: Delayed reversal of vertebral artery blood flow following percutaneous transluminal angioplasty for subclavian steal syndrome. *Neuroradiology* 26:189–198, 1984.

55. Vitek JJ: Subclavian artery angioplasty and the origin of the vertebral artery. *Radiology* 170:407–409, 1989.

56. Kachel R, Endert G, Basche S, et al: Percutaneous tarnsluminal angioplasty (dilatation) of carotid, vertebral, and innominate artery stenoses. *Cardiovasc Intervent Radiol* 10:142–146, 1987.

57. Mathias K: Stents in supraaortic vessels (abstract). *Cardiovasc Intervent Radiol* 17:64, 1994.

58. Bonn J, Gardiner GA, Shapiro MJ, et al: Palmaz vascular stent: initial clinical experience. *Radiology* 174:741–745, 1990.

59. Breall JA, Groossman W, Stillman IE, et al: Atherectomy of the subclavian artery for patients with symptomatic coronary-subclavian steal. *J Am Coll Cardiol* 21:1564–1567, 1993.

60. Ackerman H, Diener HC, Sebolt H, et al: Ultrasonographic follow up of subclavian stenosis and occlusion: natural history and surgical treatment. *Stroke* 19:431–435, 1988.

CHAPTER
8

Endovascular Reconstruction of the Superior Vena Cava and Subclavian Veins

Charles P. Semba
Michael D. Dake

Conventional therapy for patients with symptomatic venous occlusion of the axillary, subclavian, or innominate vein or superior vena cava (SVC) consists of long-term anticoagulation.[1,2] However, anticoagulation alone is rarely successful in restoring patency to the obstructed vein, so relief of symptoms is usually dependent upon the development of collateral venous pathways. Often patients have upper extremity pain and edema due to obstructive venous hypertension that persists despite therapeutic anticoagulation.[3,4] With refinement in endovascular techniques, restoring venous patency and resolution of venous congestion can be achieved by using three techniques: catheter-directed thrombolysis, balloon angioplasty, and endoluminal stenting. The purpose of this chapter is to provide an overview of the endovascular management of stenoses and occlusions of the central veins of the upper thorax.

ETIOLOGIES

Subclavian Vein Thrombosis

Deep venous thrombosis (DVT) of the upper extremity central veins accounts for approximately 7% to 10% of all DVT.[5] Subclavian vein thrombosis usually presents with progressive unilateral upper extremity pain and swelling. The entire forearm and hand may become swollen. The limb may appear slightly cyanotic, and numerous small prominent superficial shoulder and upper anterior chest wall veins may become apparent due to venous congestion and the distention of collateral veins. The diagnosis of DVT can usually be confirmed with a Doppler evaluation of the subclavian and axillary veins. However, isolated DVT central to the jugular vein and underneath the clavicle and sternum may be missed with an ultrasound examination. If ultrasound is inconclusive, then upper extremity venography may be necessary to confirm the presence or absence of DVT. The venographic features of subclavian vein thrombosis are straightforward: occlusion of the subclavian vein with the presence of numerous collateral veins and occasionally, an intraluminal filling defect (Figure 8.1). The SVC may be reconstituted via collateral venous pathways, such as the jugulovenous arch and the intercostal and lateral thoracic veins. The azygos and hemizygous veins may be seen, especially if the innominate veins or SVC are occluded (Figure 8.2).

Subclavian vein thrombosis can be categorized as primary or secondary (Table 8.1).

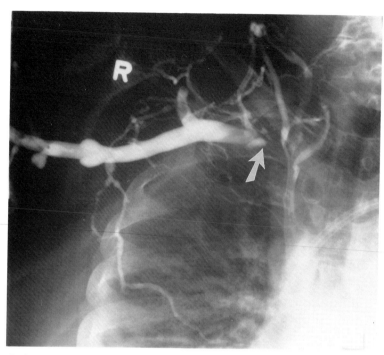

Figure 8.1 Subclavian vein thrombosis. Upper extremity venogram shows occlusion of the right subclavian vein (arrow) and development of supraclavicular and anterior chest wall venous collaterals.

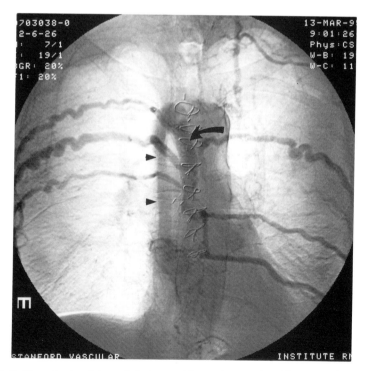

Figure 8.2 Thrombosis of the subclavian and innominate veins. Numerous intercostal veins provide collateral drainage into the azygos vein (arrow) which subsequently drains into the SVC (arrowheads).

TABLE 8.1 Subclavian Vein Thrombosis—Etiologies

Primary
    Effort vein thrombosis (Paget-Schroetter syndrome)
Secondary
    Benign
        Central venous catheter
        Dialysis fistula–related stenosis
        Pacemaker leads
        Radiation fibrosis
        Hypercoagulable state
    Malignant
        Primary mediastinal tumors
        Pancoast tumor with invasion
        Breast cancer with local invasion
        Metastatic disease

Primary Subclavian Vein Thrombosis

Primary thrombosis of the subclavian vein occurs when there is mechanical impingement on the vein at the thoracic inlet. This "nutcracker" phenomenon is also known as *primary axillosubclavian vein thrombosis, effort vein thrombosis,* or *Paget-Schroetter syndrome.*[6] As the subclavian vein enters the thorax, it is bordered by the clavicle superiorly, the first rib inferiorly, the scalenus anticus tendon posteriorly, and the subclavius tendon anteriorly. With certain types of repetitive arm motion, such as abduction of the arm and shoulder, the subclavian vein becomes intermittently compressed between the scalenus tendon and first rib. Intimal injury to the vein wall and subsequent DVT occurs with the repetitive compressive trauma. Other skeletal anomalies such as a cervical rib, an exostosis for the first rib at the site of insertion of the scalenus tendon, or callous formation at the thoracic inlet from a clavicular fracture can lead to impingement of the subclavian vein.[7]

The diagnosis of effort vein thrombosis should be suspected when unilateral arm edema and pain develop over a period of days to weeks in a young, active, and otherwise healthy individual. Effort vein thrombosis more commonly occurs in men and usually involves the dominant upper extremity. Usually there is no associated neurologic or arterial deficit. Occupational or recreational activity that involves repetitive arm abduction, as in auto mechanics, window washers, weight lifters, and swimmers, may increase the risk of effort vein thrombosis.

Venography is required to confirm the diagnosis and to determine the extent of thrombosis. When performing the venogram, it is preferable to inject the ipsilateral basilic vein, because it is in direct continuity with the axillary vein. Injecting the cephalic vein may miss a large clot in the brachial or axillary vein. The venogram is performed with the affected arm in neutral position at the patient's side and repeated with the arm abducted 90° and the head turned to the contralateral side (modified Adson's maneuver) (Figure 8.3). The abnormal venous narrowing is classically detected in the segment of the subclavian vein between the clavicle and anterior portion of the first rib. The appearance of the lesion can range from a focal web to a localized filling defect caused by exuberant intimal hyperplasia from the repetitive trauma to an acute clot that obscures the underlying venous abnormality (Figure 8.4).

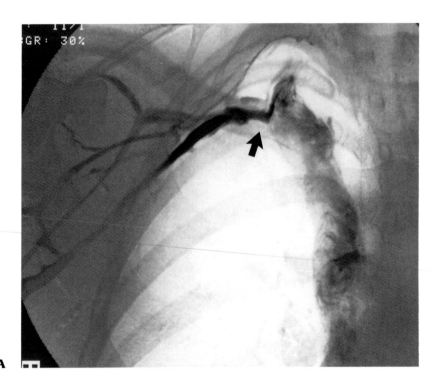

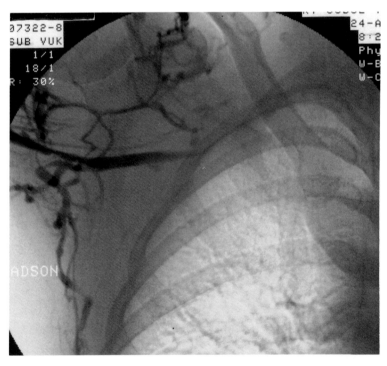

Figure 8.3 Impingement on the right subclavian vein. A. With the arm in the neutral position, a stenosis is noted at thoracic inlet (arrow). B. Modified Adson's maneuver leads to occlusion of the subclavian vein. Repetitive injury to the vein can lead to thrombosis.

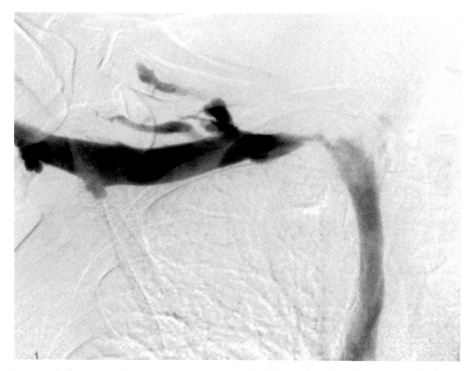

Figure 8.4 Paget-Schroetter syndrome. Stenosis of the right subclavian vein at the thoracic inlet was found to be secondary to intimal hyperplasia at the time of surgical resection of the first rib.

Secondary Subclavian Vein Thrombosis

Direct puncture of the subclavian vein for placement of central venous access catheters is the most common predisposing factor for the development of secondary subclavian vein thrombosis.[8] Patients typically present with the acute onset of unilateral arm edema on the same side as the catheterized subclavian vein. There are three general situations in which catheter-related DVT occurs: (1) thrombosis of a normal subclavian vein due to the acute venous injury caused by the thrombogenicity of the inserted catheter, (2) thrombosis of a small diameter vein due to near occlusion of the catheter, and (3) the development of thrombosis due to endothelial trauma caused by the catheterization process several weeks to months after the central line has been removed (Figure 8.5).

Pacemaker leads can lead to subclavian vein and SVC occlusion.[9,10] Due to the smaller profile of pacer leads, the incidence of DVT is less than with central venous catheters. Endothelial injury caused by a temporary subclavian dialysis catheter and/or aggressive formation of intimal hyperplasia from chronic arterialization of the vein ipsilateral to a dialysis fistula can also result in subclavian vein stenosis or occlusion.[11,12]

Superior Vena Cava Syndrome

Occlusion of the associated central veins of the thorax and/or the SVC can produce a striking constellation of clinical findings referred to as the *SVC syndrome*. The classic SVC syndrome consists of facial, periorbital, neck, and bilateral upper extremity edema, dilated superficial veins over upper anterior and lateral chest wall, dysphagia, dyspnea, and cognitive dysfunction due to cerebral venous hypertension.[13,14] The quality of life for most of these patients is extremely poor due to impaired ability to use the arms, inability to lie flat due to increase in venous congestion, and the profound facial edema. In severe cases, the trachea can be obstructed.

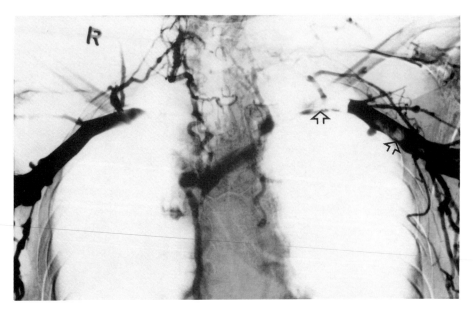

Figure 8.5 Central line–induced thrombosis of the subclavian vein. A bilateral upper extremity venogram reveals bilateral subclavian vein occlusions with acute intraluminal thrombus on the left (open arrows). This patient has had prior central venous lines.

Since SVC syndrome can be caused by benign or malignant etiologies (Table 8.2), any patient who presents with SVC syndrome should undergo a detailed history and physical examination, chest radiograph, and thoracic computed tomography (CT) scan to exclude a malignancy. Patients with newly detected Hodgkin's lymphoma or other radiosensitive tumors are initially treated with radiation and/or chemotherapy. In our experience, these patients usually do not require intervention in the acute setting since prompt oncologic therapy usually relieves the extrinsic compression on the SVC. Occasionally, patients with a *treated* mediastinal malignancy can present with SVC syndrome several months after therapy due to radiation-induced fibrosis of the central veins.

INDICATIONS FOR ENDOVASCULAR INTERVENTION

The primary indication for an endovascular intervention is to treat patients who have persistent incapacitating symptoms of upper extremity and/or head and neck edema and pain despite adequate anticoagulation. The symptoms are frequently incapacitating or associated with the full-blown SVC syndrome. The decision to exclude a patient from undergoing an endovascular intervention should be tailored to the intervention planned. For example, although a patient may have a contraindication for anticoagulation and/or fibrinolytic therapy, venography may reveal an isolated, critical SVC stenosis. Such a lesion could be treated with balloon angioplasty and/or stenting without the need for anticoagulation or fibrinolysis.

In dealing with patients with an underlying malignancy, the physician must weigh the quality-of-life issues versus the potential for a complication. The patient needs to be made aware that the endovascular intervention is merely palliative and has no effect on the malignancy. In the vast majority of patients with malignancies, the aim is to preserve the self-respect and dignity of the patient, while alleviating the pain and suffering. Although these patients may have a terminal condition, death is not imminent and most patients wish to live their remaining months to years in relative comfort. For benign disease or treated malignancies in remission, we are far more aggressive in initiating therapy.

TABLE 8.2 Etiology of SVC Obstruction—Etiologies

Benign
  Central venous catheters
  Pacemaker leads
  Dialysis fistula-related stenoses
  Radiation fibrosis
  Mediastinal fibrosis
  Histoplasmosis
Malignant
  Bronchogenic carcinoma
  Primary mediastinal tumors
  Lymphomas
  Thyroid carcinoma
  Metastatic disease

GENERAL INTERVENTIONAL STRATEGIES

Before planning any intervention, a detailed venogram must be performed to define the underlying anatomy and the amount of thrombus. The principal endovascular interventions used for upper extremity venous obstruction are catheter-directed thrombolysis, balloon angioplasty, and endoluminal stenting. The interventionalist should be familiar with and able to perform all of these techniques. The procedures are performed in the angiography suite using high-resolution image intensifies with digital subtraction capabilities.

Venography

Venography remains the gold standard for the diagnosis of upper extremity venous disease. It is not usually performed as part of the initial evaluation, but rather, in preparation for an endovascular intervention. The patient is placed on the angiography table in a supine position. As previously mentioned, a venogram is performed via the *basilic* vein to evaluate the entire deep venous system of the upper extremity, including the innominate vein and SVC. For patients with SVC syndrome, bilateral upper extremity venography is necessary to fully evaluate the central venous system. This study usually reveals high-grade stenoses or occlusion of both innominate veins and/or the SVC (Figure 8.6). In patients with a patent dialysis fistula, the venogram can be performed by directly accessing the fistula.

In a patient with profound upper extremity edema, puncturing the basilic vein may be difficult. The vein may be several centimeters below the skin surface and impossible to detect with standard tourniquet techniques. One method to facilitate localization of the basilic vein is to find a small hand vein and perform venography with an upper arm tourniquet in place. Under direct fluoroscopic guidance, the contrast-filled basilic vein can be punctured. However, in patients with marked arm edema, the hands are often edematous, thus rendering access to a peripheral vein nearly impossible. Another method used to enter the basilic vein involves the use of ultrasound guidance with a 5- or 7-MHz transducer. Recently, a dedicated ultrasound device (Site Rite; Dymax Inc., Pittsburgh, PA) for venous access guidance has become available.[15] This device has a 9-MHz probe which is extremely helpful in locating a small, compressible, basilic vein medial to the brachial artery above the antecubital fossa. If the basilic vein is several centimeters below the skin surface, deeper access can be gained with a 21-G needle 5 cm in length, an 0.018-inch guidewire, and subsequently, a transition dilator (4-Fr or 5-Fr micropuncture set; Cook, Inc., Bloomington, IN).

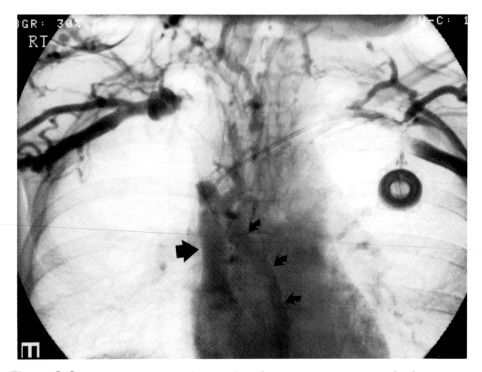

Figure 8.6 Superior vena cava syndrome. Bilateral upper extremity venography demonstrates bilateral subclavian and innominate vein thrombosis in a patient with a left subclavian port catheter. Collateral veins drain into the azygos vein (curved arrows) which subsequently empties into the SVC (large arrow).

Diagnostic venography is rarely performed from a femoral or jugular vein approach. In selected cases, the femoral and jugular veins are used as adjunctive access sites for entry into occluded central venous segments.

Catheterization of the Venous Obstruction

After the diagnostic venogram, the basilic vein access is converted to a vascular sheath (5 Fr or 6 Fr). A 5-Fr end-hole catheter with a simple curve or hockey-stick configuration and a 0.035-inch steerable hydrophilic guidewire (Glidewire; Terumo Corp, Tokyo, Japan) are used to traverse the stenotic or occluded venous segment. A stenosis is much easier to traverse than a complete venous occlusion.

For organized, fibrotic occlusions that are woody and firm to tactile sensation, a coaxial system of catheters is often required to provide extra stiffness. A 7- or 8-Fr braided guiding catheter can be fitted with a Touhy-Borst sidearm adapter to allow coaxial placement of a 5-Fr end-hole catheter and guidewire. The guiding catheter provides greater stability and reduces the amount of catheter buckling that occurs when attempting to traverse a firm occlusion. When there is SVC occlusion with extension of thrombus into both brachiocephalic (innominate) veins, both subclavian veins must be individually catheterized and navigated. Both catheters are advanced through the SVC obstruction into the right atrium. For access into a chronic, fibrotic occlusion of the SVC, the right femoral or right internal jugular approach may be necessary to gain a better mechanical advantage for lesion traversal.

After an occluded venous segment is traversed, an intraluminal catheter position is documented. Thrombolytic therapy is instituted to soften or remove any acute thrombus and reveal any underlying anatomic abnormality. Whenever possible, the basilic vein access site is used to initiate catheter-directed thrombolysis because it is the simplest and most comfortable approach for the patient. Femoral catheterization requires strict bed rest and is often uncomfortable, especially if the infusion continues for two or more days.

Catheter-directed Venous Thrombolytic Therapy

Catheter-directed thrombolysis has three major advantages over systemic fibrinolytic therapy: (1) a high concentration of the drug is delivered directly to the thrombus and is thus more efficient; (2) lower overall doses of the fibrinolytic agent are required; and (3) direct access to the diseased segment of vein for additional adjunctive interventions such as angioplasty and stenting is provided. We prefer urokinase (Abbokinase; Abbott Laboratories, Abbott Park, IL) as the thrombolytic agent rather than streptokinase or tissue plasminogen activator because it is easy to use and permits a consistent response, reliability, and a large margin of safety.[16] Thrombolysis is contraindicated in patients with bleeding disorders, neoplastic involvement of the central nervous system, sepsis, or within 14 days of a major operative procedure or 1 yr of a hemorrhagic stroke.

There are two major infusion systems for thrombolysis: coaxial and multisidehole. Both systems work equally well. The specific infusion system used is a matter of personal preference. The coaxial system is the simpler of the two techniques. After the occlusion is crossed with a 0.038-inch ID, 5-Fr end-hole catheter, a specially designed 0.035-inch infusion guidewire is advanced coaxially through the catheter. These infusion wires are designed to drip urokinase through an end-hole (Sos wire; USCI, Billerica, MA or Cragg wire; Boston Scientific, Natick, MA) or along a designated portion of the distal wire (Katzen infusion wire; Boston Scientific). The infusion wire is inserted through the catheter and secured with a Touhy-Borst sidearm adapter. From the basilic vein approach, the 5-Fr catheter is pulled back over the wire so that its tip is positioned at the most peripheral edge of the thrombus and the infusion wire is located approximately two-thirds of the way into the thrombus. The urokinase is simultaneously infused through both the infusion wire and the end-hole of the 5-Fr catheter. Use of a 6-Fr sheath allows systemic heparin infusion around the indwelling 5-Fr catheter.

The multisidehole catheter systems consist of either a single-lumen multisidehole catheter (Mewissen catheter; Boston Scientific or Pulse Spray Catheter; AngioDynamics, Inc., Glen Falls, NY), or a multilumen multisidehole catheter (EDM catheter; Mallinckrodt, Inc., St. Louis, MO). The single-lumen, multisidehole catheter uses an occluding wire that prevents the infusate from leaking out of the end-hole and forces it to weep out the sideholes. The multilumen multisidehole catheter has two ports—one drips fluid out of the guidewire end-hole and the other port communicates with the other lumens and sideholes. An advantage of the multilumen catheter is its 4.7-Fr profile, which allows infusion of heparin through the sidearm of a 5-Fr sheath. The main disadvantage to the multilumen catheter is that it only has a 0.018-inch central lumen. With tough, elastic occlusions, an 0.018-inch guidewire occasionally does not provide enough stiffness to allow passage of the thrombolysis catheter across the occluded segment.

Urokinase is available in 250,000 IU vials and must first be reconstituted with 5 cc of sterile water. The urokinase is then added to 250 cc of normal saline in a ratio of 500,000 IU urokinase/250 ml 0.9% NaCl (2,000 IU urokinase/ml). For each thrombolysis system, two bags of the urokinase solution are needed. For example, with the 5-Fr coaxial systems, one bag of urokinase is used for the end-infusion and the other for the infusion wire. As many as six infusion pumps may be needed in cases of bilateral subclavian vein thrombolysis. Four pumps would be used for the urokinase infusions and two would be used to infuse heparinized saline to maintain patency of the basilic vein sheaths.

For catheter-directed thrombolysis, total urokinase doses usually range from 100,000 to 200,000 IU/hr. Since there are two urokinase infusions for each access site, the total urokinase dose is split between the infusion sites; for example, 50,000 IU/hr through the end-hole catheter and 50,000 IU/hr through the thrombolysis wire (total dose = 100,000 IU/hr). For bilateral subclavian vein coaxial infusions, the total dose needs to be split among the four urokinase lines: 50,000 IU/hr in each end-hole catheter and 50,000 IU/hr in each infusion wire (for a total of 200,000 IU/hr). The maximum recommended total dose of urokinase is 4,400 IU/kg/hr. In patients who are susceptible to fluid overload (e.g., dialysis or congestive heart failure patients), the concentration of urokinase can be doubled in the mixes (4,000 IU/ml) to reduce the total volume of fluid infused per hour. We do not usually lace, pulse-spray, or bolus dose the occluded venous segment with urokinase at the start of the thrombolysis procedure. The patients are given 5,000 units of heparin intravenously (IV) and started on a heparin infusion at 1,000 units/hr at the same time the urokinase infusions are initiated.

The skin entrance sites of the thrombolysis catheters are covered with cotton gauze and secured to the skin with a clear adhesive dressing. The sheaths are sutured to the skin. We do not routinely use intensive care unit monitoring for patients undergoing venous thrombolysis. The patients are sent to a floor where the nursing staff is experienced in managing intravascular sheaths and thrombolytic regimens and familiar with access site complications. If this type of nursing care is unavailable, it will be necessary to monitor the patient in an ICU environment.

During urokinase infusion, the partial thromboplastin time (PTT) and fibrinogen levels are checked every 4 to 8 hr. The PTT is maintained between 60 and 90 sec by titrating the heparin infusion. A fibrinogen level below 100 mg percent indicates a systemic fibrinolytic state and increases the risk of hemorrhagic complications. In our experience, the urokinase infusion regimens described above rarely lower fibrinogen levels below 150 mg percent. Furthermore, since systemic heparin can directly interfere with the assay for fibrinogen, the fibrinogen levels obtained during systemic heparinization may be unreliable.

Following overnight infusion with urokinase, the patient is returned to the angiography suite for repeat venography. At best, there will be complete lysis of the occlusion without any underlying stricture; however, this is most unusual. More often, there is an underlying lesion (extrinsic compression or chronic organized material) which, in the absence of further intervention, will serve as a nidus for recurrent thrombosis. Therefore, angioplasty and stenting are frequently required to maintain the patency of the vessel lumen. If the venogram shows partial but incomplete clot lysis, the urokinase infusion is continued for as long as 72 hr.

Following successful thrombolysis, all patients are given 325 mg of aspirin a day and systemically anticoagulated with warfarin for at least 6 months. To minimize the length of hospital stay, 10 mg of warfarin is administered during the first 2 days of the thrombolysis procedure and then titrated with 1 to 10 mg dose daily, until steady-state levels are achieved. The target international normalized ratio (INR) is between 2.0 and 3.0.

Complications during urokinase infusion include access site hematoma or infection, idiosyncratic reactions to urokinase, heparin-induced thrombocytopenia, bleeding, and catheter dislodgment. The risk of clinically significant pulmonary emboli is extremely rare. Idiosyncratic reactions to urokinase consist of shaking chills and tachycardia, usually without associated hypotension. This reaction may be falsely interpreted as an anaphylactic reaction, seizure activity, or even a cardiac arrest. It is presumably caused by a natural by-product of the urokinase purification and isolation process. The reaction is usually self-limited, or it can be treated with 50 mg of meperidine (Demerol) and 50 mg of diphenylhydramine (Benadryl) intravenously. The use of H_2 blockers and steroids is controversial.[17] The reaction usually lasts 5 to 10 min. Interestingly, in most situations the patient can continue to receive the urokinase without subsequent reaction.[18] In our practice, this idiosyncratic reaction is more commonly associated with urokinase boluses than with continuous infusions.

Venous Angioplasty and Stenting

The primary role of balloon angioplasty (percutaneous transluminal angioplasty [PTA]) is to create a larger vessel lumen prior to stent placement. Yet, PTA alone can be effective in veins with benign, short focal stenoses. High-pressure balloons (Blue Max or Olbert Balloon; Boston Scientific) that can produce dilatation pressures of 12 to 20 atm are often needed. Unfortunately, PTA as a stand-alone procedure is often ineffective in diseased veins because of venous recoil or extrinsic compression on the vein. Therefore, a stent may be necessary.

There are three metallic stents that have been used for endoluminal venous reconstruction: (1) the rigid, balloon-expandable, stainless steel Palmaz stent (Johnson and Johnson Interventional Systems, Inc., Warren, NJ); (2) the longitudinally flexible, self-expanding, stainless steel Wallstent (Schneider, Inc., Minneapolis, MN); and (3) the rigid, self-expanding Gianturco-Rösch Z-stent (Cook, Inc.). None of these stents is perfect and all have their individual advantages and disadvantages. In addition, none of these stents is currently approved by the FDA for use in central thoracic veins. Therefore, appropriate consent and approval by the institutional review board should be obtained.

The Palmaz stent is a rigid, stainless steel cylinder which is mounted on an angioplasty balloon and deployed by balloon expansion. One important advantage of this stent is its outstanding hoopstrength. A second advantage is the ability to precisely place this stent because it does not significantly shorten with expansion. A second advantage is the ability to precisely place this stent because it does not significantly shorten with expansion. It is currently available in 10 to 40 mm lengths. The Palmaz 308 stent is probably our favorite stent for reconstructing the SVC due to its exceptional hoopstrength and its ability to create a luminal diameter as large as 16 mm. The stent is usually deployed into the SVC from a right femoral vein approach with a long 9- or 10-Fr sheath. One disadvantage of this stent is that it can be permanently deformed it if is situated between two points of compression. Therefore, the Palmaz should not be placed in the subclavian vein at the thoracic inlet.[19]

The Wallstent is a longitudinally flexible stent, which makes it easier to advance through the curved innominate and subclavian veins. It is available in 20 to 90 mm lengths and 5 to 24 mm diameters. While it has less hoopstrength than the Palmaz stent, it is useful for treating long stenoses or steeply curved portions of vein. Its relatively low profile (7 Fr to 8 Fr) makes insertion from a basilic vein approach feasible. One of the disadvantages of the Wallstent is that it foreshortens with expansion; thus, it is more difficult to precisely position the proximal and distal portions of the stent.

The Z-stent is self-expanding, possesses excellent hoopstrength, and is available in very large diameters (up to 35 mm).[20] The constrained stent is pushed from a delivery sleeve into the delivery catheter and then advanced to the target area with a Teflon pusher rod. It is deployed by fixing the pusher rod and retracting the delivery catheter to unsheath the stent.

The choice of stent is largely a matter of preference, but there are anatomic considerations that should be recognized. In general, stents should not be placed in the basilic, cephalic, and axillary veins due to the low short-term patency rates in these vessels.[21] The drawback of venous stenting is restenosis due to intimal hyperplasia or tumor ingrowth. Unfortunately, no stent has overcome either of these problems. In the subclavian and innominate veins and the SVC, the decision to place a stent depends on whether the etiology is benign or malignant and whether there is short or long segment disease. Long segment venous disease responds poorly to PTA alone, and often requires the adjunctive use of a stent. For malignant venous occlusions, we have found that stenting is extremely useful because there is usually a significant component of extrinsic venous compression. Because patients with malignant venous obstruction typically have a short life expectancy, long-term patency rates are not a decisive factor. By treating the central venous obstruction and relieving the venous hypertension, patients often receive rapid and dramatic resolution of their edema and pain and a significantly improved quality of life.

Complications associated with the use of stents include stent embolization during deployment, stent migration following deployment, or direct extrinsic damage to the stent in vivo from external compression. Stents can embolize or migrate into the right ventricle or pulmonary artery. While there are usually no immediate clinical sequelae, stents can become endothelialized in the heart or lung if they are not retrieved. The objective of stent retrieval is to capture the device and remove it or deploy it in a "safe harbor" site such as the external iliac vein.

Retrieving a Palmaz stent from the heart or pulmonary artery can be difficult due to the motion of the heart and vigorous pulsatile blood flow. Stent retrievals are best attempted by using a steerable catheter and guidewire. The guidewire is passed inside the long axis of the stent. An angioplasty balloon is advanced coaxially over the wire into the central lumen of the stent. The balloon is partially inflated to capture the Palmaz stent, which is then gently pulled into the inferior vena cava (IVC) and deployed in the iliac vein.

Because the Wallstent can be easily compressed if its ends are free-floating, it is possible to loop snare the Wallstent. Tightening the loop snare around the Wallstent will create an "hourglass" deformity. The Wallstent will then "fold over" on itself at the site of the loop snare once traction is placed on the stent. The doubled-over Wallstent can then be pulled into a 12-Fr sheath and removed.

Attempts to retrieve a longstanding, embolized stent may be impossible by percutaneous techniques since endothelialization occurs between the stent and the myocardium or vessel wall. The stent will not move freely even with the use of snares. In this situation, extraction can only be done through open heart surgery.

INTERVENTIONS FOR SPECIFIC ETIOLOGIES

Effort Vein Thrombosis (Paget-Schroetter Syndrome)

Machleder has proposed an algorithm for evaluation and treatment of effort vein thrombosis.[6,7] Following venography, the patient undergoes catheter-directed thrombolysis to clear out any occlusive thrombus, and repeat venography is performed to determine the extent of the underlying venous abnormality (Figure 8.7). If there is a relatively normal-appearing vein with good flow, the patient is given anticoagulants and followed clinically. In most cases, the underlying vein is stenotic. In this situation, surgical resection of the first rib is performed to relieve the mechanical compression. Angioplasty is not done initially since the venous stenosis is usually due to extrinsic compression by tendinous or bony structures. In Machleder's series, 50 patients with effort vein thrombosis were treated with thrombolysis, followed by anticoagulation for 3 months and subsequent transaxillary resection of the first rib. No stents were used. If follow-up venography showed a persistent subclavian vein stenosis, PTA was performed and resolution of symptoms occurred in 64% of patients over a 3-yr follow-up period.[7]

In spite of the algorithm outlined by Machleder, there is abundant anecdotal experience for balloon dilating an obstructing focal web in the subclavian vein uncovered following thrombolysis. The intermediate and long-term results appear to be good. In general, stenting should never be used as a first line of treatment in this entity and is only reserved for surgical failures. If the subclavian vein restenoses or occludes following first rib resection, and PTA is unsuccessful at reestablishing an adequate lumen, then a stent could be beneficial.

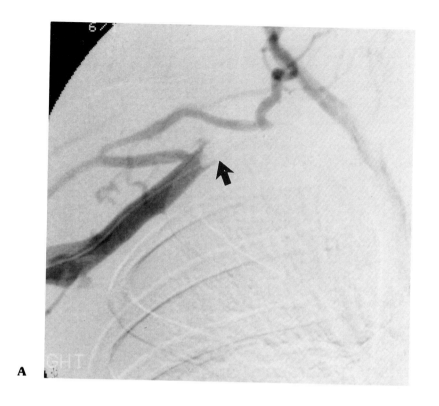

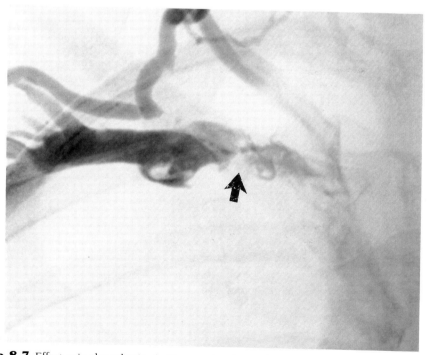

Figure 8.7 Effort vein thrombosis. **A.** Venography shows thrombosis of the right subclavian vein (arrow) at the thoracic inlet. **B.** Following overnight catheter-directed thrombolysis, venography reveals an irregular, stenotic vein (arrow) at the region of maximal impingement. The entrapment was treated with a supraclavicular first rib resection.

Central Venous Catheter-induced Thrombosis

Iatrogenic injury to the subclavian vein secondary to central venous lines is becoming a widely recognized and growing cause of upper extremity DVT. Horattas reviewed 19 clinical series on upper extremity DVT and found an incidence of 5% to 28%. Approximately 40% of these cases were associated with subclavian venous catheterization. In addition, clinically detectable pulmonary emboli occurred in 12% of patients with upper extremity DVT.[22] Therefore, central venous instrumentation is far from being a benign procedure and carries a significant long-term risk for venous thrombosis, even following removal of the indwelling line.

The initial treatment for patients who sustain an axillosubclavian DVT on the side ipsilateral to an indwelling catheter is usually based on a desire to preserve central venous access, while preventing further propagation of thrombus. In most cases, the need for long-term central venous access outweighs the immediate need for thrombolytic therapy. Therefore, in most cases, patients are initially treated with anticoagulation in order to preserve catheter function while allowing collateral venous pathways to open up and reduce the upper extremity venous hypertension.

If symptoms related to the venous thrombosis do not improve or worsen despite anticoagulation, catheter-directed thrombolysis is attempted. Unfortunately, our experience with catheter-directed thrombolysis has shown a high failure rate if the indwelling central line is not removed. This is presumably due to the presence of a large catheter in a relatively small subclavian vein, the development of intimal hyperplasia around the catheter, and/or the inherent thrombogenicity of the catheter itself. Therefore, if the central line is no longer needed, we generally advocate removal of the catheter followed by anticoagulation. If the patient's symptoms do not improve, a trial of urokinase therapy can be initiated.

Dialysis Fistula-related Occlusions

Development of venous outflow stenosis is a common problem for upper extremity dialysis fistulas. Kanterman et al. recently evaluated 215 patients with upper extremity dialysis fistulas who underwent diagnostic fistulography and venography.[23] While the overwhelming majority of fistula-related stenoses occur at or near the venous anastomosis, approximately 10% of the lesions occur in the subclavian vein or more centrally. The majority of these patients have had one or more temporary dialysis catheters placed in the subclavian vein, and catheter-related injury of the vein may predispose to stricture formation. Patients usually present with either progressive onset of unilateral arm edema or problems with dialysis such as high pressures or long recirculation times.

Most endovascular procedures related to dialysis fistulas are performed on an outpatient basis. After a butterfly needle or angiocatheter is placed directly into the fistula, contrast is injected to define the venous anatomy to the level of the right atrium. Balloon angioplasty is usually performed if there is a high-grade stenosis ($\geq 50\%$ diameter) of the subclavian or innominate vein or the SVC, with the presence of extensive supraclavicular and mediastinal venous collaterals. The angioplasty balloon should be sized to approximate the diameter of the native vein. If there is persistent elastic recoil of the vein following balloon deflation, repeat angioplasty is performed with a slightly larger balloon. If the patient experiences severe pain with balloon inflation or the balloon cannot be fully inflated, a larger balloon should not be used.

Stents are reserved for cases in which balloon angioplasty has failed. The type of stent chosen can be critical since a Palmaz stent can be permanently crushed if placed at the thoracic inlet. In general, following a failed response to aggressive balloon dilation, the Wallstent is our preferred stent due to its longitudinal flexibility and ability to recoil if compressed at the thoracic inlet. The diameter of the Wallstent should be as large as the native vein. In certain cases, the venous lesion can be so resistant to expansion that the Wallstent cannot create an adequate vessel lumen despite adjunctive PTA. This problem can usually be avoided by predilating the lesion with a balloon, but if complete balloon expansion cannot be achieved, it is unlikely that the stent will fully expand. If this situation is encountered, a second Wallstent can be placed inside the first to increase the radial force on the vein or a Palmaz stent can be deployed in the center of the Wallstent. Again, caution must be exercised since the Palmaz stent can be permanently deformed if compressed at the thoracic inlet.

If the vein is occluded, the decision whether or not to use a thrombolytic agent depends on the tactile sensation of the occlusion when probing with a guidewire. In our experience, occluded veins are extremely elastic, fibrotic, and difficult to dilate and rarely have a significant volume of acute thrombus. Therefore, we usually do not use thrombolysis, but proceed directly to PTA and stent placement.

There are only a few clinical reports on the long-term results of endovascular treatment of dialysis-related central venous lesions (Figure 8.8). Shoenfeld et al. placed 25 stents in 19 patients and demonstrated a 68% primary patency rate and a 93% secondary patency rate at 17 months follow-up. However, they did not compare the results of PTA versus PTA plus stenting.[24] Kovalik et al. compared the results of PTA alone in 30 patients versus PTA plus Wallstent placement in 11 patients and obtained at least 9 months of follow-up on all patients.[25] For nonelastic lesions, PTA alone fared significantly better than PTA plus stenting (mean patency rates: 13.1 months versus 5.2 months, respectively). For elastic lesions that were associated with recoil, stents proved to be more durable than PTA alone (mean patency rates: 2.9 months versus 8.6 months, respectively). Therefore, it appears that stent placement should be reserved for elastic central venous lesions in which PTA alone is ineffective.

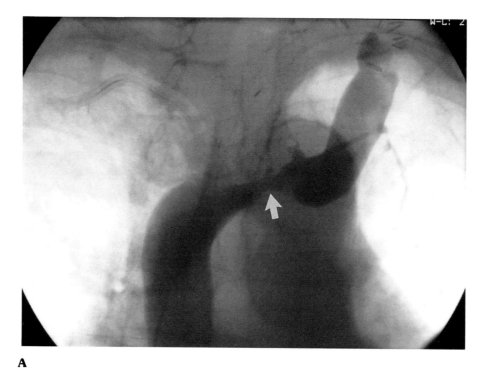

A

Figure 8.8 Dialysis-fistula–related stenosis. A. Venogram shows high-grade stenosis of the left innominate vein (arrow). B. Following page.

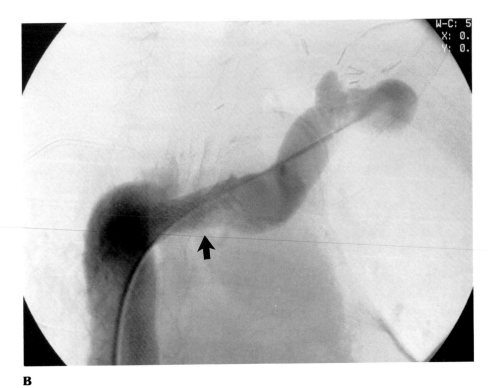

B

Figure 8.8 B. The stenosis was treated with balloon angioplasty and placement of a Palmaz stent. Control venogram reveals a good technical result (arrow).

Pacemaker Lead-induced Thrombosis

Pacemaker leads pose a unique problem since the lines often endothelialize to the vein and are not easily removed. Patients with central venous thrombosis associated with pacemaker wires can undergo thrombolytic therapy, PTA, and stenting with the leads in place. Care must be taken not to fracture the pacer leads during PTA and/or stent placement. Although the pacer lead will be compressed between the outer surface of the balloon and/or stent and the wall of the vein, there have been no reported instances of lead fracture or pacer failure following endovascular intervention.[9,10]

Superior Vena Cava Syndrome

The SVC syndrome can be caused by both benign and malignant etiologies that narrow or occlude the SVC or both innominate and subclavian veins with or without involvement of the SVC. Long-term anticoagulation is the traditional medical therapy for benign causes. For malignant etiologies, anticoagulation is supplemented with corticosteroids and radiation therapy. Unfortunately, a number of patients with both benign and malignant causes for SVC syndrome may not improve despite the initiation of standard medical therapy. Although surgical bypass is an option in patients with benign disease, it is usually not possible in patients with a malignant etiology. Endovascular therapy provides an alternative in patients who do not respond to standard medical therapy.

Patients with an isolated benign stenosis of the SVC can occasionally be treated with PTA alone, but in most patients with an isolated SVC stenosis, stenting will be required to obtain a good endovascular result. Stenoses of the SVC caused by a malignancy will invariably require placement of a stent. We favor the balloon-expandable Palmaz stent. This stent can be deployed precisely and possesses more hoopstrength than the Wallstent. However, if there is concomitant narrowing of the innominate veins, especially as they curve to enter the SVC, the Wallstent is used since the rigid Palmaz stent is more difficult to position along a curve. Because the Wallstent foreshortens during deployment, precise positioning is more difficult than with the Palmaz stent.

Occlusion of the SVC almost always requires PTA and stenting with or without adjunctive thrombolytic therapy (Figure 8.9). Furui et al. successfully placed Gianturco-Rösch Z-stents in 16 patients with malignant SVC obstruction with complete resolution of symptoms in 13.[26] The three patients who were not responsive to the interventional therapy had complete circumferential encasement of the SVC so that the stent could not reestablish a sufficiently large vessel lumen. Rösch et al. placed Z-stents in 22 patients with SVC syndrome. Complete resolution of symptoms occurred in 21 patients, with follow-up ranging from 1 to 16 months or to the time of death.[27]

Involvement of both subclavian and innominate veins requires bilateral catheter-directed thrombolysis to remove as much occlusive thrombus as possible. Stents should be used only in an area of residual critical stenosis. We have treated 46 patients with

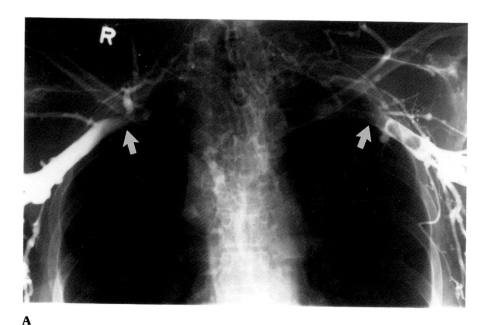

A

Figure 8.9 Superior vena cava syndrome. **A.** Bilateral upper extremity venogram shows complete occlusion of both subclavian (arrows) and innominate veins and the SVC. **B** and **C.** Following page.

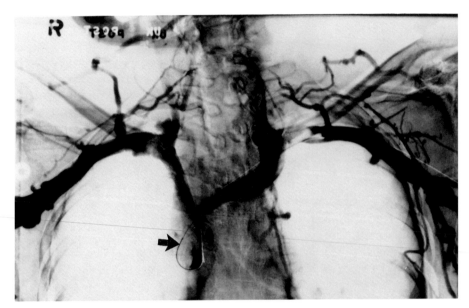

B

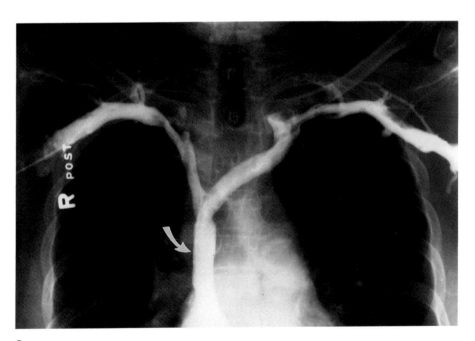

C

Figure 8.9 B. Following catheter-directed thrombolysis, there is partial restoration of venous flow, but persistent obstruction of the SVC (arrow). C. The venous drainage is fully restored after one additional session of thrombolysis and placement of a Palmaz stent in the SVC (arrow).

SVC syndrome, 31 with malignant and 15 with benign causes. Both the innominate and subclavian veins were involved in 34 patients.[28] Thrombolysis alone was used in only seven patients; angioplasty and stenting were required in 39. The overall technical success rate was 96%, with a clinical success rate of 93%. For patients with SVC syndrome due to malignancy, the primary patency rate was 83%, with a mean survival rate of 6 months. For patients with benign disease, the primary patency was 86% at 1 yr.

Stenting at the junction of the SVC and left innominate vein remains difficult and technically challenging. If both the SVC and the right innominate vein need stenting, it becomes necessary to cover the junction of the left innominate vein and the SVC with a stent. This is usually not a critical short-term factor. However, if there is further tumor ingrowth and compression of the SVC, it is difficult to gain access to the SVC through the stents from a left arm approach. The chief problem comes from attempting to advance a catheter and guidewire through the meshwork of the stent itself. In utter frustration, we have successfully used a diamond-tipped atherectomy device (Rotoblator; Boston Scientific) to drill through the stainless steel struts of the stent to gain access into a failing SVC stent from a basilic vein approach.

Postprocedure Therapy

In patients undergoing palliative SVC reconstruction who have a tumor-induced hypercoagulable state, warfarin is ineffective for DVT prophylaxis.[29] These patients should receive lifelong subcutaneous unfractionated heparin (5,000 mg twice a day) or low-molecular-weight heparin (Lovenox; Rhone-Poulenc Rorer Pharmaceuticals, Collegeville, PA).

MISCELLANEOUS ADJUNCTIVE TECHNIQUES

Atherectomy

The Simpson directional atherectomy device (Atherocath; Mallinkrodt, Inc.), can be used as an intravascular biopsy tool, especially in a patient in presumed remission who presents with SVC occlusion several months after radiation therapy.[30] The biopsy specimen can be useful to confirm recurrent invasive malignancy. False negatives can occur if there is extrinsic compression of the SVC without direct tumor invasion. A femoral vein approach is typically used due to the large diameter of these devices (7 to 10 Fr).

Rotational atherectomy (Rotoblator, Boston Scientific) has been used in our practice only to cut through the stainless steel struts of a Palmaz stent placed in the SVC. Since the burr requires passage over a 0.010-inch guidewire, it is not feasible to use this device for primary recanalization of an occluded SVC.

Intravascular Ultrasound

Intravascular ultrasound (IVUS) is used as an adjunct in the diagnosis of vascular disease. An 8-Fr, 20-MHz probe (CVIS; Boston Scientific) is used for examination of the veins only if it is necessary to measure the diameter of the vascular lumen or to determine if the deployed stent is fully apposed to the wall of the vein. Although ultrasound can image intraluminal filling defects seen on venography, the findings are nonspecific, and organized thrombus cannot be distinguished from tumor ingrowth. The availability of IVUS is not critical for endovascular reconstruction of the central thoracic veins.

Endoluminal Stent/Grafts

These devices combine both stents and standard surgical graft material such as polyester (Dacron) or polytetrafluoroethylene (PTFE; Gortex) and have been used experimentally in the arterial circulation for the treatment of occlusive disease, aneurysms, or traumatic arteriovenous fistulas involving the aorta or iliac arteries.[31] In principle, the stents are used to anchor graft material to the vessel wall. While there is no experience in the use of these devices for SVC reconstruction, it is possible that such technology may prove beneficial in the future. The stents could be used to buttress the elastic recoil while the graft material could serve as a mechanical barrier to reduce hyperplastic tissue or tumor ingrowth through the meshwork of the stent. A bifurcated system could provide an endovascular solution to the treatment of disease at the SVC–left innominate vein junction.

REFERENCES

1. Hull RD, Pineo GF: Current concepts of anticoagulation therapy. *Clin Chest Med* 16:269–280, 1995.

2. Lensing AW, Prins MH, Davidson BL, et al: Treatment of deep venous thrombosis with low-molecular weight heparin: a meta-analysis. *Arch Intern Med* 155:60–67, 1995

3. Becker DM, Philbrick JT, Walker FB: Axillary and subclavian venous thrombosis: prognosis and treatment. *Arch Intern Med* 151:1934–1943, 1991.

4. Burihan E, de Figueiredo LF, Francisco JJ, et al: Upper extremity deep venous thrombosis: analysis of 52 cases. *Cardiovasc Surg* 1:19–22, 1993.

5. Black MD, French GJ, Rasuli P, et al: Upper extremity deep venous thrombosis: underdiagnosed and potentially lethal. *Chest* 103:1887–1890, 1993.

6. Machleder HI: Evaluation of a new treatment strategy for Paget-Schroetter syndrome: spontaneous thrombosis of the axillary-subclavian vein. *J Vasc Surg* 17:305–315, 1993.

7. Makhoul RG, Machleder RI: Developmental anomalies at the thoracic outlet: an analysis of 200 consecutive cases. *J Vasc Surg* 16:534–542, 1992.

8. Wechsler RJ, Spirn PW, Conant EF, et al: Thrombosis and infection caused by thoracic venous catheters: pathogenesis and imaging findings. *Am J Roentgenol* 160:467–471, 1993.

9. Spitell PC, Hayes DL: Venous complications after insertion of a transvenous pacemaker. *Mayo Clin Proc* 67:258–265, 1992.

10. Mazzetti H, Dussaut A, Tentori C, et al: Superior vena cava occlusion and/or syndrome related to pacemaker leads. *Am Heart J* 125:831–837, 1993.

11. Criado E, Marston WA, Jacques PF, et al: Proximal venous outflow obstruction in patients with upper extremity arteriovenous dialysis access. *Ann Vasc Surg* 8:530–535, 1994

12. Gaylord GM, Taber TE: Long-term hemodialysis access salvage: problems and challenges for nephrologists and interventional radiologists. *J Vasc Intervent Radiol* 4:103–107, 1993.

13. Escalante CP: Causes and management of superior vena cava syndrome. *Oncology* 7:61–68, 1993.

14. Abner A: Approach to the patient who presents with superior vena cava obstruction. *Chest* 103:394S–397S, 1993.

15. Skolnick ML: Role of sonography in the placement and management of jugular and subclavian central venous catheters. *Am J Roentgenol* 163:291–295, 1994.

16. Comerota AJ, Aldridge SC: Thrombolytic therapy for deep venous thrombosis: a clinical review. *Can J Surg* 36:359–364, 1993.

17. Vidovich RR, Heiselman DE, Hudock D: Treatment of urokinase-related anaphylactoid reaction with intravenous famotidine. *Ann Pharmacother* 26:782–783, 1992.

18. Matsumoto AH, Selby JB, Tegtmeyer CJ, et al: Recent development of rigors during infusion of urokinase: is it related to an endotoxin? *J Vasc Intervent Radiol* 4:433–438, 1994.

19. Bjarnason H, Hunter DW, Crain MR, et al: Collapse of a Palmaz stent in the subclavian vein. *Am J Roentgenol* 160:1123–1124, 1993.

20. Rösch J, Uhida BT, Keller FS, et al: Interventional management of large venous obstructions. In Strandness DE, van Breda A (eds): *Vascular Diseases—Surgical and Interventional Therapy*. New York, Churchill Livingstone, 1994, pp 999–1015.

21. Vorwerk D, Günther RW, Mann H, et al: Venous stenosis occlusion in hemodialysis shunts: follow-up results and stent placement in 65 patients. *Radiology* 195:140–146, 1995.

22. Horattas MC, Wright DJ, Fenton AH, et al: Changing concepts of deep venous thrombosis of the upper extremity—report of a series and review of the literature. *Surgery* 104:561–567, 1988

23. Kanterman RY, Vesely TM, Pilgram TK, et al: Dialysis access grafts: anatomic location of venous stenosis and results of angioplasty. *Radiology* 195:135–139, 1995

24. Shoenfeld R, Hermans H, Novick A, et al: Stenting of proximal venous obstructions to maintain hemodialysis access. *J Vasc Surg* 19:532–539, 1994.
25. Kovalik EC, Newman GE, Suhocki P, et al: Correction of central venous stenoses: use of angioplasty and vascular Wallstents. Kidney Int 45:1177–1181, 1994.
26. Furui S, Sawada S, Kuramoto K, et al: Gianturco stent placement in malignant caval obstruction: analysis of factors for predicting outcomes. *Radiology* 195:147–152, 1995.
27. Rösch J, Uchida BT, Hall LD, et al: Gianturco-Rösch expandable Z-stents in the treatment of superior vena cava syndrome. *Cardiovasc Intervent Radiol* 15:319–327, 1992.
28. Kee ST, Dake MD, Semba CP, et al: Catheter-directed thrombolysis and endovascular stent placement as therapy for central venous obstruction (abstract). *Radiology* 197(P):234, 1995.
29. Naschitz JE, Yeshurun D, Lev LM: Thromboembolism in cancer: changing trends. *Cancer* 71:1384–1390, 1993.
30. Dake MD: The cause of superior vena cava syndrome: diagnosis with percutaneous atherectomy. *Radiology* 174(3):957–959, 1990.
31. Dake MD, Miller DC, Semba CP, et al: Transluminal placement of endovascular stent-grafts for the treatment of descending thoracic aortic aneurysms. *N Engl J Med*:1729–1734, 1994.

C H A P T E R
9

Transcatheter Therapy of Tumors of the Thoracic Vertebral Body

Mary E. Jensen
Jacques E. Dion

A host of pathologic processes can involve the vertebral column and its contents. These include primary or metastatic neoplasms, degenerative changes, trauma, congenital lesions, or vascular abnormalities. The spinal cord and its dural covering can be compressed or invaded by disease entities that involve the adjacent bone. This chapter focuses on therapeutic strategies and techniques utilized by the interventional radiologist in the treatment of tumors and tumor-like processes involving the vertebrae of the thoracic spine.

THERAPEUTIC GOALS

Patients with tumors of the bony spinal canal usually present with pain and/or a neurologic deficit. The therapeutic strategy is patient-specific, dictated by the nature of the lesion, the symptoms and clinical exam, and the desired outcome. Embolization is rarely a curative procedure for vertebral body tumors; rather, it is palliative or employed as an adjunct to surgery.[1–6] It is the physician's responsibility to discuss the various therapeutic options and relative risks of the embolization procedure with the referring clinician and the patient, in order to optimize the treatment plan.

In most cases, the primary goal of embolization is to devascularize the tumor without compromising circulation to the spinal cord or nerve roots. In resectable lesions, embolization facilitates surgical removal by reducing blood loss and shortening the operative time. A surgical procedure with less bleeding provides improved visualization, allowing more exact dissection of tissue adjacent to the delicate neural structures. In some cases, embolization allows extirpation of otherwise inoperable lesions by devascularizing inaccessible or unresectable portions of the tumor. Identification of the spinal cord arteries as part of the angiographic protocol is also important in operative planning, particularly when the parent artery to the tumor will probably be sacrificed.

With palliative procedures, the goal of embolization is to devascularize the lesion and cause tumor shrinkage. As the lesion shrinks in size, decompression of adjacent neural tissue occurs with a decrease in the patient's pain and/or neurologic dysfunction. Endovascular therapy can also be combined with chemotherapy or radiation to treat unresectable tumors.

VASCULAR ANATOMY OF THE VERTEBRAL BODY AND SPINAL CORD

Prior to an endovascular intervention, a thorough understanding of the regional vascular anatomy of the thoracic spinal column is necessary.[7-11] The T3 to T11 thoracic vertebrae are supplied by branches of paired posterior intercostal arteries that arise from the dorsal aspect of the descending thoracic aorta (Figure 9.1A). Shortly after originating from the aorta, these vessels run along the anterior border of the vertebral body, giving rise to two or more small anterior central branches which penetrate the cortical bone.[7] As the intercostal artery takes a more posterior course, it passes through a space bounded superiorly and inferiorly by the necks of adjacent ribs, medially by the vertebral body, and laterally by the superior costotransverse ligament. It subsequently gives rise to the dorsospinal artery which runs medially along the posterolateral aspect of the vertebral body to ultimately supply the paraspinous musculature, bone, dura, and neural structures. The dorsospinal artery branches into the spinal artery which enters the intervertebral foramen, and the dorsal artery which supplies the posterior paraspinous muscles. A small branch of the dorsal artery, called the posterior laminar artery, supplies the dorsal aspect of the lamina.[7] The main posterior intercostal artery continues obliquely across the intercostal space where it enters the costal groove along the inferior border of each rib and becomes part of the neurovascular bundle.

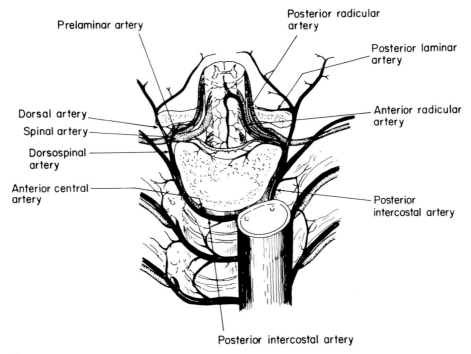

A

Figure 9.1 A. Cross-sectional view of the lower thoracic spine. The paired intercostal arteries arise from the aorta and run along the anterolateral surface of the vertebral body, giving off anterior central arteries to the adjacent vertebra. The dorsospinal artery arises from the posterior intercostal artery and courses posteriorly and laterally. From this vessel arises the spinal artery which runs through the neural foramen and divides into the posterior central artery (B), the prelaminar branches, and anterior and posterior radicular arteries. The continuation of the dorsospinal artery, the dorsal artery, ultimately supplies the dorsal surface of the lamina via the posterior laminar artery, and the paraspinous musculature. B and C. Following pages.

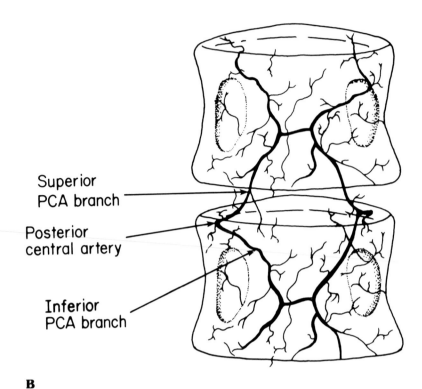

Superior
PCA branch

Posterior
central artery

Inferior
PCA branch

B

Anterior external
venous plexus

Basivertebral
plexus

Anterior internal
venous plexus

Anterior spinal
vein

Intervertebral
vein

Radicular
vein

Posterior spinal
vein

Posterior internal
venous plexus

Posterior external
venous plexus

C

Figure 9.1 B. Posterior view of adjacent vertebral bodies. At each intervertebral level, the bilateral spinal arteries give off a posterior central artery (PCA). Each PCA branches into a superior and inferior branch which courses medially toward the center of the corresponding vertebra where it connects with its counterparts. Ultimately, each vertebra is fed by four separate branches, two superior and two inferior, from two PCAs arising at adjacent levels. This duality of blood supply requires that adjacent PCAs are examined during the angiographic evaluation of any vertebral tumor. C. The venous drainage of the thoracic spine consists of a series of intra- and extraspinal concentric venous rings, each connected by longitudinal veins. The spinal cord (next page)

The anatomy is identical for the twelfth vertebral body and rib although the vessels originating from the aorta are known as the subcostal arteries. The first two thoracic vertebrae and ribs are supplied by branches of the superior (supreme) intercostal arteries which arise from the costocervical arteries and anastomose with the third intercostal arteries. Because of this connection, the superior intercostal artery may be visualized on injection of either the costocervical trunk or the third intercostal artery.[9,10]

The spinal artery may enter the neural foramen as a single vessel or arise as multiple independent branches.[8] If it enters as a single vessel, the spinal artery first gives rise to the posterior central branch which supplies the dorsal surface of the vertebral body, the posterior longitudinal ligament, and the regional dura. Each posterior central branch divides at the level of the intervertebral disc into superior and inferior branches to support two adjacent vertebrae (Figure 9.1B). Every vertebral body is supplied by two superior and two inferior branches, all of which converge at the dorsal central cavity to connect with their counterparts.[7] Therefore, each vertebral body is supplied by four arteries arising from two adjacent intervertebral levels. The next branch of the spinal artery is the prelaminar branch which follows the inner surface of the vertebral arch to supply the ventral surface of the lamina, ligamentum flavum, and adjacent dura.[7]

The spinal artery terminates as anterior and posterior radicular branches supplying the dorsal and ventral roots. However, at certain levels the radicular arteries also supply the spinal cord in addition to the nerve roots. The main anterior spinal supply in the thoracic region is the artery of Adamkiewicz. This vessel arises from a left intercostal artery in 80% of individuals, and between T9 and L2 in 85%.[10] A second anterior spinal artery usually arises from the superior intercostal artery, supplying the spinal cord at the cervicothoracic junction. The posterior spinal arteries receive one to two tributaries from the radicular arteries at each vertebral level in the upper thoracic region. However, below T4 and T5, there is usually only one posterior radicular branch for every two vertebral levels.[9,10]

Completing the vertebral anastomotic network are communications between adjacent vertebrae and intercostal arteries. Longitudinal pretransverse anastomoses are located dorsal and ventral to the transverse processes at each vertebral level and provide extraspinal communications between consecutive dorsospinal arteries. Each intercostal artery is connected to the adjacent vessels by prevertebral and paravertebral branches, another important source of collateral supply to the vertebrae. On occasion, the bronchial artery may supply a branch to the anterior spinal artery.

The venous drainage of the thoracic spine consists of a series of intra- and extraspinal concentric venous rings, each connected by longitudinal veins (Figure 9.1C). The central spinal cord parenchyma drains into the longitudinally oriented anterior and posterior spinal veins which are located on the ventral and dorsal surface of the cord, respectively. These veins subsequently join the anterior and posterior radicular veins, which are located along the ventral and dorsal roots. Minute valves, unique to the radicular veins, prevent passive congestion of the spinal cord in cases of increased epidural venous pressure.[8] The radicular veins ultimately coalesce and join the intervertebral vein, which is located in the neural foramen.

---

drains into the anterior and posterior spinal veins, which coalesce with the radicular veins and empty into the intervertebral veins. The main drainage of the vertebral body is via the basivertebral plexus, which drains into the anterior internal venous plexus located between the dura and the posterior aspect of the vertebral body, and the anterior external venous plexus located along the anterior border of the vertebral body. The lamina and posterior elements are drained by the posterior internal venous plexus and the posterior external venous plexus. Branches of the anterior and posterior internal venous plexuses coalesce at the neural foramen to form the intervertebral vein which exits the canal with the nerve root.

The vertebral body venous drainage is mainly through the basivertebral plexus, a "Y"-shaped tunnel through the cancellous bone. The basivertebral plexus exits the vertebral body posteriorly and drains into the anterior internal plexus. Other basivertebral veins drain into the anterior external plexus through channels terminating along the lateral and anterior surfaces of the vertebral body.[9–11]

The internal and external vertebral venous plexuses are valveless and consist of longitudinal veins interconnected by transverse veins. The anterior internal plexus is located within the epidural space on either side of the posterior longitudinal ligament. The smaller posterior internal plexus is situated anterior to the ligamenta flava and bony vertebral arches. It receives blood from perforators through the ligaments, the posterior external plexus located around the vertebral laminae, and the transverse, spinous and articular processes.

The anterior and posterior internal plexuses are the main tributaries of the intervertebral vein. The intervertebral vein exits the neural foramen to drain into the superior intercostal, posterior intercostal, or subcostal veins. The first posterior intercostal veins usually drain into the innominate veins. The left innominate vein receives the superior intercostal vein, while the same vein on the right frequently empties into the azygos vein. The right fifth through twelfth posterior intercostal veins usually drain into the azygos vein. The left fifth through eighth posterior intercostal veins empty into the accessory azygos vein, while the ninth through twelfth veins enter the hemiazygos vein.[11]

PATIENT SELECTION AND PREPARATION

Appropriate candidates for endovascular or percutaneous therapy are patients with vascular neoplasms of the vertebral body and/or the bony posterior vertebral elements who have pain, neurologic dysfunction, and/or vertebral body collapse. While obtaining informed consent, the procedure and its attendant risks of pain, paralysis, bladder/bowel incontinence, sensory loss, and sexual dysfunction must be clearly articulated to the patient. In uncooperative individuals, or during procedures where extreme pain is anticipated (such as alcohol injection), general anesthesia is often required. With the use of general anesthesia, the ability to identify an immediate neurologic complication is precluded. Although monitoring somatosensory evoked potentials can be helpful, it is only useful in evaluating the integrity of the posterior columns of the spinal cord.

All patients should undergo a neurologic evaluation by a nurse and a physician prior to procedure. This examination should focus on truncal and lower extremity strength and sensation. Most patients are sedated with a combination of an anxiolytic such as midazolam (Versed; Roche Pharmaceuticals, Inc., Manati, PR), and an analgesic such as fentanyl (Elkins-Sinn, Cherry Hill, NJ). Throughout the procedure, continuous physiologic monitoring (electrocardiogram, blood pressure, and oxygen saturation) is standard policy.

Patients who will be undergoing a direct percutaneous puncture of the tumor are usually required to lie on their abdomen. The prone position decreases respiratory excursion and may affect oxygenation. Therefore, prior to the procedure, the patient should be checked for respiratory tolerance while in this position.

All procedures are recorded using high-resolution digital subtraction angiography (DSA). Superior contrast resolution, the availability of roadmapping functions, pixel shifting capabilities to minimize motion artifact, and near instant review of angiographic runs all make DSA far superior to cut-film technology.

Following embolization of a vertebral body lesion, increased pain and/or paralysis can occur, and both are more common when liquid agents or very small particles are used. Since acute tumoral swelling may occur and result in neurologic decompensation, postprocedural management should include at least a 24-hr stay in a suitable intensive care unit with frequent neurologic evaluations. For patients on a non-neurosurgical service it is recommended that the neurosurgical team be consulted prior to the embolization. Lack of proper surgical support can lead to permanent neurologic dysfunction in patients who develop swelling and an acute cord or nerve root compression syndrome.

Patients are often receiving steroids prior to their embolization procedure. If symptoms worsen after the procedure, a transient increase in the steroid dosage is recommended. For patients who were not receiving steroids prior to the procedure, 10 mg of dexamethasone (Decadron, Elkins-Sinn Inc, Cherry Hill, NJ) is given intravenously immediately prior to the embolization. Dexamethasone is continued every 6 hr but rapidly tapered over 2 days. Mannitol is a drug frequently used in the treatment of increased intracranial pressure, and may be used in the treatment of acute spinal cord edema. Discussion with the neurosurgical team should be done prior to mannitol administration since emergency surgical decompression may be the more appropriate therapy. A 1.0 gm/kg bolus of mannitol followed by a second bolus of 0.25–0.5 gm/kg is the usual dose.[12]

Pain control is usually achieved with nonsteroidal anti-inflammatory agents, but small doses of narcotics may occasionally be necessary. The need for parenteral analgesics is usually limited to 1–2 days. We have found that the routine use of prophylactic antibiotics is not necessary.

ANGIOGRAPHIC PROTOCOL

The same angiographic protocol applies for all treatment candidates regardless of tumor type, indication, or therapeutic approach. Because of its midline location, the thoracic spine derives its blood supply from bilateral sources and the rich anastomotic reserve from adjacent vessels. In the upper thoracic level the costocervical trunks, bronchial arteries, and superior intercostal arteries must be evaluated. Investigation of the paired intercostal arteries at the involved level and at least the two levels above and below the tumor site is necessary in mid to lower thoracic lesions. Additional levels may need to be studied depending upon the extent of the lesion. In cases where selective angiography for defining tumor vessels is fruitless, a flush aortogram with filming over the involved vertebra may point to an unrecognized or aberrant vascular supply. Identification of the intrinsic blood supply of the spinal cord and nerve roots is also necessary before embolization and/or surgery (Figure 9.2).

PROVOCATIVE TESTING

Originally described by Doppman et al.[13] in an animal model, the spinal Wada test is a provocative maneuver to try to determine if embolization of a vascular bed might lead to a permanent neurologic deficit. By injecting a short-acting barbiturate directly into the artery of Adamkiewicz of an animal, the authors noted suppression of gray matter neuronal synaptic activity, resulting in flaccid paralysis. The administration of intraarterial lidocaine resulted in inhibition of nerve conduction through white matter spinal tracts, and provoked a brief period of flaccidity followed by hyperreflexia and thigh muscle fasciculations. All animals demonstrated normal ambulation and climbing ability after recovery from general anesthesia.

Because the radiculomedullary arteries supplying the spinal cord and nerve roots are in close proximity to the branches feeding the vertebral body, proximal emboliza-

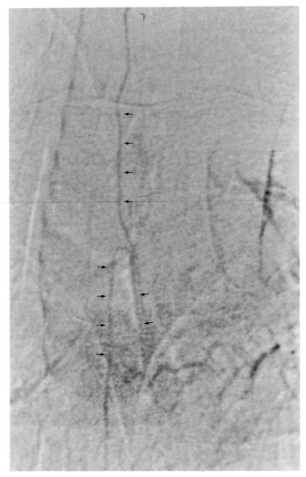

Figure 9.2 This patient with a metastatic lesion to T2 was referred for potential embolization. Injection of the left T4 intercostal artery shows filling of the anterior spinal artery (arrowheads) seen best in the late arterial phase. Careful examination of the diagnostic angiogram prior to embolization is essential in order to avoid spinal cord complications. Embolization of this vessel was not performed.

tion with a penetrating agent (i.e., liquid agents or very small particles) places the patient at greater risk for a neurologic complication. Therefore, provocative testing with lidocaine and a short-acting barbiturate has been recommended in this setting. In general, we reserve the spinal Wada test for embolization procedures in which a penetrating agent will be used. The potential neurologic effects of the spinal Wada test are transient, lasting approximately 5 to 10 min before restoration of function is noted.

MATERIALS AND METHODS

A variety of catheters, guidewires, and embolic agents have been used in the embolization of vertebral body lesions.[14–18] When using coaxial systems involving microcatheters, the guiding catheter is positioned in the origin of the parent artery that supplies the lesion. Because of the small size of the intercostal arteries, and their orientation from the posterior aspect of the aorta, a 4- to 6-Fr guiding catheter (0.035–0.038 inch internal diameter [I.D.]) with a modified Cobra, Simmons I, or

Mikaelsson shape is usually used. A sidearm adaptor is placed on the guiding catheter hub. The microcatheter is advanced through the hemostatic valve on the adaptor into the guiding catheter lumen. The dead space between the guiding catheter and microcatheter is infused continuously with heparinized saline through the sideport on the sidearm adaptor. A three-way stopcock placed on the sideport allows injection of contrast material for serial angiograms or roadmapping without disturbing the saline flush or the positioning of the microcatheter. Injection of contrast through the sideport is often difficult with smaller lumen guiding catheters when the microcatheter is in place.

The microcatheter can be advanced over a steerable guidewire or flow-directed in situations of high flow (i.e., [AVM]s). Even though some tumors are highly vascular, the regional blood flow is not increased enough in neoplasms to make use of flow-directed catheters practical. Therefore, the guidewire system is most frequently used for treating tumors involving the vertebral bodies. In addition, the internal diameter of steerable microcatheters is typically larger than that of their flow-directed counterparts, and is more compatible with a wider variety of embolic agents.

In some cases, direct percutaneous puncture of the tumor can be done. In tumors where a liquid embolic agent such as alcohol is utilized, an 18G–22G spinal needle may be used. For thicker embolic solutions such as methyl methacrylate, a larger bore needle, such as an 11G Jamshedi bone biopsy needle (Cook, Inc., Bloomington, IN), is usually required.

Commonly used particulate agents include polyvinyl alcohol (PVA) (Contour; Interventional Therapeutics Corp., Fremont, CA), microfibrillar collagen (Avitene; Alcon, Inc., Woburn, MA), and gelatin powder or sponge (Gelfoam; Upjohn Co., Kalamazoo, MI). Liquid embolic materials include tissue adhesives (N-butyl-cyanoacrylate) Histoacryl; B. Braun Melsungen AG, Melsungen, Germany), dehydrated alcohol (Tera Pharmaceuticals, Inc., Buena Park, CA), sodium tetradecyl sulfate (Sotradecol, Elkins-Sinn, Inc., Cherry Hill, NJ), or methyl methacrylate (CMW Laboratories Limited, Blackpool, England). Occasionally, larger mechanical embolic agents such as platinum microcoils (Target Therapeutics, Inc., Fremont, CA; Cook, Inc.) may be used for protection of distal vascular territories or as the terminal occlusive devices after use of more penetrating agents.

The choice of embolic agent is based upon the vascular characteristics of the tumor and the desired therapeutic goal. In many cases, the desired outcome can be achieved with several different types of embolic materials. The choice of which specific agent to use is left to the preference and personal experience of the interventionalist. Each agent is associated with potential risks and benefits that must be considered in each individual case.

Factors affecting the choice of an embolic agent include the therapeutic goal, location of the tumor, size of the feeding vessel, position of the catheter tip, blood flow, and the presence and location of radiculomedullary arteries. The greatest penetration of the tumor bed is achieved by liquid agents or very small particles. However, these agents carry an increased risk of neurologic impairment or tissue necrosis. Particles that measure 150 to 350 μm in size often provide adequate distal penetration while sparing the vasa nervosum of spinal nerves and capillary bed of adjacent soft tissues.

To allow the operator to monitor vessel runoff, stagnation of blood flow, and for reflux of the embolic agent, particles should be suspended and delivered in contrast material.[19] Liquid agents can also be opacified with contrast material, although dilution of the agent will occur. Powdered metrizamide (Amipaque; Winthrop, New York, NY) was once added to liquid agents for opacification when a full strength embolic agent was required, but this product is no longer commercially available. The addition of tantalum powder to tissue adhesives will render these agents fluoroscopically visible.

Chemoembolization with mitomycin C capsules or doxorubicin has also been reported in the palliative treatment of various metastases. Reports of improvement in clinical symptoms and pain have been described,[20,21] but further study is necessary to determine the long-term effects of this type of therapy.

EMBOLIZATION TECHNIQUES

The desired endpoint of embolization is the angiographic obliteration of the tumor blush while sparing the vascular supply to the adjacent normal tissues. In order to achieve this goal, meticulous technique is paramount, especially during catheter manipulation and the injection of the embolic material.[22] After identification of the arterial supply, the microcatheter is advanced into each feeding artery and a magnified study is performed to define the angioarchitecture, identify the tumor neovascularity, and search for vessels potentially supplying the spinal cord (Figure 9.3A–C). The vascular supply to the spinal cord is from terminal radiculomedullary branches which are inconstant at some levels, particularly along the posterior axis. The rich collateral circulation seen throughout the brain is not as evident in the spinal cord. When collaterals do exist, they usually arise from small segmental pial branches.

Excessive guidewire or catheter manipulation, or wedging the catheter tip in the artery can induce vasospasm, altering blood flow to the lesion, thereby preventing safe and effective embolization. If vasospasm occurs, it can be relieved by the application of topical nitroglycerin (one–two inches of Nitropaste) or the administration of intra-arterial vasodilators (i.e., 30–60 mg of papaverine). Removal of the catheter and a "tincture of time" will also often alleviate the vasospasm.

The embolic agent is injected by hand into the arterial stream in small, pulsed aliquots. The operator monitors the flow of the embolic agent away from the catheter

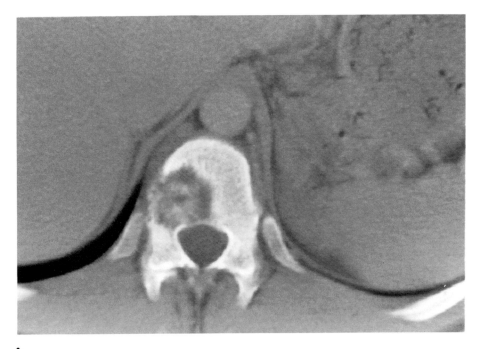

A

Figure 9.3 A. An 18-yr-old male was found to have metastatic osteoblastoma to the T12 vertebra. He was referred for cisplatinum infusion directly into the tumor bed. **B** and **C**. Following pages.

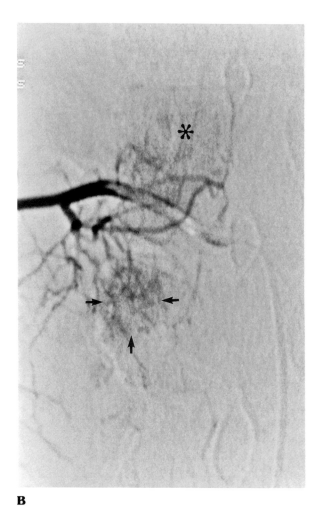

B

Figure 9.3 B. Injection of the T-11 intercostal artery shows the normal vascular blush of the T-11 vertebra (asterisk) and tumor blush at the T-12 vertebra from dorsospinal branches (arrows).

tip and into the tumor bed, evaluating for reflux of the embolic material around the catheter tip or stagnation of flow in the feeding vessel. The embolization is complete when the tumor blush is no longer visualized. Care should be taken not to wedge the catheter tip during the embolization procedure. Forcible injection of contrast or embolic material into a closed vascular system can result in vessel rupture or in opening of previously unseen anastomoses, with inadvertent embolization of adjacent normal tissue.[23]

Larger anastomoses or side branches feeding normal tissue can be spared in one of three ways: (1) the catheter tip is placed distal to the origin of the anastomosis and no reflux of embolic material occurs; (2) proximal embolization with particles larger than the anastomotic vessels is used; or (3) the proximal lumen of the anastomosis is blocked with a gelatin sponge pledget or platinum microcoil to prevent embolic material from entering, followed by particulate embolization of the tumor from the main trunk of the feeding vessel.

In some instances, normal tissue is supplied by the distal portion of an artery which feeds the tumor bed proximally. In this situation, the microcatheter is advanced to a point distal to the tumor branch take-off and the normal vascular territory is protected

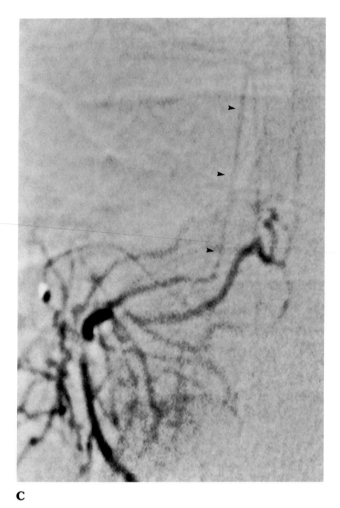

C

Figure 9.3 C. Superselective angiography of the dorsospinal artery shows a radiculomedullary artery arising from the spinal artery to supply the conus. Infusion was not performed at this level due to the potential complication of spinal cord toxicity.

with a Gelfoam pledget or microcoil. The catheter tip is then withdrawn to a point proximal to the tumor branches and embolization is performed (Figure 9.4A–D).

After embolization, the proximal portion of the main feeding vessel may be occluded using a Gelfoam pledget to enhance thrombosis within the tumor bed. Microcoils have also been used for the same purpose but these agents may cause permanent vascular occlusion, preventing reembolization in cases of tumor recurrence.

Upper thoracic lesions may recruit small feeders from the vertebral artery. These vessels are usually too small to select with a microcatheter. If superslective emboliza-

Figure 9.4 This 9-yr-old female presented with progressive numbness and paresis. A. CT scan shows a lytic, expansile lesion involving the left pedicle and posterior elements of T-1 with cortical thinning and canal encroachment. B. T2-weighted sagittal MR shows posterior impingement of the canal by a heterogeneous mass of mixed signal intensities. Internal septations are noted (arrowheads). Although the majority of the mass is located posteriorly from C-7 to T-2, a small portion of the vertebral body (asterisk) is also involved. These findings are consistent with an aneurysmal bone cyst (next page). C and D. Following pages.

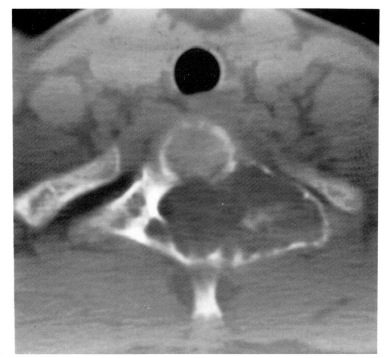

A

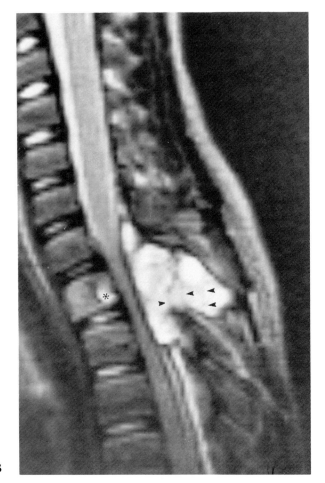

B

199

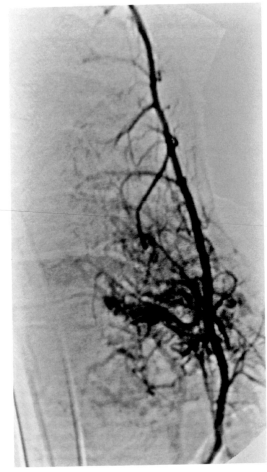

C

Figure 9.4 C. Selective injection of the left ascending cervical artery shows a dense tumor stain involving several proximal branches with a normal arterial appearance distally. **D.** Following page.

tion is precluded, embolization can be performed from the parent artery, if an occlusion balloon is inflated distal to the most distal feeding artery.[24] A permanently attached silicone or latex balloon mounted on the end of a microcatheter is floated to a point distal to the tumor feeders. With the patient fully heparinized, the balloon is inflated with contrast to the point of vertebral artery occlusion. Neurologic testing is performed every 5 min for a total of 30 min to rule out immediate or delayed cerebral ischemia. Once the patient has passed the test occlusion, a second microcatheter is advanced into the vertebral artery and positioned proximal to the tumor feeders. Embolization is performed through this catheter until the tumor blush is eliminated. In order to prevent escape of residual embolic agent into the intracranial circulation, copious flushing of the dead space behind the balloon prior to balloon deflation is mandatory. This flushing is done through the microcatheter and the guiding catheter. The balloon is then deflated, and a check angiogram of the intracranial circulation is performed to rule out distal embolization. When the vertebral artery is to be sacrificed at surgery, the previously described procedure can be done with detachable balloons. Instead of deflating the balloon following embolization, the balloon is detached and a

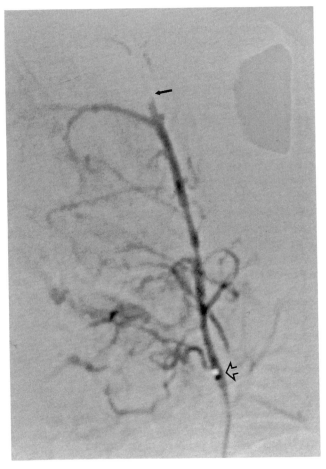

D

Figure 9.4 D. The microcatheter was advanced past the tumor feeders and the distal territory was protected with a Gelfoam pledget (arrow). The microcatheter was then withdrawn to a point proximal to the feeders (open arrow) and embolization with polyvinyl alcohol particles (300–500 μm) was performed. No significant tumor blush remained and the tumor was excised with minimal blood loss.

second safety balloon is placed in the proximal portion of the vertebral artery (Figure 9.5A–D).

When neither selective catheterization nor parent artery occlusion is desired, tolerated, or indicated, some tumors can be approached by percutaneous or intraoperative direct puncture technique.[25] Advantages of the direct puncture technique include the potential for: (1) delivery of the embolic agent to the capillary bed with a more complete embolization; (2) establishment of a good surgical cleavage plane with the adjacent normal tissue; (3) staining of the tumor which allows separation of pathologic from normal tissue; and (4) a lower complication rate. Disadvantages include: (1) the potential need for general anesthesia for intraprocedural pain management; (2) the possibility of retrograde reflux into the parent artery; and (3) passage of a large needle through regions containing vital neurovascular structures, although this risk can be minimized by using a transpedicular route for needle insertion.

The direct puncture technique has been used in patients with vertebral body metastases and primary tumors.[26] We have utilized this technique to facilitate direct injec-

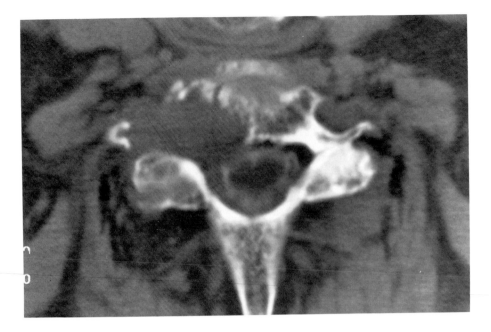

A

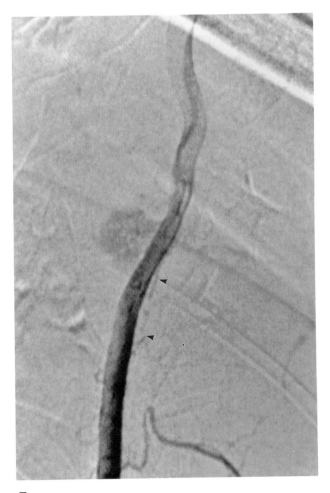

B

Figure 9.5 A. A 67-yr-old female with right arm pain was found by CT to have a breast metastasis of C6 involving the right pedicle with extension into the vertebral body. B. Lateral angiography of the right vertebral artery shows narrowing of the vessel with a tumor blush supplied by a branch too small to catheterize. C and D. Following pages.

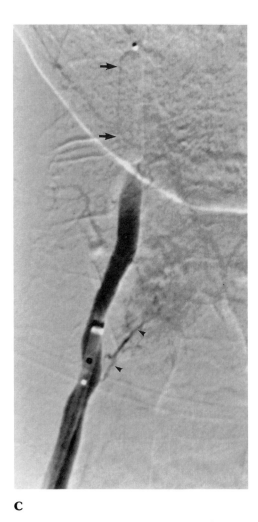

C

Figure 9.5 C. A temporary balloon occlusion test was performed at the C4 level (arrows). The patient tolerated the test occlusion, and the balloon was subsequently detached. **D**. Following page.

tion of methyl methacrylate to stabilize compression fractures caused by either neoplastic processes (Figure 9.6A–F) or osteoporosis.

With the patient in the prone position and under neuroleptic analgesia, the vertebral body to be treated is identified. The overlying skin is sterilely prepared and draped. The C-arm fluoroscopy tube is angled so that one pedicle is isolated in an anteroposterior (AP) "bull's-eye" position. The skin, underlying tissues, and periosteum are anesthetized with 1% lidocaine and a small dermatotomy is made. An 11G Jamshedi bone biopsy needle is advanced through the chosen pedicle using both AP and lateral position fluoroscopy. The stylet tip of the needle trocar is advanced to the midportion of the vertebral body. The stylet is withdrawn and contrast (Omnipaque 300) is injected during 1–2 frames per second filming to identify the venous anatomy and exclude subligamentous or endplate extravasation. The stylet is replaced and its tip advanced if positioning within an intravertebral venous structure is noted on contrast injection. Once satisfactory positioning is documented, the methyl methacrylate is prepared. We use a slow-set Codman cranioplasty kit (CMW Laboratories Limited). The kit contains a powder pouch and a liquid ampule. The powder is mixed with 1 tsp of barium sulfate and 1 gm of tungsten powder to increase its opacification under fluo-

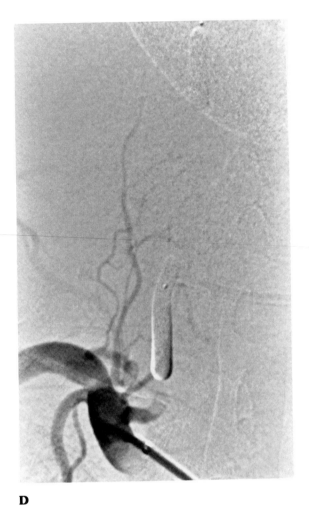

D

Figure 9.5 D. Embolization of the tumor from the stump was performed using PVA particles (150–250 μm) followed by placement of a second balloon just distal to the vertebral artery origin.

roscopy. The powder is divided into two equal portions and one portion is set aside. One half of the liquid agent is removed from the ampule. One portion of the powder is placed in a plastic bowl and a small amount is removed and set aside. The liquid is mixed with the powder until a thin, cake-glaze consistency is reached. If the mixture is too thin, then the powder that was initially removed is gradually added until the desired consistency is reached. The material is poured into a 20-cc syringe which is then used to backload 1-cc Luer-lock syringes. Backloading the smaller syringes keeps the Luer-lock tip clean for tight attachment to the Jamshedi hub. The stylet is removed and the dead space of the trocar is filled with methyl methacrylate using an 180-gauge spinal needle. The methyl methacrylate is then injected under fluoroscopic control, using the 1-cc syringes. Instillation of the material is performed until the vertebral body hemisphere is filled or further injection becomes impossible. Careful evaluation of the image during injection is required to exclude subligamentous extravasation or embolization to the epidural venous plexus. In our experience, treatment of the contralateral hemivertebra in an identical manner is usually necessary, because the methyl methacrylate rarely crosses the midline. the second portion of powder and liquid is used for the contralateral hemivertebra.

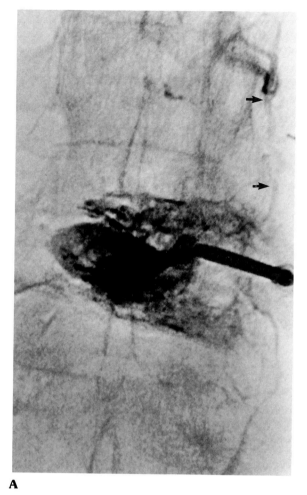

A

Figure 9.6 Same patient as Figure 9.8, 2 months after his second transarterial embolization. The patient complained of lower back pain without radicular radiation. The pain was felt to be secondary to the vertebral body collapse from the renal cell metastasis. The vertebral body was directly punctured with an 11-G bone biopsy needle placed transpedicularly on the right. A. Anteroposterior (AP) oblique. B, C, D, and E. Following page.

COMPLICATIONS

Embolization of vertebral body lesions carries a very low morbidity and mortality rate (less than 1%) when performed by an experienced interventionalist.[1-6] Some patients experience transient fever, or localized pain, both of which are self-limiting and usually abate in 1–2 days. If nontarget capillaries or distal muscular branches are embolized, tissue necrosis may occur. More severe complications, such as nerve root injury, paralysis, bowel-bladder incontinence, or sexual dysfunction have been reported. With transpedicular percutaneous puncture, bleeding, fracture of the pedicle, pulmonary embolization, subligamentous extravasation of methyl methacrylate, or migration of embolic material into the epidural venous plexus may also result. Paravertebral puncture with transgression of the pleural surface can also result in pneumothorax.

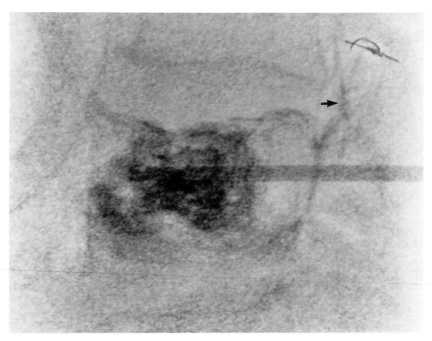

B

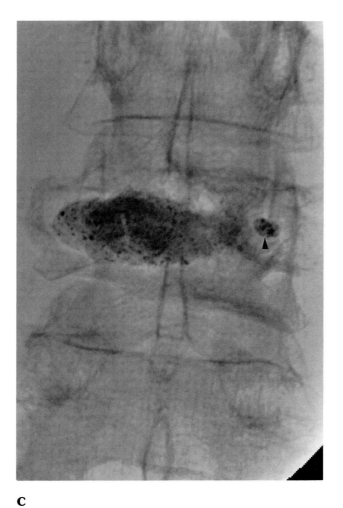

C

Figure 9.6 B. Lateral and C. AP views during contrast injection show extensive vertebral body tumor blush with subsequent filling of paravertebral veins (arrows). D, E, and F. Following pages.

206

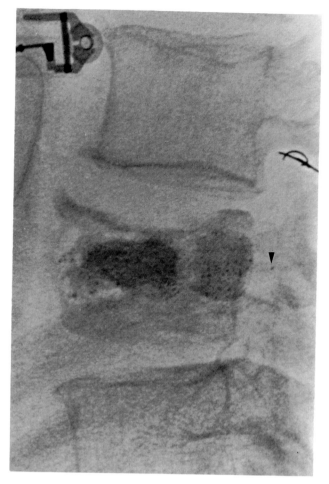

D

Figure 9.6 D. Lateral plain film following methyl methacrylate injection shows filling of the vertebral body with material. The methyl methacrylate was too viscous to pass into the vertebral veins. A methyl methacrylate plug (arrowheads) was pushed into the needle track during needle withdrawal to prevent hemorrhage. E and F. Following page.

PRIMARY BONE TUMORS

Hemangiomas

Hemangiomas are slowly-growing, benign hamartomas, usually discovered incidentally on radiographs or at autopsy. Most arise from the thoracic and lumbar vertebrae, but occasionally the cervical spine is involved. Although the majority of vertebral body hemangiomas remain clinically silent, they can produce pain and, rarely, spinal cord compression.[27–29] Impingement on the spinal cord may be secondary to epidural extension of the tumor, narrowing of the spinal canal from bony hypertrophy of the vertebra, and thickening of the neural arch, compression fracture of the involved vertebral body, or rarely, epidural hemorrhage.[30]

Hemangiomas that compress the spinal cord are most likely to arise from the midthoracic region, involve the entire vertebral body, extend into the neural arch, and have an extraosseous soft tissue component. Intrathecal contrast with CT evaluation or MRI will outline extension of the tumor into the epidural space.[27]

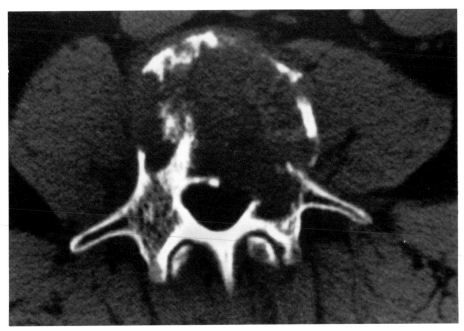

E

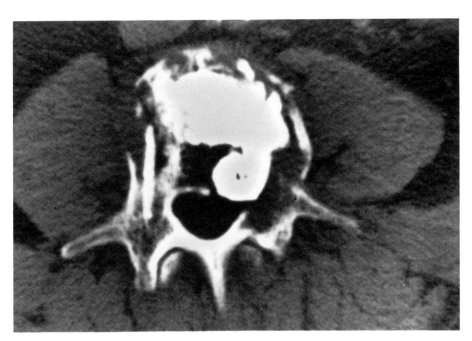

F

Figure 9.6 E. Pre- and F. post-treatment CT scans show methyl methacrylate within the tumor bed in addition to the needle track. No extravasation into the spinal canal is noted. His pain was markedly improved.

Plain radiographs demonstrate a characteristic vertebral trabeculation ("corduroy cloth") pattern or coarse "honeycomb" appearance within the vertebral body involved with a hemangioma. Most cases involve only the vertebral body, with 10–15% showing concomitant involvement of the posterior elements.[31] The overall density of the bone is also decreased. The bony cortex may be thinned or bulge outward, but the cortex usually remains intact unless extension into the paraspinal or epidural spaces occurs (Figure 9.7A). Axial computed tomography (CT) images will show the striations in cross-section, interspersed with a stroma of soft tissue or fat, giving the bone a "polka-dot" pattern.[30]

Unlike most bony lesions, the intraosseous portions of vertebral hemangiomas demonstrate a mottled, increased signal intensity on both T1 and T2 magnetic resonance (MR) images, with intervening, scattered low to isointense areas corresponding to the trabeculations.[32] Correlation with histopathologic sections indicates that the shortened T1 signal reflects the adipose-laden stroma interspersed between thin-walled vessels and bony trabeculae. The increased signal on T2 images is less easily explained, and may arise from the more cellular components of the tumor. Extraosseous portions of the tumor are composed mainly of angiomatous and fibrous elements, accounting for an intermediate soft tissue signal on T1 and an increased signal on T2.[27]

Selective angiography of asymptomatic hemangiomas shows minimal hypervascularity with no extension of the vascular blush outside the vertebra. In contrast, compressive lesions demonstrate dilated feeding arteries, extreme hypervascularity with dense, homogeneous staining, and opacification extending beyond the normal hemivertebral territory to involve the entire vertebral body, the paraspinal soft tissues, and/or the extradural space (Figure 9.7B).

The treatment of symptomatic vertebral hemangiomas is controversial. Therapeutic modalities include embolization, surgical resection, and radiotherapy.[33] Some investi-

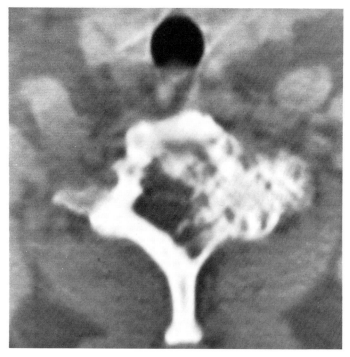

A

Figure 9.7 This 45-yr-old woman presented with neck pain. A. Axial CT scan through the C7 vertebral body shows a "honeycomb" expansile lesion of the left vertebral body, pedicle, transverse process, and lamina that is encroaching on the spinal canal. B and C. Following pages.

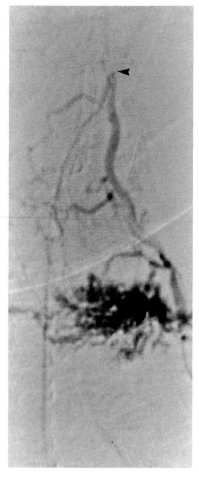

B

Figure 9.7 B. An angiogram of the ascending cervical artery shows dense tumor blush from multiple muscular branches. The normal tissue located distal to the tumor feeders was protected with a Gelfoam pledget (arrowhead). C. Following page.

gators feel the risk of radionecrosis outweighs the questionable benefits from radiotherapy.[34] Others consider radionecrosis unlikely at fractionated doses of less than 40 Gy, and have found good results in patients whose symptoms are slowly progressive or limited to pain.[35] With total vertebral involvement, laminectomy in conjunction with radiotherapy has demonstrated a 93% recovery rate without recurrence in one series.[36]

Embolization alone may alleviate acute neurologic decompensation from spinal cord compression from a vertebral hemangioma[28,35,37] but relief may only be transient.[38] Excellent pain palliation has been achieved with embolization alone, although no long-term studies are available.[28,39] The risk of vertebral body embolization is very low if the regional vascular supply to the cord is identified and avoided.[28,40] Arterial feeders may also arise from the thyrocervical and costocervical trunks and the superior intercostal arteries should be included in the angiographic evaluation for upper thoracic vertebral body lesions.

Most authors agree that surgical biopsy or resection should not be performed without preoperative embolization[28,29,33,38,40] (Figure 9.7C). In addition, if surgery is contraindicated, the patient may benefit from embolization prior to radiotherapy.

Any of the above described treatment modalities can result in collapse of the involved vertebral body, making stabilization of the vertebral column necessary. One

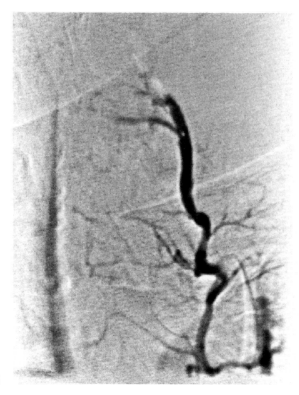

C

Figure 9.7 C. Following particulate embolization, no residual tumor blush is seen.

method used for stabilization involves intraoperative transosseous injection of methyl methacrylate, following percutaneous transarterial embolization.[41] Direct fluoroscopically guided puncture of the vertebral body with intraosseous injection of the acrylic cement has been described as a method to treat pain[42,43] and to stabilize a fracture related to a hemangiomatous lesion.[44] Although no long-term studies are available involving this technique, one short-term study showed a rapid regression of pain within 24 to 48 hr, with continued relief over a period of 11 to 17 months.[42]

Tumors with an inaccessible blood supply may also benefit from the use of a direct puncture technique for embolization. One recent report[45] indicated that instillation of alcohol using a percutaneous transpedicular approach showed promise in the treatment of compressive hemangiomas. These authors suggest that this approach may be preferable to a transarterial embolization. However, collapse of the affected vertebrae following devascularization can occur in these patients, requiring surgical stabilization of the vertebral column.

Aneurysmal Bone Cysts

Aneurysmal bone cysts are benign, expansile, vascular bone tumors occurring in children, adolescents, and young adults.[46] They comprise 1.4% of all bone tumors and occur in the spine in up to 20% of cases.[47,48] Patients usually present with complaints of pain and swelling, and vertebral lesions are often accompanied by paresis and sensory abnormalities of the extremities.[48,49] An expansile, osteolytic lesion with a well-defined transition zone and a peripheral shell of thin cortical bone is the classic plain film appearance.[46] Multiple internal septations are often present.[49] In 60% of patients with vertebral tumors, the epicenter is located in the neural arch with extension to the vertebral body via the pedicles[48] (Figure 9.4A). Encroachment on the spinal canal is common.[46] The lesion may also extend to contiguous vertebrae.

CT may show a thin rim of calcium not evident on plain radiographs. CT also helps to exclude calcified tumor matrix characteristic of other primary bone or soft tissue tumors. The extent of the tumor and its relationship to the adjacent thecal sac and neural structures is well demonstrated by MR imaging (Figure 9.4B), while both CT and MR imaging may show fluid-fluid levels within the lesion because of the layering of solid blood components.[46] Gadolinium-enhanced MR imaging may aid in differentiation from other fluid-fluid level containing tumors by demonstrating enhancement of internal septations.[48]

Arteriography (Figure 9.4C) often shows arteriovenous shunting, diffuse tumor staining in the late arterial phase, and indistinct pools of contrast in cystic areas.[50] Yet, none of these angiographic findings are necessarily characteristic of an aneurysmal bone cyst,[47] which often lack a true major feeding vessel. A distinct arterial supply to and venous drainage from the tumor may or may not be identified.[39,47]

Complete surgical excision of the aneurysmal bone cyst is the most effective, and preferred, method of treatment although such an approach is problematic in difficult locations such as the sacrum, spine, or pelvis or in large lesions. When excision of the tumor would cause severe disability, curettage (intralesional excision) with bone grafting may be performed. Although an overall recurrence rate of 19% following curettage has been reported,[49] lesions in the vertebrae have a lower rate than those in the long bones. Radiotherapy has been used to treat inoperable lesions or to alleviate pain, but tumor recurrence and complications such as radiation induced myelopathy and sarcomatous change render it a less desirable option.[39,47,51]

Transarterial embolization has been described as preparatory for surgical resection[46,47,50,52] (Figure 9.4D), for treatment of clinical symptoms,[39,53] and as definitive therapy.[46,53–55] Embolization should be considered as the treatment of choice when the extent of involvement by the tumor is such that total excision or radical curettage is too risky, reconstruction is difficult or, operative and perioperative morbidity could involve neural elements or compromise the stability of the spine.[54]

The availability of an appropriately sized vascular supply and the identification of spinal cord feeders determines the feasibility of transarterial embolization. In several reports[46,50,52.54] presurgical embolization with polyvinyl alcohol or Gelfoam aided the adequate excision of the tumor by decreasing blood loss and improving visualization. In several small series where vertebral tumors were treated palliatively with transarterial embolization with polyvinyl alcohol particles,[39,46,54] Gelfoam sponge,[53] ethanol,[39] or a combination of agents,[56] pain control and partial or complete regression of the tumor occurred in the majority of patients.[39,46,56,57] Regression was determined by cessation of growth or tumor shrinkage, and radiographic evidence of progressive ossification. In addition to particulate and liquid embolic agents, the use of coils has also been described. Prior to tumor embolization, coils have been placed distal to vessels supplying the tumor in order to protect the normal, distal vascular bed.[39,52,56] Coils have also been used for proximal vessel occlusion following tumor embolization to enhance the extent and duration of the peripheral arterial occlusion.[39,53,56] The presence of coils has been known to interfere with attempts at repeat embolization[39, 54] by limiting access to the main feeding vessel.

The potential problem caused by coils can be avoided by using Gelfoam pledgets in place of coils. The microcatheter tip is placed at the site of embolization and flushed with heparinized saline. A Gelfoam sponge pad is flattened with the cylindrical portion of a 10-cc syringe and 1-mm-wide by 3-mm-long strips are cut with a razor blade. The pledgets are tightly rolled and placed within the Luer-lock stem of a 1-cc syringe filled with contrast. The syringe is attached to the hub and the pledget is quickly injected into the microcatheter. Continued pressure on the syringe results in expulsion of the pledget into the vessel, evidenced by the appearance of contrast and the sudden ease of injection. If the injection is not performed quickly, the pledget can swell in the microcatheter, resulting in catheter blockage or rupture. Multiple pledgets can be injected until vessel occlusion is seen. Dissolution of the pledget occurs within several days to 6 wks, reestablishing flow to the excluded territory.

Percutaneous injection of aneurysmal bone cysts involving the pelvis and the humerus has been reported.[52] The cystic cavities were filled with Ethibloc (Ethicon, Hamburg, Germany), a radiopaque fibrosing agent composed of alcohol and vegetable protein. Follow-up studies demonstrated tumor shrinkage and progressive ossification. We have not seen this approach reported in the treatment of vertebral tumors. While direct puncture may seem tempting in patients with limited arterial access, one must be mindful of the potentially disastrous complications if the sclerosing material were to leak into the spinal canal.

Embolization of aneurysmal bone cysts using particulate agents is associated with a morbidity of 0–2%. The complication rate increases when liquid agents are used, particularly ethanol.[56] Complications associated with the use of ethanol consist mainly of inducing ischemia in adjacent neural structures or causing tissue necrosis. Local pain, fever, and nausea have also been observed in the first few days after any embolization procedure.[39] Some authors[54] advocate the use of provocative testing with sodium amytal and the monitoring of somatosensory evoked potentials prior to and during all embolizations. We have not found such testing and monitoring necessary when particles alone are used for embolization. Because excellent results have been reported with the use of particulate agents, we do not feel that ethanol or tissue adhesives are appropriate first-choice agents.

Remission of clinical symptoms generally occurs within days to weeks after embolization, with evidence of ossification apparent within 2–4 months.[39,52] The reappearance of pain is a major predictor of recurrent tumor growth[39] and additional embolizations may be performed as necessary.

Other Primary Bone Tumors

Other rare tumors, such as osteoblastomas,[58] osteoid osteomas,[59] hemangiopericytomas,[60] and giant cell tumors[61] may exhibit vascularity, and can be embolized in a similar manner as hemangiomas or aneurysmal bone cysts.[60–63]

METASTATIC BONE TUMORS

Certain metastatic tumors to the vertebral axis are highly vascular, particularly primary renal (Figure 9.8A–H) or thyroid malignancies. Other metastatic lesions may also exhibit varying degrees of tumor neovascularity such as lesions that originate from the breast (Figure 9.5) or liver, and squamous cell carcinoma primaries. As with primary bone tumors, presurgical embolization facilitates surgery by devascularizing the tumor bed, decreasing blood loss, and improving visibility at the surgical site, thus allowing for a more thorough resection.

Many reports on the surgical resection of vascular metastatic tumors to the vertebral body recommend preoperative embolization to decrease blood loss.[61,64–67] In one series, the major perioperative complications were related to excessive blood loss in patients without preoperative embolization.[65]

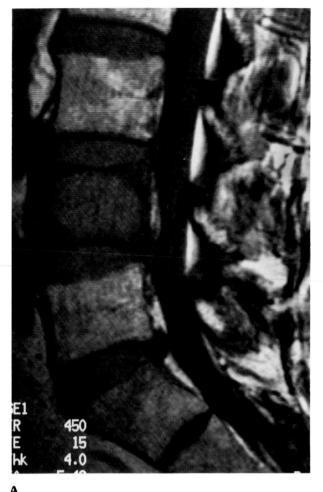

A

B

Figure 9.8 This 57-yr-old male presented with left leg pain. A. T1-weighted MR image shows hypointensity of the L4 vertebral body consistent with metastasis from known renal cell carcinoma. B. Selective injection of the L4 lumbar arteries shows a dense tumor stain fed mainly by proximal branches of the left L4 artery. The left L4 artery was selectively catheterized with a microcatheter and embolization was performed with PVA particles (150–250 μm) suspended in contrast and combined with sodium tetradecyl sulfate in a 2:1 mixture. C, D, E, F, G, and H. Following pages.

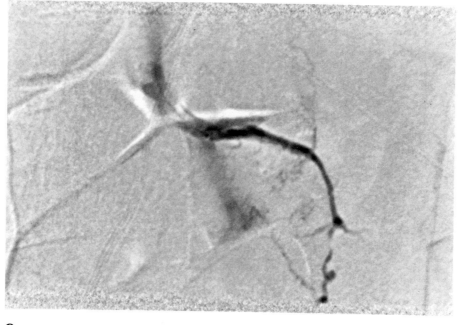

C

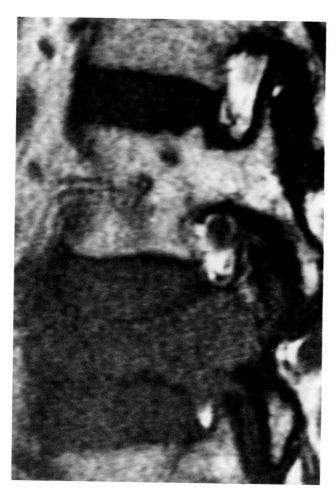

D

Figure 9.8 C. The postembolization angiogram shows minimal residual blush. Although the pain was alleviated, it returned 9 months later. D. A repeat MR study showed collapse of the L4 vertebral body. At angiography, the L4 lumbar vessels could not be cannulated. E, F, G, and H. Following pages.

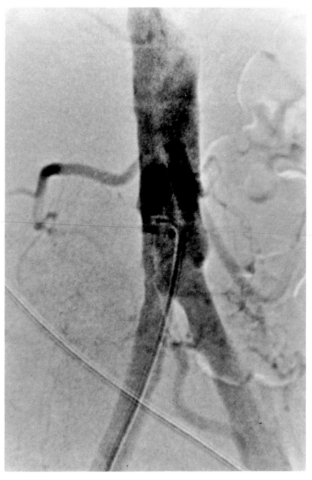

E

Figure 9.8 E. Aortography showed occlusion at the vessel origins presumably from the previous embolization. F, G, and H. Following pages.

Reports attempting to quantify the actual amount of blood loss are few. In one study,[66] 24 patients underwent surgical decompression of vertebral body metastases. Twenty patients were treated with preoperative embolization and had an average blood loss of 1,850 cc at surgery. The four patients without preoperative embolization had an average blood loss of greater than 3,500 cc. Olerud et al.[67] found that the average blood loss in surgery performed after embolization was decreased by two-thirds. In another report,[61] the estimated blood loss in seven of nine surgical procedures in patients who were embolized preoperatively ranged from 300 to 800 ml. No transfusions were required in these patients. More extensive resections in two other patients necessitated postoperative transfusion despite preoperative embolization. In this series, embolization with microfibrillar collagen (20–180 μm in size) was used as the embolic agent. We have found that adequate embolization can be performed with particles 150–250 μm in size with similar beneficial effects, while lowering the risk of compromising circulation to the spinal cord.

In patients in whom surgery is not an option, embolization has been shown to be an effective palliative measure to aid in pain control, relieve nerve root or cord compression[68] and slow tumor growth. In some instances, increased calcification follow-

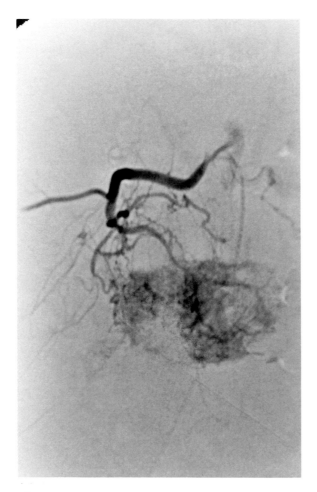

F

Figure 9.8 F. Indirect supply to the L4 vertebral body was noted from the right L3 lumbar artery. A provocative test using lidocaine, 30 mg was performed and no neurologic changes were elicited. **G** and **H**. Following pages.

ing embolization suggesting partial bone healing has been demonstrated.[69] As with hemangiomas, using a direct puncture technique to instill methyl methacrylate into the tumor has resulted in pain reduction in 80% of patients in one study[70] and in 73% of patients in another[71] (Figure 9.6). CT-guided percutaneous alcohol injection has also been reported to be effective at reducing pain, but vertebral body collapse may occur.

The embolization techniques for treatment of metastatic lesions are similar to those described for primary bone tumors. The anterior spinal artery must be identified and avoided when performing transarterial embolization. In presurgical cases, embolization is performed only with particulate agents. Surgical removal of the tumor should be done as soon as possible after the embolization procedure to minimize the recanalization of embolized vessels, or the opening of collateral arteries. For palliative measures, a tumoricidal or chemotherapeutic agent may be mixed with other embolic materials or used alone to aid in tumor shrinkage.

In those cases where the tumor and spinal cord share the same arterial supply, direct puncture embolization may be effective.[72] For preoperative lesions, liquid or par-

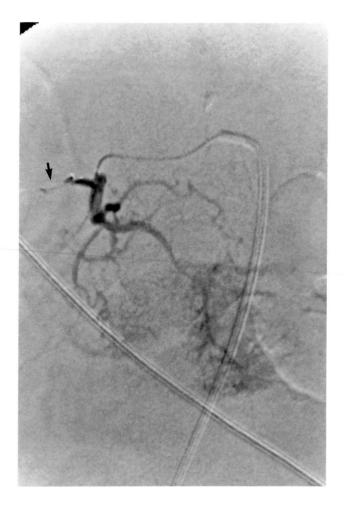

G

Figure 9.8 G. The muscular branch was protectively embolized with microcoils (arrow), prior to proximal embolization with PVA particles (45 to 150 μm) suspended in contrast combined with absolute ethanol in a 1:1 mixture. H. Following page.

ticulate agents or soft embolic materials such as NBCA, should be used so as to not interfere with the surgical resection. Direct puncture and installation of methyl methacrylate (vertebroplasty) to stabilize compression fractures and reduce pain has been very successful.[70,71,73] Needle placement can be done under fluoroscopic control[26] or CT guidance.[42] Neural and vascular structures need to be identified and avoided. Prior to embolization, an injection of contrast should be performed to evaluate for reflux of contrast into the spinal circulation or extravasation into the surrounding tissues. If either of these two findings is identified, the needle should be repositioned and the contrast injection repeated.

A potential complication associated with embolization includes a rapid increase in the tumor size secondary to swelling. Acute tumoral edema causing neurologic dysfunction may necessitate immediate surgical decompression. In those patients embolized for pain palliation, vertebral body collapse can occur over several weeks. Certain precautions, such as avoiding activities that increase axial loading of the spine or the use of external bracing, should be employed.

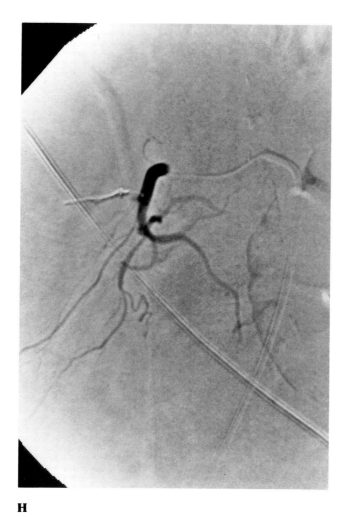

H

Figure 9.8 H. No residual tumor blush is seen. The patient's radicular pain resolved.

SUMMARY

In summary, this chapter outlines the potential uses for embolization techniques in the treatment of various vertebral body tumors. It does not pretend to be an exhaustive compilation of all the literature previously published concerning this topic. Instead, it should serve as an impetus to further discussion and evaluation of these lesions, to improve embolization techniques and to promote outstanding patient care.

REFERENCES

1. Latchaw RE, Gold LH: Polyvinyl foam embolization of vascular and neoplastic lesions of the head, neck, and spine. *Radiology* 131:669–679, 1979.
2. Valvanis A: Preoperative embolization of the head and neck: indications, patient selection, goals and precautions. *AJNR* 7:943–952, 1986.
3. Russell EJ: Functional angiography of the head and neck. *AJNR* 7:927–936, 1986.
4. Mehta BA, Jack CR Jr, Boulos RS, et al: Interventional neuroradiology: Henry Ford Hospital experience with transcatheter embolization of vascular lesions in the head, neck, and spine. *Henry Ford Hosp Med J* 34:19–30, 1986.

5. Platzbecker H, Dohler K: Embolization in the head and neck region. *Acta Radiologica Suppl* 377:25–26, 1991.

6. Jensen ME: Endovascular treatment of vascular pathology of the head and neck. *Semin Intervent Radiol* 11:21–36, 1994.

7. Crock HV, Yoshizawa H: *The Blood Supply of the Vertebral Column and Spinal Cord in Man*. New York, Springer-Verlag, 1977.

8. Rothman RH, Simone FA: *The Spine*, ed 2. Philadelphia, WB Saunders, 1982, pp 39–48.

9. Gray H: *Gray's Anatomy*, ed 35. London, Longman, 1975, pp 646, 839–840, 700–704.

10. Netter FH: *The CIBA Collection of Medical Illustrations. Volume 1, Nervous System, Part 1, Anatomy and Physiology*. West Caldwell, NJ, CIBA, 1986, pp 64–66.

11. Lundell C, Kadir S: Inferior vena cava and spinal veins. In Kadir S: *Atlas of Normal and Variant Angiographic Anatomy*. Philadelphia, WB Saunders, 1991, pp 187–202.

12. Greenberg J: *Handbook of Head and Spine Trauma*. New York, Marcel Dekker, 1993, p 227.

13. Doppman JL, Girton M, Oldfield EH: Spinal wada test. *Radiology* 161:319–321, 1986.

14. Berenstein A, Kricheff II: Catheter and material selection for transarterial embolization: technical considerations. I. Catheters. *Radiology* 132:619–630, 1979.

15. Berenstein A, Kricheff II: Catheter and material selection for transarterial embolization: technical considerations. II. Materials. *Radiology* 132:631–639, 1979.

16. Kunstlinger F, Brunelle F, Chaumont P, et al: Vascular occlusive agents. *AJR* 136:151–156, 1981.

17. Dion JE: Principles and methodology. In Vinuela F, Halbach VV, Dion JE (eds): *Interventional Neuroradiology*. New York, Raven Press, 1992, pp 1–15.

18. Lasjaunias P, Berenstein A: Technical aspects of surgical neuroangiography. In Lasjaunias P, Berenstein A: *Surgical Neuroangiography*, Vol 1. Berlin, Springer-Verlag, 1987, pp 1–56.

19. Kerber CW: Catheter therapy: fluoroscopic monitoring of deliberate embolic occlusion. *Radiology* 125:538–540, 1977.

20. Kato T, Ryosuke N, Mori H, et al: Arterial chemoembolization with mitomycin C microcapsules in the treatment of primary or secondary carcinoma of the kidney, liver, bone and intrapelvic organs. *Cancer* 48:674–680, 1981.

21. Courtheoux P, Alachkar F, Casasco A, et al: Chemoembolization of lumbar spine metastases. A preliminary study. *J Neuroradiol* 12:151–162, 1985.

22. Kerber CW: Flow-controlled therapeutic embolization: a physiologic and safe technique. *AJR* 134:557–561, 1980.

23. Seeger JF, Gabrielsen TO, Latchaw RE: Some technique-dependent patterns of collateral flow during cerebral angiography. *Neuroradiology* 8:149–155, 1974.

24. Theron J, Cosgrove R, Melanson D, et al: Embolization with temporary balloon occlusion of the internal carotid or vertebral arteries. *Neuroradiology* 28:246–253, 1986.

25. Casasco A, Herbreteau D, Houdart E, et al: Devascularization of craniofacial tumors by percutaneous tumor puncture. *AJNR* 15:1233–1239, 1994.

26. Laredo JD, Bellaiche L, Hamze B, et al: Current status of musculoskeletal interventional radiology. *Radiol Clin North Am* 32:377–398, 1994.

27. Laredo JD, Reizine D, Bard M, et al: Vertebral hemangiomas: radiologic evaluation. *Radiology* 161:183–189, 1986.

28. Raco A, Ciappetta P, Artico MN, et al: Vertebral hemangiomas with cord compression: the role of embolization in five cases. *Surg Neurol* 34:164–168, 1990.

29. Picard L, Bracard S, Roland J, et al: [Embolization of vertebral hemangiomas. Technique–indications–results.] *Neurochirurgie* 35:289–293, 1989. (French)

30. Schnyder P, Fankhauser H, Mansouri B: Computed tomography in spinal hemangioma with cord compression. Report of two cases. *Skeletal Radiol* 15:372–375, 1986.

31. Youchum TR, Lile RL, Schultz GE, et al: Acquired spinal stenosis secondary to an expanding thoracic vertebral hemangioma. *Spine* 18:299–305, 1993.

32. Ross JS, Masaryk TJ, Modic MT, et al: Vertebral hemangiomas: MR imaging. *Radiology* 165:165–169, 1987.

33. Fox MW, Onofrio BM: The natural history and management of symptomatic and asymptomatic vertebral hemangiomas. *J Neurosurg* 78:36–45, 1993.

34. Benati A, Da Pian R, Mazza C, et al: Preoperative embolization of a vertebral hemangioma compressing the spinal cord. *Neuroradiology* 7:181–183, 1974.

35. Gross CE, Hodge CJ, Binet EF, et al: Relief of spinal block during embolization of a vertebral body hemangioma. *J Neurosurg* 45:404–406, 1976.

36. Nguyen JP, Djindjian J, Pavlovitch JM, et al: [Vertebral hemangiomas with neurologic symptoms. Treatment. Results of the "Société Française de Neuro-Chirurgie" series.] *Neurochirurgie* 35:299–303, 1989. (French)

37. Heckster REM, Luyendijk W, Tan TI: Spinal cord compression caused by vertebral hemangioma relieved by percutaneous catheter embolization. *Neuroradiology* 3:160–164, 1972.

38. Nguyen JP, Djindjian M, Gaston A, et al: Vertebral hemangiomas presenting with neurologic symptoms. *Surg Neurol* 27:391–397, 1987.

39. DeCristofaro R, Biagini R, Boriani S, et al: Selective arterial embolization in the treatment of aneurysmal bone cyst and angioma of bone. *Skeletal Radiol* 21:523–527, 1992.

40. Smith TP, Koci T, Mehringer CM, et al: Transarterial embolization of vertebral hemangioma. *JVIR* 4:681–685, 1993.

41. Nicola N, Lins E: Vertebral hemangioma: retrograde embolization-stabilization with methyl methacrylate. *Surg Neurol* 27:481–486, 1987.

42. Gangi A, Kastler BA, Dietemann JL: Percutaneous vertebroplasty guided by a combination of CT and fluoroscopy. *AJNR* 15:83–86, 1994.

43. Galibert P, Deramond H: [A new method for the treatment of some spinal lesions. Percutaneous acrylic vertebroplasty.] *Chirurgie* 116:326–335, 1990. (French)

44. Galibert P, Deramond H, Rosat P, et al: [A treatment method for certain spinal angiomas: percutaneous vertebroplasty with acrylic cement.] *Neurochirurgie* 33:166–168, 1987.

45. Heiss JD, Doppman JL, Oldfield EH: Brief report: relief of spinal cord compression from vertebral hemangioma by intralesional injection of absolute ethanol. *NEJM* 331:508–511, 1994.

46. Cory DA, Fritsch SA, Cohen MD, et al: Aneurysmal bone cysts: imaging findings and embolotherapy. *AJR* 153:369–373, 1989.

47. Dysart SH, Swengel RM, van Dam BE: Aneurysmal bone cyst of a thoracic vertebra. *Spine* 17:846–848, 1992.

48. Caro PA, Mandell GA, Stanton RP: Aneurysmal bone cyst of the spine in children. MRI imaging at 0.5 tesla. *Pediatr Radiol* 21:114–116, 1991.

49. DeDios AM, Bond JR, Shives TC, et al: Aneurysmal bone cyst: a clinicopathologic study of 238 cases. *Cancer* 69:2921–2931, 1992.

50. Disch SP, Grubb RL, Gado MH, et al: Aneurysmal bone cyst of the cervicothoracic spine: computed tomography evaluation of the value of preoperative embolization. *Neurosurgery* 19:290–293, 1986.

51. Adamsbaum C, Kalifa G, Seringe R, et al: Direct Ethibloc injection in benign bone cysts: preliminary report on four patients. *Skeletal Radiol* 22:317–320, 1993.

52. Konya A, Szendroi M: Aneurysmal bone cysts treated by superselective embolization. *Skeletal Radiol* 21:167–172, 1992.

53. Chuang VP, Soo CS, Wallace S, et al: Arterial occlusion: management of giant cell tumor and aneurysmal bone cyst. *AJR* 136:1127–1130, 1981.

54. DeRosa GP, Graziano GP, Scott J: Arterial embolization of aneurysmal bone cyst of the spine. *J Bone Joint Surg* 72A:777–780, 1990.

55. Boriani S, DeCristofaro R, Ruggieri P, et al: Selective arterial embolization in the treatment of lesions of the musculoskeletal apparatus. Chirurgia Degli Organi di Movimento. 76:99–112, 1991.

56. Rossi C, Ricci S, Boriani S et al: Percutaneous transcatheter arterial embolization of bone and soft tissue tumors. *Skeletal Radiol* 19:555–560, 1990.

57. Szendroi M, Cser I, Konya A, et al: Aneurysmal bone cyst. A review of 52 primary and 16 secondary cases. *Arch Orthop Trauma Surg* 111:318–322, 1992.

58. Kroon HM, Schurmans J: Osteoblastoma: clinical and radiologic findings in 98 new cases. *Radiology* 175:783–790, 1990.

59. Crouzet G, Mnif, Vasdev A, et al: [Osteoid osteoma of the spine: radiological aspects and value of arteriography. Four cases.] *J Neuroradiol* 16:145–159, 189. (French)

60. Ciappetta P, Celli P, Palma L, et al: Intraspinal hemangiopericytomas: report of two cases and review of the literature. *Spine* 10:27–31, 1985.

61. Broaddus WC, Grady MS, Delashaw JB Jr, et al: Preoperative superselective arteriolar embolization: a new approach to enhance resectability of spinal tumors. *Neurosurgery* 27:755–759, 1990.

62. Cizmeli MO, Ilgit ET, Ulug H, et al: A giant paraspinal hemangiopericytoma and its preoperative embolization. *Neuroradiology* 34:81–83, 1992.

63. Boriani S, Capanna R, Donati D, et al: Osteoblastoma of the spine. *Clin Orthop Relat Res* 278:37–45, 1992.

64. King GJ, Kostuik JP, McBroom RJ, et al: Surgical management of metastatic renal carcinoma of the spine. *Spine* 16:263–271, 1991.

65. Sundaresan N, Choi IS, Hughes JE, et al: Treatment of spinal metastases from kidney cancer by presurgical embolization and resection. *J Neurosurg* 73:548–554, 1990.

66. Gellad FE, Sadato N, Numaguchi Y, et al: Vascular metastatic lesions of the spine: preoperative embolization. *Radiology* 176:683–686, 1990.

67. Olerud C, Johsson H Jr, Lofberg AM, et al: Embolization of spinal metastases reduces preoperative blood loss. 21 patients operated on for renal cell carcinoma. *Acta Orthop Scand* 64:9–12, 1993.

68. O'Reilly GV, Kleefield J, Klein LA, et al: Embolization of solitary spinal metastases from renal cell carcinoma: alternative therapy for spinal cord or nerve root compression. *Surg Neurol* 31:268–271, 1989.

69. Soo CS, Wallace S, Chuang VP, et al: Lumbar artery embolization in cancer patients. *Radiology* 145:655–659, 1982.

70. Kaemmerlen P, Thiesse P, Bouvard H, et al: [Percutaneous vertebroplasty in the treatment of metastases. Technic and results.] *J Radiologie* 70:557–562, 1989. (French)

71. Weill A, Chiras J, Simon JM, et al: Spinal metastases: indications for and results of percutaneous injection of acrylic surgical cement. *Radiology* 199:241–247, 1996.

72. Chiras J, Cognard C, Rose M, et al: Percutaneous injection of an alcoholic embolizing emulsion as an alternative preoperative embolization for spine tumor. *AJNR* 14:1113–1117, 1993.

73. Cotten A, Dewatre F, Cortet B, et al: Percutaneous vertebroplasty for osteolytic metastases and myeloma: effects of the percentage of lesion filling and the leakage of methyl methacrylate at clinical follow-up. *Radiology* 200:525–530, 1996.

Endovascular Stents
and Stent-Grafts in the
Management of Thoracic
Aortic Dissections
and Aneurysms

Michael D. Dake
Charles P. Semba
Stephen T. Kee

The results of surgical treatment of thoracic aortic aneurysms and aortic dissection have steadily improved over the past 20 to 30 years due to advances in diagnostic and surgical techniques.[1-6] Despite this progress, a less invasive approach to treatment is desirable, especially in high-risk patients. Patients with severe neurologic, cardiovascular, pulmonary, or renal dysfunction may not tolerate aortic replacement under general anesthesia and extracorporeal bypass. Transluminal endovascular stent or stent-graft placement offers an alternative treatment that may prove to be less invasive, expensive, and morbid, with a shorter hospital recuperation time than traditional operative therapy.

Recent medical literature documents the effectiveness of uncovered vascular stents for the treatment of stenotic disease involving the coronary, renal, and brachiocephalic arteries.[7-11] Stents have proved especially beneficial in managing hemodynamically significant angioplasty-induced dissection flaps.[12] Similarly, the clinical feasibility, safety, and utility of endovascular stent-grafts have been documented for the management of abdominal aortic, descending thoracic aorta, and subclavian artery aneurysms, as well as arteriovenous fistulae and femoral occlusive disease.[13-17]

The development of stents and stent-grafts provides two more tools for dealing with the perplexing complexities of a variety of thoracic aortic pathologies. In this chapter, the use of endovascular techniques in the management of thoracic aortic aneurysms and aortic dissections will be explored. Much of the clinical experience discussed is preliminary. However, these initial results suggest that these less invasive procedures may provide safe, effective therapy for highly selected patients who have limited surgical opportunities and may play significant roles in the future management of complicated thoracic aortic disease.

ENDOVASCULAR TREATMENT
OF THORACIC AORTIC ANEURYSMS

An aneurysm of the thoracic aorta is a life-threatening condition. It occurs when there is progressive damage to the medial layer of the aorta leading to degenerative weakening of the vessel wall and subsequent aortic dilatation and aneurysm formation. The most common cause for medial injury is atherosclerosis. Although the most frequent location of a thoracic aortic aneurysm is the descending aorta, isolated aneurysmal involvement of the ascending aorta or transverse aortic arch or extension of the disease process to the entire thoracic aorta or thoracoabdominal segment is not uncommon.[18] Aneurysmal dilatation of the thoracic aorta is usually asymptomatic, often attracting initial clinical attention when it is serendipitously discovered as an unsuspected mass on a routine chest radiograph. When symptoms do occur, they may be related to leakage from or rupture of the aneurysm, or progressive enlargement of the aneurysm with associated compression of adjacent tissues.[19] As many as 20% of patients with an aneurysm of the thoracic aorta either present with or are discovered to have, a second aneurysm, frequently affecting the abdominal aorta.

Rupture of a thoracic aortic aneurysm is catastrophic and almost uniformly fatal. Studies of the natural history of untreated thoracic aortic aneurysms estimate a 50% 5-yr and 70% 10-yr mortality rate.[20] The 5-yr survival for these patients is worse than that reported for patients with untreated abdominal aortic aneurysms.[21,22] Actual rupture of a thoracic aortic aneurysm is responsible for nearly half of the mortality.[1,21] Other causes of fatality are usually related to coexisting medical disease, principally hypertension and diffuse cardiovascular pathology.

Conventional treatment for a thoracic aortic aneurysm is surgical repair. Operative therapy is urgently indicated if an aneurysm is 6 cm or greater in diameter (especially when serial imaging studies show progressive enlargement of the aneurysm), there is sudden onset of aortic regurgitation, or acute chest or back pain develops. Traditional surgery involves resection and replacement of the aneurysm with prosthetic graft material. If the aneurysm originates distal to the left subclavian artery and terminates above the celiac trunk, surgical resection can often be performed without the need for extracorporeal circulation.[2,23] However, in elective operations performed by experienced cardiothoracic surgeons on patients with good cardiac reserve, the surgical mortality rate is still 12–15%.[2,3] Even when patients are excellent surgical candidates, there is considerable morbidity, with paraplegia reported in 5–12%.[2,3,23] The difficult nature of the surgical challenge is underscored by reports documenting an operative mortality rate of 50% or greater in patients with significant cardiopulmonary disease or those requiring emergency treatment.[1,3]

The concept of transluminal placement of a prosthetic tube within the thoracic aorta to serve as a permanent conduit to exclude an aneurysm was first investigated by Alexis Carrel in 1912.[24] Although other investigators had experimented with metal and glass tubes within the femoral arteries and abdominal aorta, Carrel was the first to test the feasibility of permanent intubation of the thoracic aorta as a means of excluding an aneurysm. After surgically exposing the thoracic aorta in a canine model, he transluminally introduced various tubes and secured the implants with ligatures. Of 11 animals, there were 9 primary successes (7 in the glass tube group and 2 in the aluminum tube group). Survival ranged from 5 to 97 days.

In 1969, Dotter coined the term "stent-graft" in a report describing his investigations with transluminally placed endovascular devices in a series of canine superficial femoral arteries.[25] His work established the practicality of this technique. A number of investigators followed his proposal with feasibility research in animal models of abdominal aortic aneurysms.[26–31] In 1991, the first clinical cases of endovascular stent-graft placement for abdominal aortic aneurysms were reported by Parodi and colleagues.[13] They used polyester graft material sutured to a balloon-expandable stent that was deployed above the aneurysm.

Our initial experience with transluminal endovascular stent-graft technology suggests that it can provide a safe and effective treatment modality to manage highly selected patients with aneurysms of the descending thoracic aorta.[14] Over a 3-yr period, we have placed endovascular stent-grafts in 54 patients with descending thoracic aortic aneurysms. Our first patient was treated in July 1992. All of the patients had aneurysms originating distal to the left subclavian artery and terminating above the celiac axis. All were high-risk patients for traditional surgical repair and most had undergone prior cardiac or aortic surgery. Aortic pathology was due to a variety of etiologies; however, atherosclerosis was responsible for most of the aneurysms.

Each case has its own unique anatomic considerations, and consequently all the stent-graft devices were custom fabricated to address each patient's particular aneurysm morphology and aortic dimensions. However, the basic principles outlined below apply to all cases.

Clinical and Anatomic Considerations

Thoracic aortic aneurysms caused by atherosclerosis, trauma, dissection, infection, and prior surgery have been treated using endovascular techniques. To assess the suitability of the aneurysm for treatment with a stent-graft, all patients at our institution undergo an extensive preprocedural workup, including aortography and spiral computed tomography (CT) with three-dimensional reconstructions.

The spiral CT data allow measurement of the necessary dimensions to custom-build the prosthesis, including its diameter (based upon the proximal and distal neck dimensions) and its overall length. Conventional aortography is used to help evaluate the relationship of the aneurysm to the left subclavian and celiac arteries, the relative degree of aortic arch curvature, and the size and tortuosity of the iliac and femoral arteries.

An aneurysm that arises 15–20 mm distal to the origin of the left subclavian artery is highly desirable to ensure secure anchoring of the stent-graft without inadvertently covering the ostium of this vessel. If this distance is less than ideal, a more favorable proximal neck may be artificially created by surgically transposing the left subclavian artery onto the left common carotid artery prior to the stent-graft procedure. This has been required in 4 (7.4%) of the first 54 cases at our institution. Similarly, it is optimal for the aneurysm to terminate 15–20 mm proximal to the origin of the celiac artery to avoid occluding this vessel. To limit unnecessary exclusion of intercostal arteries, the overall length of the stent-graft is kept to a minimum.

If the size of the pelvic vessels is not sufficient to accommodate introduction of the stent-graft delivery system (less than 9 mm), an alternative vascular access is obtained via the distal infrarenal abdominal aorta. After surgically exposing the infrarenal aorta through a retroperitoneal approach, a noncalcified, relatively normal segment of the vessel is identified by digital palpation. A purse string suture is introduced around the anticipated catheterization site and the aorta is subsequently punctured using the standard Seldinger technique. After introduction of a stiff guidewire, the delivery system is introduced over a tapered dilator. This approach has been required in 6 (11.1%) of our 54 cases because of small or otherwise inadequate iliac and/or common femoral arteries.

Technical Considerations

The technical principles of endovascular stent-grafting, irrespective of the clinical application, can be simplified into three components: stents, graft materials, and delivery systems. The overall goal of the initial work has been to develop a strategy that allows placement of standard surgical graft material into the aorta to exclude blood flow into the aneurysm using interventional radiology techniques.

Stents

In general, the stent serves as a method for securing graft material into the normal proximal and distal aortic necks. Stents are currently manufactured from stainless steel, nitinol, or tantalum. Stents can be divided into two basic designs: balloon-expandable, such as the Palmaz stent (Johnson & Johnson Interventional Systems

Inc., Warren, NJ) and self-expanding stents, such as the Wallstent (Schneider USA Inc., Minneapolis, MN) and the modified Z-stent (Cook Inc., Bloomington, IN). Balloon-expandable stents are mounted on an angioplasty catheter and expanded by balloon inflation, while self-expanding stents return to a preformed shape and diameter when released from inside a constraining sheath.

After extensive testing in experimental animal models, self-expanding stents appear to be better suited for use in the thoracic aorta. This, in part, is due to the large diameters of the proximal and distal necks of thoracic aortic aneurysms, which limit the use of balloon-expanded stents. In our experience, the mean diameter of the proximal neck measured 36 mm. This is greater than the maximum diameter (25 mm) valvuloplasty balloon catheters currently marketed in the United States. In addition, as a balloon inflates within the thoracic aorta, the force associated with blood flow in the aortic arch may cause migration of the inflated balloon and misplacement of the stent-graft device. Self-expanding devices offer less resistance to flow in the aorta and can be designed to fit the vessel diameters required.

The stents that we have chosen to use consist of 0.020-inch surgical-grade stainless steel wire formed into Z-shaped elements (Figure 10.1). Individual stent bodies are 2.5 cm in length, with diameters ranging from 24 to 45 mm. On the basis of dimensions obtained from the spiral CT data, several stent bodies can be sewn together to obtain the necessary total length. Polypropylene suture (5-0) is used to attach individual stent bodies together. The Z-stent endoskeleton is used to support the full length of graft material required to bridge the aneurysm from the proximal to the distal neck. The subjacent metallic framework supports the polyester graft to avoid kinking, buckling, torsion, or collapse of the graft within the aneurysm. The Z-stent design appears to provide the appropriate hoop strength and high expansion ratio required to anchor the graft material into position and seal it snugly against the neck of the aneurysm. No hooks or anchoring wires are required to prevent migration. The mean stent-graft length used in our 54 patients was 10.2 cm.

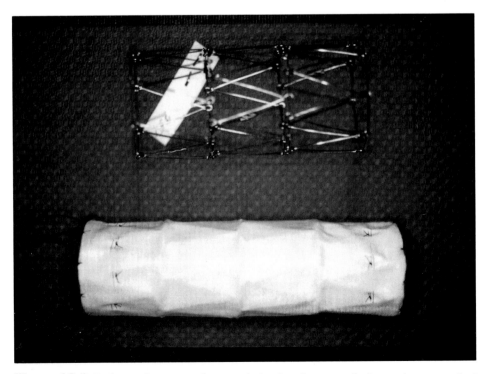

Figure 10.1 Endovascular Z-stent framework (top) and stent-graft (bottom) composed of Z-stent endoskeleton covered with woven polyester graft material.

Graft Material

The graft material used for our stent-grafts is a woven polyester (Cooley Veri-Soft, Meadox Medicals, Inc., Oakland, NJ). The crimps in the graft material are ironed out with a standard laundry iron to reduce the overall diameter of the prostheses. Woven polyester graft material is relatively nonporous and thin and resists radial stretching. A single piece of tubular graft material is cut to the appropriate length and secured around the Z-stent framework with multiple 5-0 polypropylene interrupted sutures. The cut edges of the graft material are heat-sealed to prevent fraying during handling and insertion. After fabrication of the stent-graft is complete, the entire device is gas-sterilized with ethylene oxide.

Delivery System

The delivery system we employ consists of four components: an 80-cm 24-Fr Teflon sheath (Desilet-Hoffman, Cook, Inc.) with an external hemostatic valve apparatus; a gradually tapered single-piece dilator to allow sheath introduction and advanced over an 0.035-inch-diameter extra-stiff guidewire (MediTech/Boston Scientific, Natick, MA); a 24-Fr loading cartridge to facilitate stent-graft introduction into the delivery sheath; and a 24-Fr Teflon mandril that is used as a pusher to advance the stent-graft through the delivery sheath (Figure 10.2).

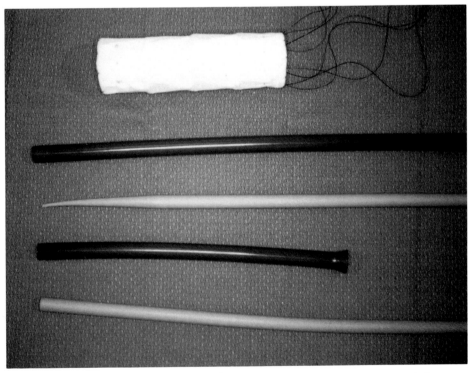

Figure 10.2 Endovascular stent-graft delivery system consisting of (top to bottom) the stent-graft device, 24-Fr delivery sheath, tapered sheath dilator, loading cartridge to facilitate device introduction, and solid mandril "pusher" to advance the stent-graft within the sheath to the desired deployment site.

Endovascular Procedure

All patients are evaluated by the cardiothoracic surgery and interventional radiology teams, and full informed consent is obtained for both conventional surgical and stent-graft procedures. All stent-graft procedures for treatment of thoracic aortic aneurysms are performed in the operating suites at Stanford University Hospital, with the patient intubated and under general anesthesia (Figure 10.3). The operating suite is prepared for aortic surgery, and the patient is prepared and draped for a left thoracotomy. After selecting the side with the pelvic arterial anatomy most likely to allow introduction of the delivery system, the groin area is prepared for surgical exposure of the femoral artery. After surgical dissection and isolation of the appropriate femoral artery, an 18-g needle is used to puncture the artery to allow introduction of a soft-tip guidewire. The guidewire is advanced into the thoracic aorta to facilitate introduction of a pigtail catheter.

High-quality fluoroscopic equipment in the operating suite is essential to provide fluoroscopic guidance and ensure accurate placement of the stent-graft device. A portable C-arm unit capable of digital acquisition, playback, and "road-mapping" is a minimum requirement. An initial aortogram is performed and reviewed. The proximal and distal necks of the aneurysm are identified, and their location is marked with external opaque markers or correlated with stationary intrathoracic landmarks (i.e., vertebral bodies). The pigtail catheter is then removed over an exchange length (260 cm) 0.035-inch extra-stiff guidewire. The patient is given intravenous heparin (300 IU/kg) to prevent thrombus formation. A transverse arteriotomy is performed and the 24-Fr dilator and delivery sheath assembly are advanced over the guidewire under fluoroscopic guidance. Once the sheath is located proximal to the neck of the aneurysm, the dilator and guidewire are withdrawn. Because the 24-Fr sheath is usually longer than

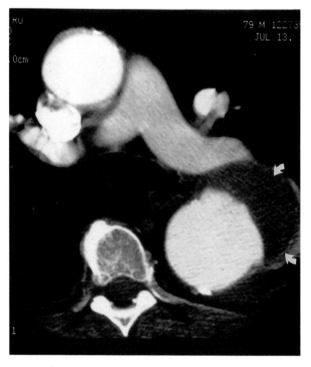

A

Figure 10.3 Eccentric atherosclerotic saccular aneurysm of the mid-descending thoracic aorta. A. Axial CT scan at the level of the main pulmonary artery bifurcation demonstrates an aneurysm of the descending thoracic aorta associated with significant mural thrombus (arrows). B, C, D, E, and F. Following pages.

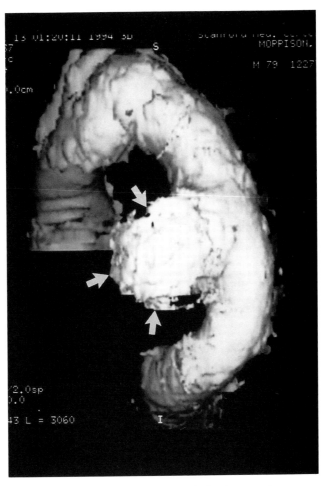

B

Figure 10.3 B. Shaded surface rendering of a spiral CT data set demonstrates the three-dimensional eccentric appearance of the aneurysm (arrows). C, D, E, and F. Following pages.

necessary, a portion of the sheath (i.e., 12 cm) can be cut off and used as the loading cartridge for the stent-graft. In addition, once the 24-Fr sheath has been introduced and satisfactorily positioned, the tip of the 24-Fr dilator can be cut off and the remainder of the dilator can be made into a pusher to deploy the stent-graft device. The 24-Fr Teflon pusher is used to introduce the stent-graft from its loading cartridge into the 24-Fr sheath. The stent-graft is then advanced by the pusher until it approaches the tip of the introducer sheath.

Due to the effect of brisk antegrade blood flow, there is a risk of inadvertent displacement of the stent-graft into a "downstream" location during its initial deployment. To reduce this risk, the arterial blood pressure is lowered to a mean of 50–60 mm Hg by an intravenous infusion of sodium nitroprusside. With the stent-graft positioned in the proximal neck of the aorta approximately one stent body length (2.5 cm) above the mouth of the aneurysm, the pusher is maintained in a stable position, and the sheath is rapidly withdrawn, allowing the self-expanding stent-graft to deploy. Immediately after deployment, the nitroprusside infusion is discontinued, allowing the blood pressure to normalize.

The pigtail catheter is reintroduced through the 24-Fr sheath and a postdeployment aortogram is performed. If the stent-graft does not completely cover the aneurysmal segment, it may be necessary to place a second device. If there is no leak into the

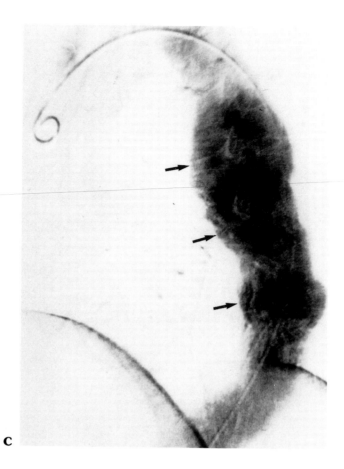

C

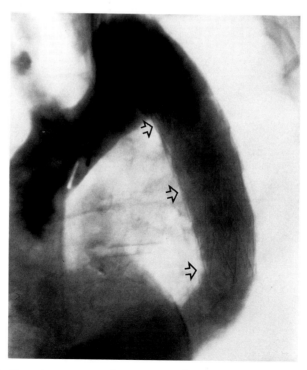

D

Figure 10.3 C. Thoracic aortogram shows aortic enlargement and luminal contour abnormalities associated with the partially thrombosed aneurysm (arrows). D. Completion thoracic aortogram following stent-graft deployment within the descending thoracic aorta. The position of the stent-graft (arrows) bridges the aneurysm from its proximal to distal necks. E and F. Following page.

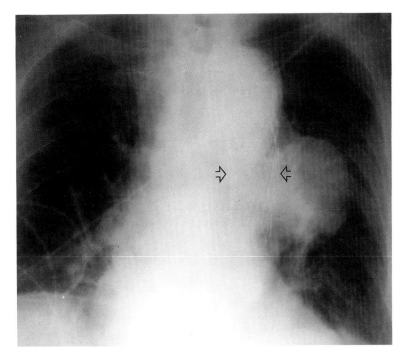

E

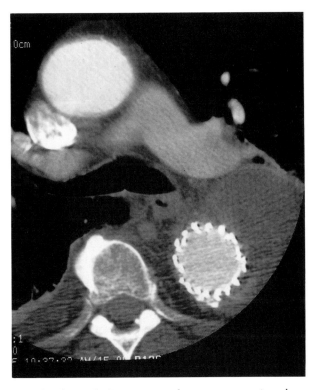

F

Figure 10.3 E. Frontal radiograph demonstrates the aneurysm projected over the left hilar region and the stent-graft (arrows) in place. F. Axial CT scan at the level of the main pulmonary artery bifurcation following stent-graft placement identifies a patent prosthesis and a thrombosed aneurysm sac surrounding the device without signs of a contrast leak or other abnormality. Following the immediate postplacement aortogram and thoracic CT scan, the patient was discharged on the third postoperative day.

aneurysmal sac on the completion aortogram, the delivery sheath is removed, and the anticoagulation effects of the heparin are reversed with protamine sulfate. The common femoral artery or aortotomy site is repaired surgically.

Postprocedural Monitoring

Patients typically spend the first 24 hr after the procedure in the intensive care unit. The next 1–2 days are often spent recuperating on a regular ward. Patients are usually discharged on the third postoperative day. No further anticoagulation is administered. Before discharge, all patients undergo a repeat aortogram and spiral CT examination to evaluate for residual aneurysm patency. After discharge, the patients have repeat spiral CT examinations 6 months after stent-graft placement, with yearly examinations thereafter.

Complications

In our first 54 cases, we had major complications in 7 (13%) patients. There has been one periprocedural death associated with iliac artery rupture during insertion of the stent-graft device. Another patient died within 30 days of the procedure, following aspiration and development of bilateral pneumonia and respiratory failure. Three patients (5.5%) developed paraplegia, one of whom died 31 days after the procedure.

There have been no cases requiring surgical conversion, and no episodes of stroke, distal embolization, or infection. Complete thrombosis of the aneurysm occurred in 50 (92.5%) of the 54 cases. The mean follow-up time for this group of 50 patients is 12.2 months, with a range of 1 to 37 months. Two late deaths occurred, 4.5 and 14 months after the stent-graft procedure. In the former, the previously thrombosed aneurysm apparently recanalized via a penetrating ulcer just distal to the stent-graft. The patient died after the aneurysm eroded into the esophagus.

Our incidence of paraplegia is not significantly different from that reported by Svensson in a review of 832 patients who underwent surgical treatment of aneurysms of the descending thoracic aorta.[32] While we do not routinely search for the anterior spinal artery preoperatively, whenever possible we try to limit the length of the stent-graft to spare any patent intercostal arteries.

The issue of which specialty should lead the practical application of endovascular technologies, including stent-graft placements, is a topic of considerable debate. The interventional radiologists, vascular surgeons, and cardiovascular surgeons should develop a collegial approach to investigate this procedure. Although this multispecialty concept may not be feasible in all institutions, the team approach is clearly advisable. It should also be emphasized that these procedures should not be undertaken by individuals without considerable expertise in catheterization techniques. A number of inserted stent-graft devices have required adjunctive percutaneous manipulations to ensure exclusion of the aneurysm (e.g., embolization of small persistent leaks, balloon angioplasty of the devices, addition of uncovered stents, etc.).

The morbidity and mortality associated with stent-graft placement compares favorably with rates reported by contemporary surgical series. Obviously, further studies and continued follow-up are required. However, the potential advantages of stent-graft treatment of highly selected thoracic aorta aneurysms include a reduction in procedural time, blood loss, length of intubation, intensive care unit confinement, total hospital stay, overall complications, and death. Documenting the effect of this procedure on these parameters, and on the long-term clinical outcome and potential cost savings, is an important future challenge.

ENDOVASCULAR TREATMENT OF AORTIC DISSECTION

Dissection of the aorta is the most frequent catastrophe affecting the aorta, estimated to occur at least twice as frequently as a ruptured abdominal aortic aneurysm.[33] It is often fatal, and if left untreated, its mortality rate reaches 83% within 1 month from onset.[34,35] Recently, several groups described their experience with uncovered stents[36-39] and covered stents or stent-grafts[40-42] in the treatment of aortic dissection created in animal models. The results of these initial studies support the feasibility of an endovascular approach to the treatment of aortic dissection. Another endovascular technique, percutaneous balloon fenestration of the dissection septum, has also been used to treat complications of complex aortic dissections.[43-45] This section will present our experience with stents, stent-grafts, and balloon fenestration, their role in managing primary aortic dissection, and the associated peripheral ischemic sequelae.

Aortic dissection results from a tear in the aortic wall with intramural hemorrhage, which causes separation of the inner one-third and outer two-thirds of the media.[46] Aortic dissection may be associated with many predisposing conditions; however, it is almost always associated with systemic hypertension.[46]

Evaluation of patients with aortic dissection currently focuses on two basic questions: (1) Does the dissection involve the ascending aorta? and (2) Is the aorta aneurysmally dilated? These diagnostic questions are usually easily addressed with CT and magnetic resonance (MR) imaging.

The answers to the above questions directly affect the overall prognosis of the patient and the therapeutic algorithm. Dissections involving the ascending aorta, either with or without distal extension, are classified as type A and account for 60% to 70% of dissections. The tear in a type A dissection usually occurs within a few centimeters of the aortic valve. Proximal extension of the dissection to the aortic valve ring or ostia of the coronary arteries can produce aortic incompetence, myocardial ischemia and left ventricular failure. Rupture into the pericardium can produce acute cardiac tamponade. These complications of type A dissections are the principal cause of fatality in these patients.[46]

Type B dissections involve only the descending aorta and usually arise from a primary tear located just distal to the origin of the left subclavian artery at the site of insertion of the ligamentum arteriosum.[46] Surgical intervention in type A dissection significantly affects prognosis, whereas surgical intervention is no better than medial therapy in reducing the mortality rate in patients with an uncomplicated type B dissection.[47-50] It should be noted that 20–50% of patients who survive the acute stage of a type B dissection with medical management will develop an aneurysm of the dissected aortic segment within 1–5 yr.[34-50]

In practical terms, there is currently no feasible endovascular alternative to adequately address the spectrum of complications associated with a type A aortic dissection. To prevent lethal proximal extension of a type A dissection in those patients without evidence of cardiac involvement, it is necessary to prevent any communication of the false lumen with the aortic valve ring, coronary artery ostia, or pericardium. It is conceivable that a stent-graft could seal the sites of intimal tears and obliterate blood flow in the false lumen, thereby eliminating further proximal extension of the dissection.

If a type A dissection extends through the transverse arch, the application of a stent-graft is more complicated due to the possible involvement of the brachiocephalic vessels. The anatomic orientation of the flap relative to these arch branches is idiosyncratic, and the hemodynamic effects are often serious. Significant technical factors limiting the application of stent-grafts in this setting are the lack of devices with diameters large enough and delivery systems flexible enough to meet the anatomic challenge presented by the curvature of the aortic arch. To date, there have been no clinical reports or animal investigations employing stent-grafts for the management of type A dissections. Thus, immediate surgical intervention appears to be the only therapeutic option currently available for the treatment of ascending aorta and aortic arch dissections.

There are essentially three main types of pathologic manifestations that can complicate an acute type B aortic dissection. These include (1) aortic rupture, which may occur acutely or as a late complication; (2) peripheral ischemia involving the renal, mesenteric, and lower extremity vasculature; and (3) aneurysmal dilatation of the false lumen of the dissection. The feasibility, safety, and effectiveness of a variety of endovascular techniques in the management of complications associated with type B aortic dissections have been the focus of considerable laboratory and clinical investigations.[36-44]

Acute aortic rupture complicating type B aortic dissections is almost universally fatal unless it is locally contained by surrounding mediastinal tissues. Theoretically, a stent-graft could be used to temporarily manage an unstable clinical situation prior to operative repair, or provide an alternative treatment option in patients who could not survive surgery. We have reported one such case where a stent-graft was successfully used to treat an acute rupture of the false lumen of a chronic dissection.[14]

Similarly, placement of a stent-graft within the true lumen could be considered beneficial as a prophylactic intervention to prevent rupture. To accomplish this goal, it would be necessary for the stent-graft to either obliterate the false lumen or cause the false lumen to thrombose by isolating it from the true lumen. A potential ideal setting for use of a stent-graft in an aortic dissection is one in which the false lumen does not have a distal reentry site and no significant branch vessel fills from the false lumen. In the laboratory, uncovered stents have been capable of obliterating the false lumen of an aortic dissection.

Reapproximation of the dissection septum against the outer wall of a dilated false lumen is not always structurally possible due to a mismatch in the anatomic dimensions.[37-39] In addition, if fenestrations exist in the dissected aortic segments above or below the stents or stent-grafts, continued flow via the uncovered fenestrations may maintain false-lumen patency. The attendant risk of progressive aneurysmal dilatation and aortic rupture would also still exist. Moreover, in the clinical setting of a chronic dissection, it may not be possible to stretch a dissection flap once it has evolved from a flaccid intimal tear into a fibrotic and thickened band, irrespective of the amount of intrinsic hoop strength of a stent or stent-graft.

However, false-lumen obliteration or thrombosis is readily obtainable in the acute setting if the entire length of the dissection is treated. Unfortunately, even in the ideal pathoanatomic situations, the desired anatomic effects extend only to the segment treated.[39,40] Obviously, there are limitations to the extent that stent-grafting of the aorta can be performed, especially when the dissection flap may extend from the thoracic aorta to the aortic bifurcation.

Unless all major vascular beds are supplied by one of the two lumens, paraplegia, or mesenteric, renal, and/or lower extremity ischemia may develop. In a review of the Stanford experience of 272 cases of acute aortic dissection, Fann et al., noted peripheral vascular ischemic symptoms in 31% of patients.[51] Other investigators have reported that compromise of an aortic branch vessel occurs in 30–50% of patients with aortic dissection.[35,52-57] Peripheral pulse deficit is the most frequent peripheral ischemic complication, occurring in 24% of the Stanford patients.[51] This is a relatively benign condition and usually responds to traditional surgical repair of the thoracic aorta.[51,55,58,59] Less is known about the frequency of peripheral ischemic complications in patients with chronic aortic dissection. A necropsy study by Roberts and Roberts found that obliteration of the true aortic lumen by the false channel produced aortic branch vessel compromise in 10 (56%) of 18 patients with a chronic type B aortic dissection.[60]

Renal and mesenteric ischemia and infarction are also major causes of morbidity and death in patients with acute aortic dissection. When the renal and/or mesenteric circulation is compromised by acute aortic dissection, significant clinical sequelae occur. At Stanford, the incidence of impaired renal and mesenteric perfusion in association with an aortic dissection was 8% and 5%, respectively.[51] In a multivariant analysis of the Stanford experience, renal and mesenteric ischemia/infarction were significant independent predictors of operative death, whereas peripheral pulse loss was not.[61] Despite a wide array of operative strategies, the operative mortality rate for patients with acute aortic dissection complicated by renal ischemia is about 50% and may reach 88% when mesenteric perfusion is impaired.[51,53,57,62]

The appropriate management of compromised perfusion to significant branch vessels of the aorta secondary to an acute dissection is yet to be established. The issue is of critical importance because renal, mesenteric, or peripheral revascularization at the same time as surgery for thoracic aortic dissection adds to the complexity of an already complex procedure. Even without the need for a secondary surgical procedure, surgical repair of an acute thoracic aortic dissection is associated with relatively high operative morbidity and mortality rates.

This is a challenging clinical problem that continues to encourage the development of new management strategies. Recently, percutaneous endovascular techniques have been developed and applied to the treatment of aortic dissection, specifically to improve the results in patients with branch vessel ischemia[43–45] It is also conceivable that a stent-graft could be developed that would provide flow to significant branch vessels via channels or graft limbs coursing from the true lumen through a thrombosed false lumen.

Clinical and Anatomic Considerations

Over a 2-yr period, 26 patients at our institution have undergone percutaneous management of peripheral ischemic complications of aortic dissection using endovascular stents and balloon fenestration techniques. The average age of the patients treated was 52 yr (range, 35 to 77 yr). The aortic dissection was considered acute if the patient's symptoms began within 14 days of the endovascular procedure. Dissection was considered as chronic if the symptoms began more than 14 days before the endovascular procedure. An acute dissection was present in 16 patients, 6 type A and 10 type B. Chronic dissections were present in 10 patients, 6 type A and 4 type B.

Twenty-one of the patients had a history of hypertension and two had Marfan's disease. Fifteen (58%) of the 26 patients had undergone at least one previous surgical procedure for repair of the aortic dissection. Six had the aortic surgery within 1 day and 3 had the surgery within 10 days of the endovascular procedure.

Patients were referred for angiographic evaluation and endovascular management because of clinical suspicion for peripheral or visceral ischemic complications caused by the dissection process. Clinical signs of lower extremity ischemia included an absent or decreased peripheral pulse, rest pain, altered sensation, or claudication. Signs of renal ischemia included hypertension resistant to medical therapy, elevated serum creatinine, oliguria, or anuria. The concern for mesenteric ischemia was raised when abdominal pain, nausea and vomiting, abnormal liver function tests, or lactic acidosis developed. Any patient who did not have arteriographic evidence of compromised arterial perfusion to the suspected ischemic territory was not considered to have ischemia related to the dissection process.

Seventeen patients had renal, 12 patients had lower extremity, and 8 patients had mesenteric ischemia. Considering the lower extremities, the kidneys, and the mesenteric vasculature each as one vascular bed, 18 patients had involvement of 1 vascular bed, 5 patients had involvement of 2 vascular beds, and 3 patients had involvement of 3 vascular beds.

Technical Considerations

In general, endovascular stent placement was performed when a dissection flap extended into a peripheral branch vessel of the aorta and caused a hemodynamically and clinically significant obstruction to blood flow. Stents were used in the branch vessels to reapproximate the obstructing dissection flap against the vessel wall, thus creating an adequate vessel lumen (Figure 10.4). This was accomplished in a manner analogous to the treatment of a dissection induced by balloon angioplasty.[12] In an aortic dissection, PTA alone is ineffective in reestablishing the vessel diameter because of the fibroelastic recoil of the dissection flap and the nature of the flow obstruction caused by the false lumen. Stents can readily overcome the elastic recoil of a flap and effectively displace the false lumen to reestablish an adequate diameter to the true lumen.

If the branch supplying an ischemic vascular bed is not directly involved by the dissection septum, it is likely that the branch arises directly off of the aortic (true or false) lumen, which is malperfused relative to the other aortic lumen. In these cases, there may not be effective admixture of flow between the two aortic lumens because of the absence of a distal "reentry" site and in insufficient number of adequate fenestrations in the dissection flap.

Percutaneous balloon fenestration of the dissection septum can be done to enlarge small fenestrations in the flap or create de novo perforations to facilitate better mixing of blood flow between the two aortic channels and improve branch vessel perfusion. However, it is theoretically possible that balloon fenestration may adversely affect flow hemodynamics. Because of this concern, complete arteriography, including catheterization of both aortic channels, and measurement of arterial pressures in multiple locations in both channels should precede the decision to create or enlarge a septal fenestration.

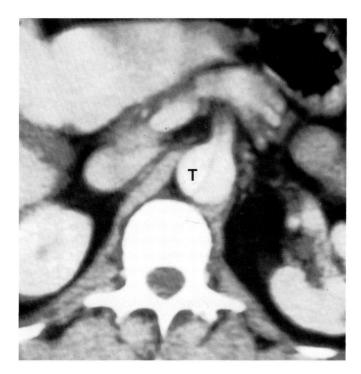

A

Figure 10.4 Endovascular stent placement to treat a branch vessel complication associated with complex type B aortic dissection. A. Axial CT image demonstrates extension of aortic dissection flap into the superior mesenteric artery (SMA). This was associated with significant abdominal pain. The true lumen (T) is more dense and located on the right side of the vessel at this level. B, C, D, E, and F. Following pages.

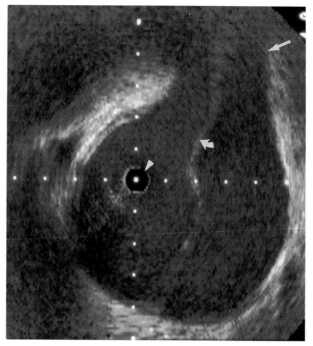

B

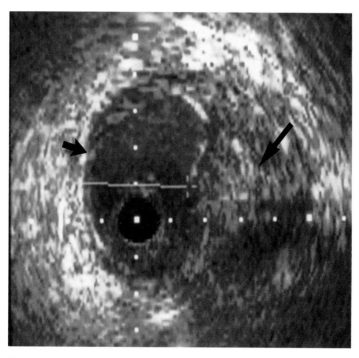

C

Figure 10.4 B. Intravascular ultrasound image obtained 36 hr after the CT scan shows the imaging catheter (arrowhead) within the true lumen and the presence of the dissection flap (curved arrow) extending from the aorta into the SMA (straight arrow) C. Intravascular ultrasound image obtained within the SMA demonstrates a deformed and narrowed true lumen (short arrow) and an engorged, thrombosed, highly echogenic false lumen (long arrow). D, E, and F. Following pages.

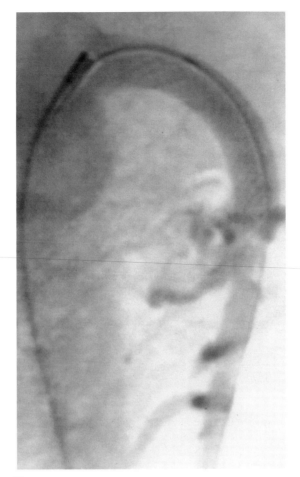

D

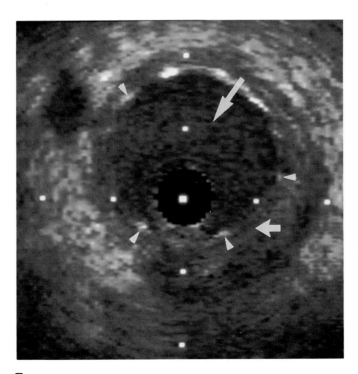

E

Figure 10.4 D. Superior mesenteric arteriogram in the lateral projection following placement of an 8-mm-diameter Wallstent shows a good result. E. Intravascular ultrasound imaging following stent placement demonstrates a more normal appearance to the true lumen (long arrow) with compression of the thrombosed false lumen (short arrow) by the stent (arrowheads). F. Following page.

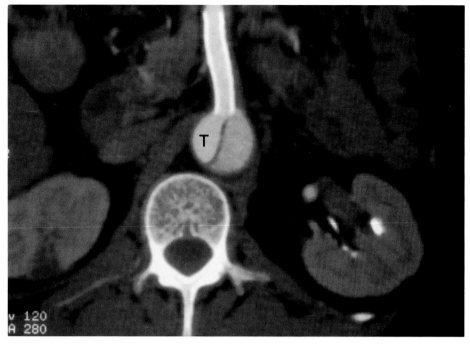

F

Figure 10.4 F. CT image at the level of the SMA stent reveals complete restoration of flow to the mesenteric bed via the true lumen (T).

Intravascular ultrasound (IVUS) has recently been used as a tool to evaluate the complexities of aortic dissection.[44] The entire extent of the thoracic and abdominal aorta can be rapidly and repeatedly visualized in real time with clear delineation of the pathologic anatomy. Use of IVUS can also reduce the need for extensive arteriographic injections of contrast media, thereby benefiting patients with acute or chronic abnormalities in renal function. Adjunctive use of IVUS can provide important supplementary pathoanatomic data including the location, extent, and integrity of the dissection septum separating the true and false channels within the aorta and its branches; the relationship of the celiac, superior mesenteric, renal, inferior mesenteric, and common iliac arteries to each aortic lumen; and the location and extent of septal fenestrations. In addition to providing valuable diagnostic information, IVUS may be indispensable in directing therapeutic endovascular interventions such as percutaneous balloon fenestration of the dissection septum.

Endovascular Procedures

All procedures are performed in the angiography suite. When the false lumen is patent, angiography and hemodynamic pressure measurements are performed on both the true and false lumens. If access into both the true and false lumens cannot be achieved through a single puncture site, an additional access site is gained. In patients with signs of renal ischemia, portions of the procedure are performed with carbon dioxide as the contrast agent in an attempt to reduce the patient's exposure to iodinated contrast media.

Percutaneous Balloon Fenestration

Percutaneous balloon fenestration of the dissection septum is performed with either IVUS or biplane fluoroscopic guidance. With either technique, percutaneous access is gained into both the true and false lumens. When using IVUS guidance, the IVUS probe is placed into the larger (usually false) lumen while a long metal cannula (Rösch-Uchida needle, Cook, Inc.) is advanced into the other lumen. The cannula and IVUS probe are positioned at the same level to allow ultrasound visualization of the cannula tip. The cannula is rotated until it points toward the center of the dissection septum. This causes tenting of the dissection flap, which can be visualized sonographically. The inner needle and 5-Fr catheter are then advanced to the tip of the cannula. Real-time imaging ensures that the subsequent transeptal advancement of the needle and sheath will be made through the middle of the intimal flap and not toward a free wall of the aorta. Only a short, 1–2 mm throw of the puncture system is necessary to push the needle and sheath through the tented intimal flap. Once transgression of the septum is confirmed by IVUS, the needle is removed. Following contrast documentation of a satisfactory position, a guidewire is passed through the sheath into the opposite lumen and the sheath is then removed. A balloon catheter is then advanced over the guidewire and positioned across the intimal flap. The fenestration created is usually enlarged to 14–20 mm using a balloon catheter (Figure 10.5). Subsequent to balloon dilatation, arteriography and hemodynamic recordings are performed to assess the effectiveness of the intervention and the necessity for creating additional septal fenestrations.

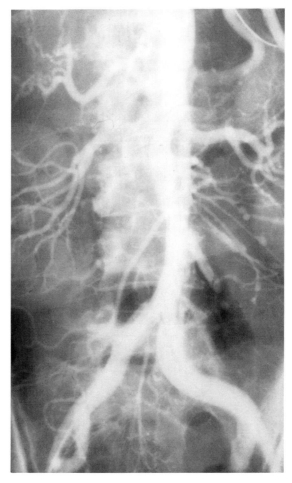

A

Figure 10.5 Percutaneous balloon fenestration of a dissection septum for treatment of a complicated aortic dissection. **A.** Flush aortogram performed with the catheter tip within the true lumen demonstrates opacification of the celiac artery branches, superior mesenteric artery (SMA), right and left renal arteries, and both iliac arteries. **B, C, D, E, F, G, H, I, J,** and **K** Following pages.

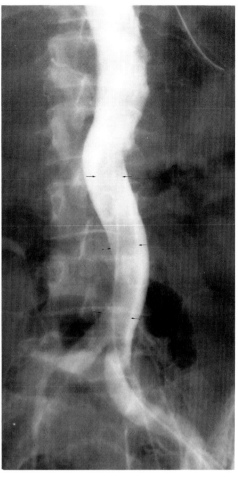

B

Figure 10.5 B. Abdominal aortogram with the catheter placed within the false lumen demonstrates no significant branch vessels. A cylindrical filling defect running longitudinally within the contrast column represents the poorly opacified true lumen (small arrows). C, D, E, F, G, H, I, J, and K. Following pages.

We have treated three patients with balloon fenestration of the dissection flap: two patients had the fenestrations created in the upper abdominal aorta and one was performed in the distal aorta.

Endovascular Stenting

A total of 23 patients were treated with endovascular stents, 4 in combination with balloon fenestration. Thirteen patients received renal stents. Of these, 12 had unilateral and 1 had bilateral stents placed. Of the unilateral renal stents, 4 were placed on the right, and 8 on the left. Seven patients were treated with lower extremity stents, 5 with unilateral and 2 with bilateral stents. Of the 5 unilateral lower extremity stents, 4 were on the right and 1 was on the left. Four patients were treated with aortic stents (Figure 10.6, p. 248), and 2 were treated with superior mesenteric artery stents. Overall, 17 patients were treated with balloon-expandable Palmaz stents, 3 with self-expanding Wallstents, and 3 with both types of stents. Several patients had stents placed in more than one vascular bed.

Of the 4 patients treated with a combination of balloon fenestration and stenting, the fenestration was performed in the proximal abdominal aorta in 3 patients and in the distal aorta in 1.

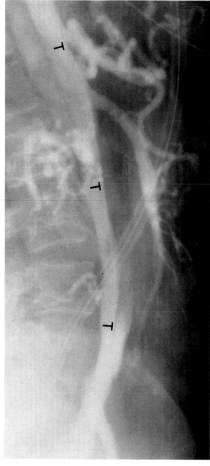

C

Figure 10.5 C. Lateral view of a true lumen injection shows the spiral extension of the dissection septum. The true lumen (T) is located anteriorly at the level of the celiac trunk and SMA, however, it courses posteriorly from the level of the renal arteries to provide flow to the kidneys and lumbar vessels. D, E, F, G, H, I, J, and K. Following pages.

Results and Complications

Technically successful revascularization was achieved in all 26 patients treated with balloon fenestration and/or stenting. One patient with an acute type B dissection, who developed paraplegia, anuria, abdominal pain, and bilateral lower extremity ischemia, died with profound irreversible metabolic acidosis and multiorgan dysfunction 14 hr after stenting and percutaneous septal fenestration. One patient died from peritonitis 3 days after the endovascular procedure. This death was probably related to irreversible effects of significant and prolonged preprocedural bowel ischemia. One patient died of cardiorespiratory arrest 14 months after therapy and 1 patient was lost to follow-up. The remaining 22 patients have had persistent clinical benefit from the endovascular procedures. No patient has required surgical revascularization of the ischemic region. Mean follow-up is 16 months (range, 3 to 48 months). One case of aortic dissection with extension into the left renal artery was treated by endovascular stent placement and complicated by a perinephric hematoma. This complication was believed to be caused by penetration of a renal artery branch by a guidewire positioned too distally during stent deployment. The patient required transfusion of 2 units of blood and per-

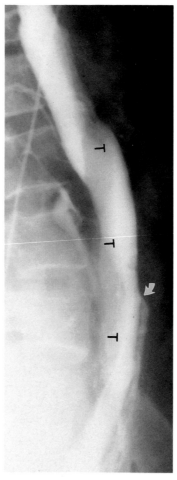

D

Figure 10.5 D. False lumen aortogram in the lateral projection demonstrates the inferior mesenteric artery (IMA) (arrow) originating from the false channel. Again evident is a negative filling defect corresponding to the true lumen (T) within the contrast opacified false lumen. The false lumen spirals from posterior to anterior as it courses caudally. E, F, G, H, I, J, and K. Following pages.

cutaneous embolization of the bleeding artery with coils. There have been no long-term sequelae of this complication.

Stent-Grafts for Aneurysms Related to Aortic Dissections

A potential application of endovascular techniques is for the treatment of aneurysms that develop in association with chronic type B dissections. These aneurysms may involve either the true or false lumen and can occur within the aorta or a branch vessel. In this setting, stent-grafts may have a future therapeutic role in eliminating the attendant risk of catastrophic rupture. This technology has already been shown to be effective in treating certain thoracic and abdominal aortic aneurysms not associated with dissection. We have used stent-grafts to treat patients with aneurysms involving either the true or false lumen of the aorta.[14] One patient had a partially thrombosed aneurysm of the aortic false lumen and a branch vessel aneurysm associated with extension of the flap into the right subclavian artery. This patient was successfully treated with two stent-grafts.

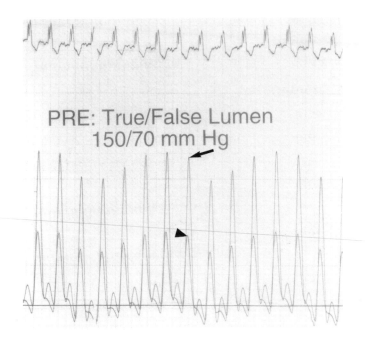

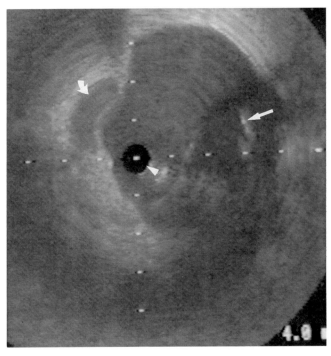

Figure 10.5 E. Simultaneous pressure recordings from within the true (straight arrow) and false (arrowhead) lumina demonstrate an 80 mm Hg pressure gradient. Clinically, this was associated with lower abdominal pain and cramping. Colonoscopy demonstrated dusky, cyanotic colonic mucosa limited to the sigmoid colon, presumably related to the low perfusion pressure in the IMA and poor collateralization from the SMA. F. Intravascular ultrasound with the imaging catheter (arrowhead) in the false lumen shows the IMA (curved arrow). The highly echogenic linear focus corresponds to a curved metallic cannula (straight arrow) in the true lumen. G, H, I, J, and K. Following pages.

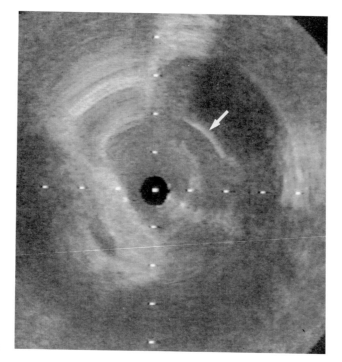

G

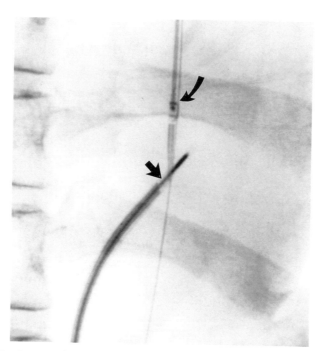

H

Figure 10.5 G. The curved cannula (straight arrow) is rotated until it tents the center of the dissection septum. H. Under direct intravascular ultrasound (curved arrow) visualization, a 5-Fr needle-sheath combination (arrow) is advanced 1–2 mm out of the cannula through the tented dissection flap and into the false lumen. I, J, and K. Following pages.

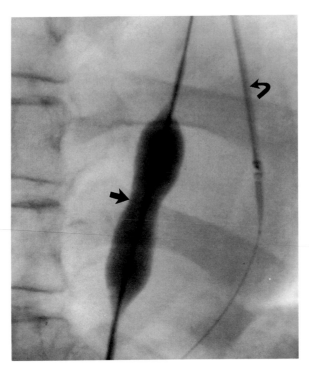

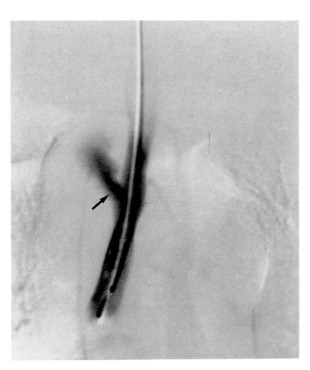

Figure 10.5 I. The needle is then removed and a guidewire is passed through the catheter, providing access across the dissection septum from the true to false lumen. The cannula and catheter are then removed and an angioplasty balloon is advanced over the wire and positioned across the dissection septum (straight arrow) using ultrasound (curved arrow) guidance. The balloon is then inflated to create the septal fenestration. J. Injection of contrast media within the true lumen after the procedure demonstrates flow through the fenestration (arrow) into the false lumen. K. Following page.

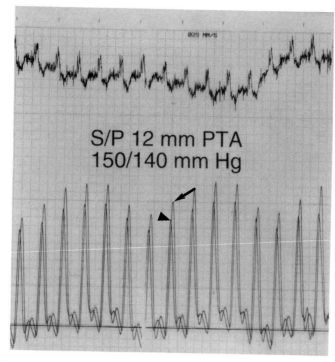

K

Figure 10.5 K. Repeat simultaneous pressure measurements within the true (straight arrow) and false (arrowhead) lumina show a residual gradient of only 10 mm Hg. Within 24 hr after percutaneous creation of the fenestration, the patient's abdominal symptoms resolved.

In general, it is anticipated that treatment of dissection-associated aneurysms will be significantly more difficult owing to the idiosyncratic and complex geometric shapes of the aneurysm necks. These noncircular, proximal and distal necks make the likelihood of obtaining a snug, watertight seal between the graft material and the aortic wall or dissection septum problematic. Stent-grafts, irrespective of their hoop strength, may not successfully impose their circular shape on the dissected luminal contour without leaving gaps or crevices capable of channeling flow into the aneurysm. The problem of residual gaps following stent-graft treatment is of particular concern in chronic aortic dissections where the flap is thick and relatively rigid. A solution to this problem in the near future is unlikely.

As previously noted, 20–50% of patients who survive the acute stage of a type B aortic dissection will develop an aneurysm of the false lumen within 1–5 yr.[34,50] In this regard, it is possible that endovascular stent-graft technology may be investigated as a prophylactic measure to prevent subsequent progressive dilatation of the false lumen. The potential merit of this concept would be further enhanced if angiographic or cross-sectional imaging findings and/or clinical criteria were capable of determining which patients with acute type B dissections were at high risk for subsequent aneurysm formation. Currently, only the presence of poorly controlled hypertension after an acute dissection is known to result in an increased incidence of aneurysmal dilatation of the aortic false lumen.[35] It is anticipated that future innovations may permit development of procedures and unique stent-graft prostheses specifically designed to address the idiosyncratic challenges presented by aneurysms related to aortic dissection.

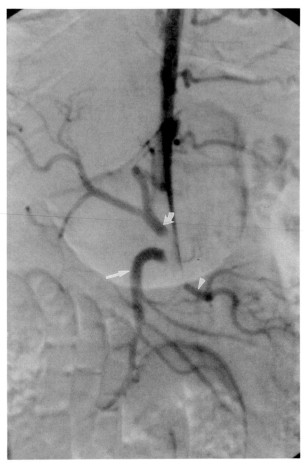

A

Figure 10.6 Aortic dissection with significant compression of the aortic true lumen by the false lumen successfully treated by placement of endovascular stents. **A.** Frontal projection of an abdominal aortogram performed with the catheter tip in the true lumen demonstrates obliteration of the true lumen by the false lumen. The celiac (curved arrow), superior mesenteric (straight arrow), and left renal arteries (arrowhead) are opacified. The patient was markedly hypertensive despite a parenteral, multidrug, antihypertensive regimen and was also complaining of severe abdominal pain. **B.** Following page.

CONCLUSION

In general, the therapeutic strategy for management of complicated aortic dissection should be based on the severity of symptoms, the ease of blood pressure control with medical therapy, the patient's age and general medical condition, the risk associated with operative or endovascular intervention, and the potential benefits of any such intervention. In acute cases, the judicious rapid use of endovascular techniques, such as stent placement and balloon fenestration of a dissection septum, appear to have a definite salutary impact on the unacceptably high mortality rate associated with compromised renal or mesenteric arterial perfusion. Stent-graft therapy in the setting of aortic rupture associated with dissection appears promising as either definitive management or an adjunctive maneuver to optimize the patient's condition before definitive thoracic aortic repair.

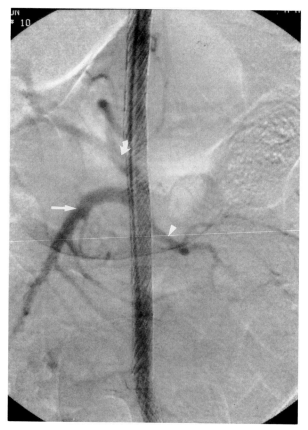

B

Figure 10.6 B. A repeat aortogram following placement of multiple overlapping Palmaz stents within the true lumen shows recanalization of the true lumen of the abdominal aorta. There is now better flow to the celiac (curved arrow), superior mesenteric (straight arrow), and renal (arrowhead) arteries.

In the setting of a chronic aortic dissection, refractory hypertension caused by renal artery stenosis should be treated vigorously because of its significant correlation with thoracic aortic aneurysm formation. Treatment of aneurysms associated with chronic aortic dissections by endovascular techniques remains a complicated challenge.

Further evaluation of these new endovascular techniques is clearly warranted in high-risk patients with aortic dissection who have appropriate clinical indications for intervention. Additional experience and longer follow-up are necessary before the full utility, the early and late complications, and the limitations of these techniques become apparent so that we may judge the long-term safety and effectiveness of these procedures.

REFERENCES

1. Pressler V, McNamara JJ: Thoracic aortic aneurysm: natural history and treatment. *J Thorac Cardiovasc Surg* 79:489–498, 1980.

2. DeBakey ME, McCollum CH, Graham, JM: Surgical treatment of aneurysms of the descending thoracic aorta: long-term results in 500 patients. *J Cardiovasc Surg* 19:571–576, 1978.

3. Moreno-Cabral CE, Miller DC, Mitchell RS, et al: Degenerative and atherosclerotic aneurysms of the thoracic aorta: determinants of early and late surgical outcome. *J Thorac Cardiovasc Surg* 88:1020–1032, 1984.

4. Desantics RW. Doroghazi RM, Austen WG, et al: Aortic dissection. *N Engl J Med* 317: 1060–1067, 1987.

5. Miller DC, Mitchell RS, Oyer PE, et al: Independent determinants of operative mortality for patients with aortic dissections. *Circulation* 70:153–164, 1984.

6. Ergin MA, Galla JD, Lansman S, et al: Acute dissection of the aorta: current surgical treatment. *Surg Clin North Am* 65:721–741, 1985.

7. Bonn J. Gardiner GA, Shapiro MJ, et al: Palmaz vascular stent: initial clinical experience. *Radiology* 174:741–745, 1990.

8. Schatz RA, Baim DS, Leon M, et al: Clinical experience with the Palmaz-Schatz coronary stent: initial results of a multicenter study. *Circulation* 83:148–161, 1991.

9. Sigwart U, Puel J, Mirkovitch V, et al: Intravascular stents to prevent occlusion and restenosis after transluminal angioplasty. *N Engl J Med* 316:701–706, 1987.

10. Rees CR, Palmaz JC, Becker GJ, et al: Palmaz stent in atherosclerotic stenoses involving the ostia of the renal arteries: preliminary report of a multicenter study. *Radiology* 181: 507–514, 1991.

11. Marks MP, Dake MD, Steinberg GK, et al: Stent placement for arterial and venous cerebrovascular disease: preliminary experience. *Radiology* 191:441–446, 1994.

12. Becker GJ, Palmaz JC, Rees CR, et al: Angioplasty-induced dissection in human iliac arteric management with Palmaz balloon-expandable intraluminal stents. *Radiology* 176:31–38, 1990.

13. Parodi JC, Palmaz JC, Barone HD: Transfemoral intraluminal graft implantation for abdominal aortic aneurysms. *Ann Vasc Surg* 5:491–499, 1991.

14. Dake MD, Miller DC, Semba CP, et al: Transluminal placement of endovascular stent-grafts for the treatment of descending thoracic aortic aneurysms. *N Engl J Med* 331:1729–1734, 1994.

15. May J, White G, Waugh R, et al: Transluminal placement of a prosthetic graft-stent device for treatment of subclavian artery aneurysms. *J Vasc Surg* 18:1056–1059, 1993.

16. Marin ML, Veith FJ, Panetta TF, et al: Percutaneous transfemoral insertion of a stented graft to repair a traumatic femoral arteriovenous fistula. *J Vasc Surg* 18:299–302, 1993.

17. Cragg AH, Dake MD: Percutaneous femoropopliteal graft placement. *Radiology* 187: 643–648, 1993.

18. Lindsay J, DeBakey ME, Beall AC: Diagnosis and treatment of diseases of the aorta. In Schlant RC, Alexander RW (eds): *The Heart*, ed 8. New York, McGraw-Hill, 1994.

19. Najafi H. Javid H, Hunter JA, et al: An update of treatment of the descending thoracic aorta. *World J Surg* 4:553–561, 1980.

20. Joyce JW, Fairbairn JF II, Kincaid OW, et al: Aneurysms of the thoracic aorta: a clinical study with special reference to prognosis. *Circulation* 29:176–181, 1964.

21. Bickerstaff LK, Pairolero PC, Hollier LH, et al: Thoracic aortic aneurysms: a population-based study. *Surgery* 92:1103–1108, 1982.

22. Estes JE Jr: Abdominal aortic aneurysm: a study of 102 cases. *Circulation* 2:258–264, 1950.

23. Crawford ES, Rubio PA: Reappraisal of adjuncts to avoid ischemia in the treatment of aneurysms of the descending thoracic aorta. *J Thorac Cardiovasc Surg* 66:693–704, 1973.

24. Carrel A: Results of the permanent intubation of the thoracic aorta. *Surg Gynecol Obstet* 15: 245–248, 1912.

25. Dotter CT: Transluminally placed coilspring endarterial tube grafts: long-term patency in canine popliteal artery. *Invest Radiol* 4:329–332, 1969.

26. Laborde JC, Parodi JC, Clem MF, et al: Intraluminal bypass of abdominal aortic aneurysm: feasibility study. *Radiology* 184:185–190, 1992.

27. Chuter TAM, Green RM, Ouriel K, et al: Transfemoral endovascular aortic graft placement. *J Vasc Surg* 18:185–197, 1993.

28. Mirich D, Wright KC, Wallace S, et al: Percutaneously placed endovascular grafts for aortic aneurysms: feasibility study. *Radiology* 170(3 Pt 2):1033–1037, 1989.

29. Lawrence DD Jr, Chansangavej C, Wright KC, et al: Percutaneous endovascular graft: experimental evaluation. *Radiology* 163:357–360, 1987.

30. Balko A, Piasecki GJ, Shah DM, et al: Transfemoral placement of intraluminal polyurethane prosthesis for abdominal aortic aneurysm. *J Surg Res* 40:305–309, 1986.

31. Yoshioka T, Wright KC, Wallace S, et al: Self-expanding endovascular graft: an experimental study in dogs. *Am J Roentgenol* 151:673–676, 1988.

32. Svensson LG, Crawford ES, Hess KR, et al: Variables predictive of outcome in 832 patients undergoing repairs of the descending thoracic aorta. *Chest* 104:1248–1253, 1993.

33. Wheat MW JR, Palmer RF: Dissecting aneurysms of the aorta. *Curr Probl Surg* 1–43, 1971.

34. Anagnostopoulos CE, Prabhakar MJS, Kittle CF: Aortic dissections and dissecting aneurysm. *Am J Cardiol* 30:263–273, 1972.
35. DeBakey ME, McCollum CH, Crawford ES, et al: Dissection and dissecting aneurysms of the aorta: 20-year follow-up of 527 patients treated surgically. *Surgery* 92:1118–1134, 1982.
36. Charnsangavej C, Wallace S, Wright KC, et al: Endovascular stent for use in aortic dissection: an in vitro experiment. *Radiology* 157:323–324, 1985.
37. Trent MS, Parsonnet V, Shoenfeld R, et al: A balloon-expandable intravascular stent for obliterating experimental aortic dissection. *J Vasc Surg* 11:707–717, 1990.
38. Kato N, Hirano T, Takeda K, et al: Treatment of acute aortic dissection with expandable metallic stent: experimental study. *J Vasc Intervent Radiol* 5:417–423, 1994.
39. Moon MR, Dake MD, Pelc LR, et al: Intravascular stenting of acute experimental type B dissection. *J Surg Res* 54:381–388, 1993.
40. Kato N, Hirano T, Takeda K, et al: Treatment of aortic dissection with a percutaneous intravascular endoprosthesis: comparison of covered and bare stents. *J Vasc Intervent Radiol* 5:805–812, 1994.
41. Yoshida H, Yasuda K, Tanabe T: New approach to aortic dissection: development of an insertable aortic prosthesis. *Ann Thorac Surg* 58:806–810, 1994.
42. Kato M, Matsuda T, Kaneko M, et al: Experimental assessment of newly devised transcatheter stent-graft for aortic dissection. *Ann Thorac Surg* 59:908–915, 1995.
43. Williams DM, Brothers TE, Messina LM: Relief of mesenteric ischemia in type III aortic dissection with percutaneous fenestration of the aortic septum. *Radiology* 174:450–425, 1990.
44. Walker PJ, Dake MD, Mitchell RS, et al: The use of endovascular techniques for the treatment of complications of aortic dissection. *J Vasc Surg* 18:1042–1051, 1993.
45. Peterson AH, Williams DM, Rodriguez JL, et al: Percutaneous treatment of a traumatic aortic dissection by balloon fenestration and stent placement. *Am J Roentgenol* 164:1274–1276, 1995.
46. Roberts WC: Aortic dissection: anatomy, consequences and causes. *Am Heart J* 101:195–214, 1981.
47. Daily PO, Trueblood HW, Stinson EB, et al: Management of acute aortic dissections. *Ann Thorac Surg* 10:237–247, 1970.
48. Jex RK, Schaff HV, Piehler JM, et al: Early and late results following repair of dissections of the descending thoracic aorta. *J Vasc Surg* 3:226–237, 1986.
49. Elefteriades JA, Hartleroad J, Gusberg RJ, et al: Long-term experience with descending aortic dissection: the complication-specific approach. *Ann Thorac Surg* 53:11–21, 1992.
50. Doroghazi RM, Slater EE, DeSanctis RW, et al: Long-term survival of patients with treated aortic dissection. *J Am Coll Cardiol* 3:1026–1034, 1984.
51. Fann JI, Sarris GE, Mitchell RS, et al: Treatment of patients with aortic dissection presenting with peripheral vascular complications. *Ann Surg* 212:705–713, 1990.
52. Jamieson WRE, Munro AI, Miyagishima RT, et al: Aortic dissections: early diagnosis and surgical management are the keys to survival. *Can J Surg* 25:145–149, 1982.
53. Cambria RP, Brewster DC, Gertler J, et al: Vascular complications associated with spontaneous aortic dissection. *J Vasc Surg* 7:199–209, 1988.
54. Slater EE, DeSanctis RW: The clinical recognition of dissecting aortic aneurysm. *Am J Med* 60:625–633, 1976.
55. Sarris GE, Miller DC: Peripheral vascular manifestations of acute aortic dissection. In Rutherford RB (ed). *Vascular Surgery*. Philadelphia, WB Saunders, 1989, pp. 842–851.
56. Leonard JC, Hasleton PS: Dissecting aortic aneurysms: a clinicopathological study. I. Clinical and gross pathological findings. *O J Med* 48:55–76, 1979.
57. Pinet F, Froment JC, Guillot M, et al: Prognostic factors and indications for surgical treatment of acute aortic dissections: a report based on 191 observations. *Cardiovasc Intervent Radiol* 7:257–266, 1984.
58. Shumacker HB Jr, Isch JH, Jolly WW: Stenotic and obstructive lesions in acute dissecting thoracic aortic aneurysms. *Ann Surg* 181:662–669, 1975.
59. Svensson LG, Crawford ES, Hess KR, et al: Dissection of the aorta and dissecting aneurysms: improving early and long-term surgical results. *Circulation* 82(suppl):IV-24–38, 1990.
60. Roberts CS, Roberts WC: Aortic dissection with entrance tear in the descending thoracic aorta: analysis of 40 necropsy patients. *Ann Surg* 213:356–368, 1991.
61. Miller DC, Mitchell RS, Oyer PE, et al: Independent determinants of operative mortality for patients with aortic dissections. *Circulation* 70(suppl):I-153–164, 1984.
62. Laas J, Heinemann M, Schaefers H-J, et al: Management of thoracoabdominal malperfusion in aortic dissection. *Circulation* 84(suppl):III-20–24, 1991.

SECTION II

NONVASCULAR INTERVENTIONS

Nonvascular Thoracic Anatomy: Normal and Frequent Variants

Peter A. Loud
Paul L. Molina

Performance of interventional procedures in the chest requires an intimate knowledge of normal anatomic relationships. Careful attention to structures near and along the path to a given lesion can minimize the risk of iatrogenic injury. This chapter briefly reviews the nonvascular thoracic anatomy relevant to the interventionalist.

CHEST WALL

The musculoskeletal structures of the chest wall provide strong yet flexible support and protection for intrathoracic contents. The 12 thoracic vertebrae increase gradually in size from the cervical to the lumbar region. Muscle groups posterior and lateral to the spine control motion of the vertebral column. Important structures traversing the paraspinal regions lateral to the vertebral bodies include the thoracic sympathetic trunks and ganglia, posterior mediastinal lymph nodes, and intercostal neurovascular bundles. The ribs articulate with the posterolateral vertebral body and transverse process and then curve around the chest at an obliquely caudal angle. The cartilaginous ends of the ribs articulate with the sternum (ribs 1–7) or fuse, forming the anterior costal margin (ribs 8–10). Ribs 11 and 12 do not generally merge with the other ribs anteriorly. The thin external, internal, and innermost intercostal muscles bridge the ribs. The intercostal spaces are thickest anteriorly and in the upper chest. Nerve roots exit the neural foramina laterally, give off dorsal and ventral rami and continue as the intercostal nerves, traveling with the intercostal arteries and veins along the inferior inner surface of the corresponding ribs between the internal and innermost intercostal muscles.

The sternum consists of the manubrium, body, and xyphoid process. The manubrium articulates with the clavicular heads superolaterally and the first ribs laterally. The first rib occasionally has an inferiorly projecting spur which can mimic a pulmonary nodule on computed tomography (CT).[1] The second rib articulates at the junction of the manubrium and sternal body. The paired internal mammary arteries and veins and lymphatics are intrathoracic in location and course along the anterior chest wall lateral to the sternum.

The scapulae overlie the upper posterior chest and are quite mobile. When the arm is elevated and rotated anteriorly, a posterior percutaneous approach to chest lesions is usually possible.

Many of the muscles overlying the upper chest control movement of the upper extremities (Figure 11.1).[2] The pectoralis major muscle originates anteriorly on the ster-

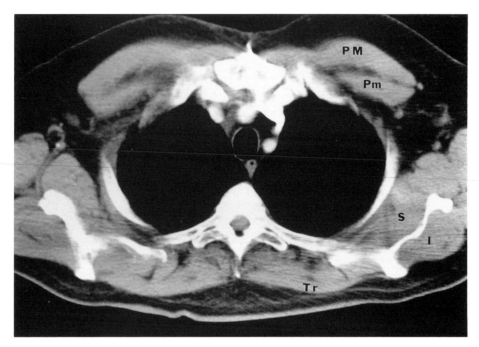

A

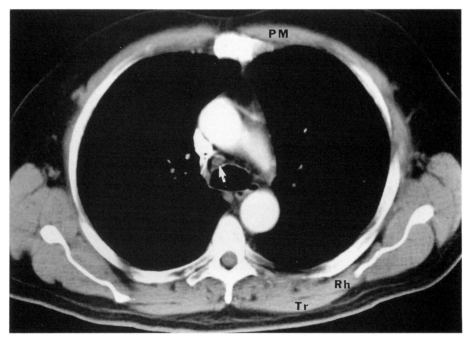

B

Figure 11.1 Normal chest wall musculature. Computed tomography images at the level of the A. manubrium, B. carina, C and D. Following page.

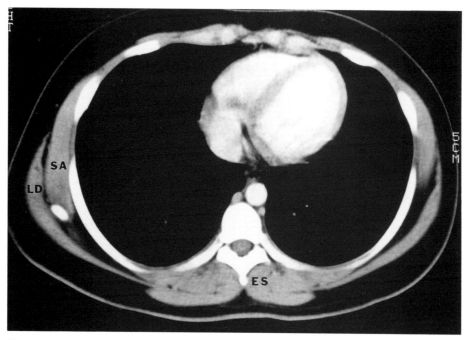

C

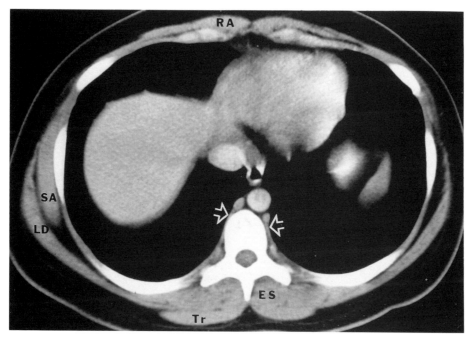

D

Figure 11.1 C. base of the heart, and **D**. diaphragm. PM, pectoralis major; Pm, pectoralis minor; S, subscapularis; I, infraspinatus; Tr, trapezius; Rh, rhomboideus; ES, erector spinae; RA, rectus abdominis; SA, serratus anterior; LD, latissimus dorsi. A normal precarinal lymph node (solid white arrow) is seen in (B). Intercostal veins (open white arrows) drain into the azygos and hemiazygous veins in (D).

num, upper ribs, and medial clavicle and inserts on the greater tuberosity of the humerus. The pectoralis minor muscle extends from the anterior third, fourth, and fifth ribs to insert on the coracoid process of the scapula. Laterally, the serratus anterior muscles extend to the ventral scapula from the lateral aspect of the upper eight or nine ribs. The latissimus dorsi muscle inserts posteriorly along the spine of the scapula and the lateral clavicle and originates from the spinous processes of the cervical and thoracic spine. The rhomboideus muscle lies beneath the trapezius muscle and extends from the spinous processes of the upper thoracic vertebrae obliquely downward to the medial scapula. The superior and inferior posterior serratus muscles extend from the spinous processes in the upper and lower back to insert on lateral ribs to aid in respiration.

PLEURA AND ITS REFLECTIONS

The thoracic cavity is lined by the parietal pleura. The parietal pleura reflects at the hila to become the visceral pleura. The visceral pleura invests the surface of the individual lobes of the lung and lines the fissures. The pleural cavity between the parietal and visceral pleura is a potential space that normally contains a small amount of pleural fluid. The close apposition of pleural surfaces permits respiration by coupling expansion and contraction of the thoracic cavity to that of the lungs. The parietal pleura is firmly attached to the thoracic wall by an underlying layer of extrapleural fat and connective tissue, and is innervated by afferent pain pathways via the intercostal and phrenic nerves. Some patients have a prominent layer of subpleural fat, which may be several millimeters thick along the posterior and lateral chest wall (Figure 11.2).

The inferior pulmonary ligaments are double pleural reflections that extend inferiorly from the hila to the medial diaphragm and tether the medial lower lobes to the mediastinum (Figure 11.3). In the upper chest, the right and left lungs and pleura often abut each other in the midline anteriorly and posteriorly, forming the anterior and posterior junction lines. These junction lines may be visible on frontal chest radiographs (Figure 11.4).

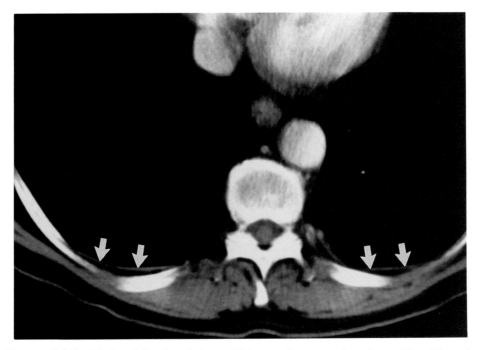

Figure 11.2 Subpleural fat. Coned-down CT image of posterior lung bases. Note bilateral subpleural fat immediately posterior to the pleura (white arrows).

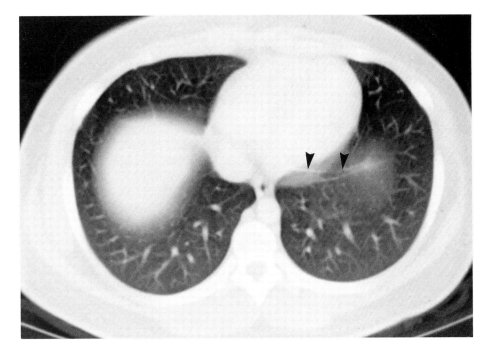

Figure 11.3 Inferior pulmonary ligament. Computed tomography image at the level of the diaphragmatic dome shows the left inferior pulmonary ligament (arrowheads).

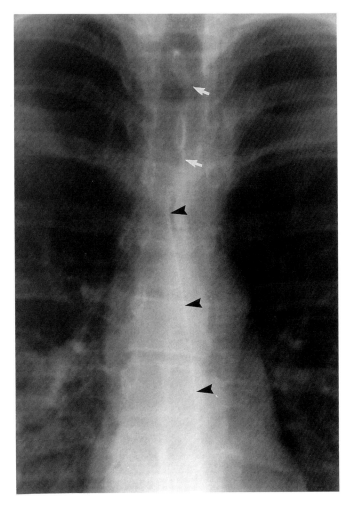

Figure 11.4 Normal junction lines. Magnified PA view of the upper mediastinum shows the normal anterior (black arrowheads) and posterior (white arrows) junction lines.

The most inferior extent of the pleural cavity, the costophrenic recess, extends close to the costal margin anteriorly to about the tenth rib in the midaxillary line, and to a level between the eleventh and twelfth ribs posteriorly. The pleural reflection may lie below the eleventh rib when the twelfth rib is rudimentary. Only in deep inspiration does the lung extend to the deepest portions of the posterior and lateral pleural recesses. In shallow respiration, the lung edge normally lies one to two intercostal spaces above the costophrenic recess.[3]

AIRWAYS AND LUNGS

The intrathoracic trachea extends 6–9 cm from the thoracic inlet to the carina.[4] It has a flat fibrous posterior wall. The remainder of the trachea is supported by horseshoe-shaped cartilaginous rings. The right lung comes into contact with and may extend behind the right side of the trachea, while the left side of the trachea is separated from lung by mediastinal fat. The normal right paratracheal stripe thickness is less than 5 mm.

The anatomy of the central bronchi is well depicted on CT (Figure 11.5).[6] The right mainstem bronchus divides into the upper lobe bronchus and bronchus intermedius. The upper lobe bronchus gives off apical, anterior, and posterior segmental bronchi. The bronchus intermedius gives off the middle lobe bronchus anteriorly and the superior segmental lower lobe bronchus posteriorly before branching into the four basal lower lobe segmental bronchi (anterior, posterior, lateral, and medial). The left mainstem bronchus is longer than the right. It bifurcates into upper lobe and lower lobe bronchi. The upper lobe bronchus gives off the lingular bronchus before supplying the upper lobe segments. The lower lobe bronchus gives off the superior segmental bronchus before branching into the three basal segmental bronchi (anteromedial, lateral, and posterior). Eight to 20 bronchial divisions are required to reach the level of

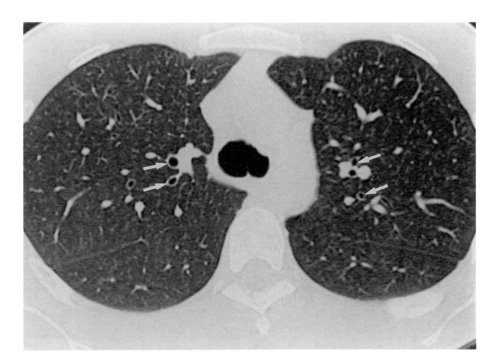

A

Figure 11.5 Normal central bronchial anatomy. Representative high-resolution CT images through the pulmonary hila. **A.** White arrows show branches of the upper lobe segmental bronchi bilaterally. **B, C,** and **D.** Following pages.

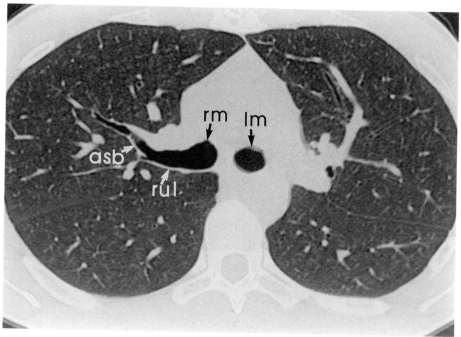

B

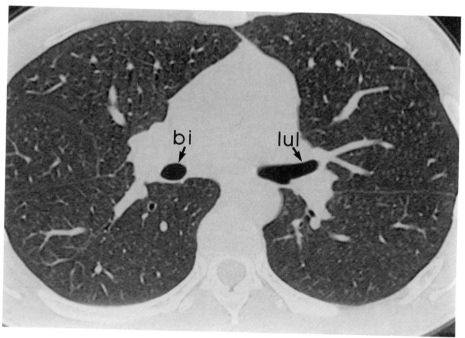

C

Figure 11.5 B. rm, right main bronchus; lm, left main bronchus; rul, right upper lobe bronchus; asb, anterior segmental bronchus of right upper lobe. C. bi, bronchus intermedius; lul, left upper lobe bronchus. D. Following page.

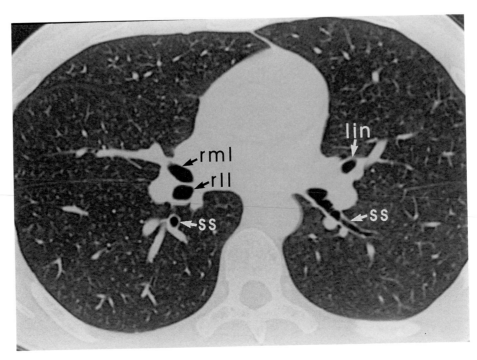

D

Figure 11.5 D. rml, right middle lobe bronchus; rll, right lower lobe bronchus; lin, lingular bronchus; ss, superior segmental bronchi of the lower lobes. Note the normally thin posterior walls of the right upper lobe bronchus and bronchus intermedius.

the terminal bronchioles, which then branch to the respiratory bronchioles, alveolar ducts, and alveoli where gas exchange occurs. The unit of lung parenchyma supplied by 3–5 terminal bronchioles is termed the *secondary pulmonary lobule*. These consist of 1–2 cm polygonal units separated by interlobular connective tissue septae.[7] Pulmonary segmental anatomy is based on the portions of lung supplied by individual segmental bronchi and pulmonary arteries.

The interlobar fissures serve as important landmarks in localizing pulmonary parenchymal lesions. The major fissures run obliquely caudad and anteriorly from the posterior upper chest to the anterior diaphragm. The horizontal minor fissure on the right delineates the middle from the upper lobe. On standard 10-mm CT images the fissures appear as bands of relative avascularity while high-resolution CT can identify the fissural line itself (Figure 11.6). Accessory fissures lined by visceral pleura are occasionally identified.[8] The most common accessory fissures include: the azygous fissure which extends from the lateral border of the right brachiocephalic (innominate) vein anteriorly to the right superior intercostal vein posteriorly; the left minor fissure which separates the lingula from the left upper lobe; the inferior accessory fissure which separates the medial basal segment from the rest of the lower lobe; and the superior accessory fissure which separates the superior segment from the remainder of the lower lobe. The inferior and superior accessory fissures occur more commonly on the right.

MEDIASTINUM

Several mediastinal connective tissue spaces have been described. These contain lymph node groups that drain the lungs and adjacent mediastinal structures. These spaces are a logical way to subdivide the mediastinum and describe the location of disease processes. Pneumomediastinography has been used to depict communication be-

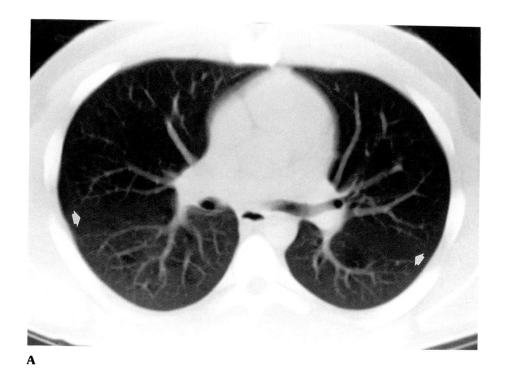

A

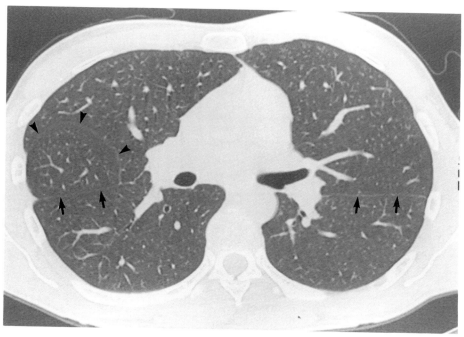

B

Figure 11.6 Normal pulmonary fissures. **A.** Conventional CT image (10 mm collimation) shows the major fissures as bands of relative avascularity (arrows). **B.** High-resolution CT image (2 mm collimation) shows the major fissures as thin lines (arrows). A portion of the minor fissure is seen as a thin curved line (arrowheads).

tween mediastinal spaces.[9] The pretracheal, prevascular, aortopulmonary window, sub-carinal and retrocrural spaces are described below.

The *pretracheal space* extends from the thoracic inlet to the carina (Figure 11.7). This space is accessible by mediastinoscopy, which permits sampling of lymph nodes in the pretracheal, paratracheal, precarinal, and anterior subcarinal regions. Bound-

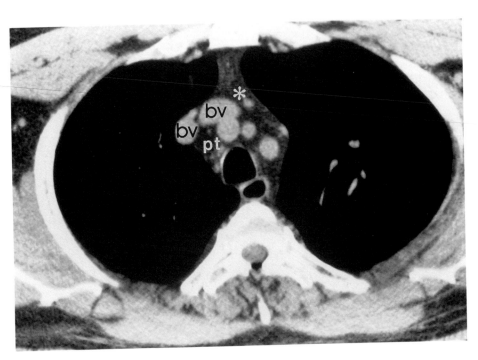

A

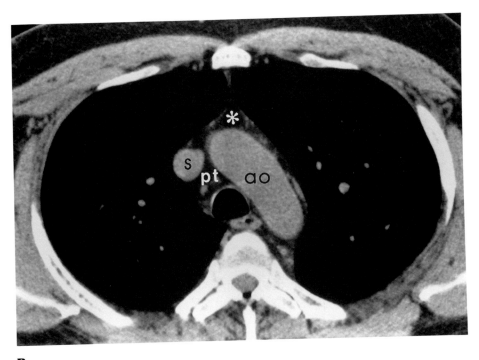

B

Figure 11.7 Pretracheal and prevascular spaces. CT images at the level of **A.** the proximal great vessels, **B.** aortic arch, and **C.** Following page.

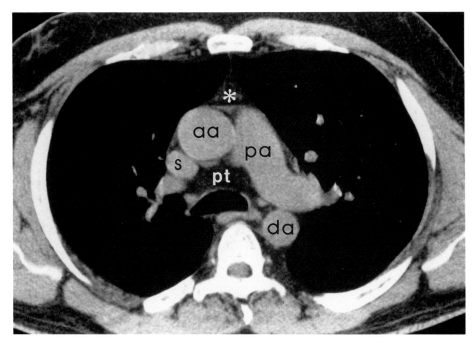

C

Figure 11.7 C. carina. The pretracheal space (pt) extends from the thoracic inlet to the carina and includes the area between the trachea and the great vessels. The prevascular space (asterisk) is bordered by aorta, main pulmonary artery, and great vessels posteriorly, the sternum anteriorly, and pleura of the upper lobes laterally. bv, brachiocephalic veins; s, superior vena cava, ao, aortic arch; aa, ascending aorta; da, descending aorta; pa, pulmonary artery.

aries of the pretracheal space include the superior vena cava and right brachiocephalic (innominate) vein on the right, the aortic arch and the left common carotid and subclavian arteries on the left, and the ascending aorta and brachiocephalic (innominate) artery anteriorly (Figure 11.7). The pretracheal space also contains the superior pericardial recess, which is usually closely applied to the posterior aspect of the ascending aorta. Pretracheal lymph nodes are usually surrounded by mediastinal fat and should not be confused with the superior pericardial recess.

The *prevascular space* in the anterior mediastinum is bordered laterally by lung and pleura of the upper lobes (Figure 11.7). It is bordered by the sternum anteriorly and by the aortic arch, great vessels, main pulmonary artery, and superior vena cava posteriorly. The prevascular space contents include the thymus, lymph nodes, brachiocephalic (innominate) veins, and internal mammary vessels. This space is continuous with the aortopulmonary window.

The *aortopulmonary window* is a small space between the undersurface of the aortic arch and the left main pulmonary artery. It is bordered medially by the trachea and laterally by the left lung (Figure 11.8). Contents include lymph nodes, the left recurrent laryngeal nerve, and the ligamentum arteriosum.

The *subcarinal space* is bordered superiorly by the carina, inferiorly by the left atrium, anteriorly by the right main pulmonary artery, posteriorly by the spine, and laterally by the right and left mainstem bronchi (Figure 11.9). The esophagus, azygos vein, and lymphatics course through this space.

The *retrocrural space* lies between the crura of the diaphragm and the spine. Structures passing through this space include the aorta, azygos and hemizygous veins, thoracic duct, and lymph nodes (Figure 11.10).

Examination of thoracic lymph nodes is a vital part of the evaluation and follow-up of bronchogenic carcinoma and other disease processes. An extensive network of

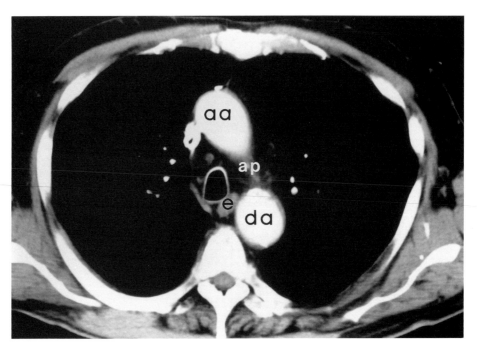

Figure 11.8 Aortopulmonary window. CT image just below the aortic arch shows fat within the aortopulmonary window (ap). This space is bordered anteriorly, posteriorly, and superiorly by aorta, inferiorly by left pulmonary artery, medially by trachea, and laterally by left lung. aa, ascending aorta; da, descending aorta; e, esophagus.

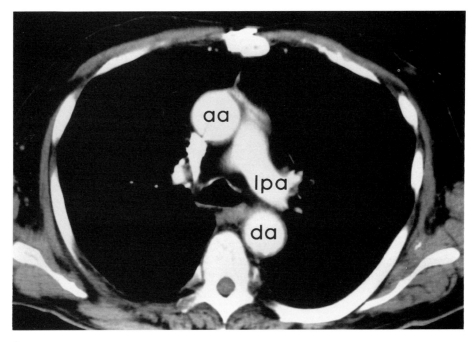

A

Figure 11.9 Subcarinal space. CT images at **A.** the level of the carina and **B.** Following page.

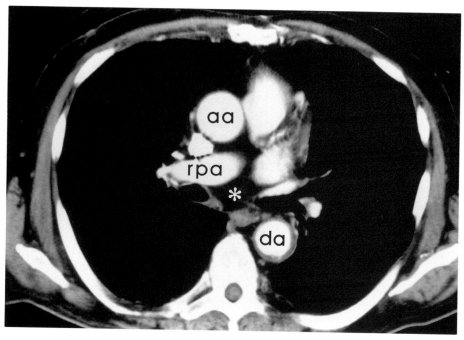

B

Figure 11.9 B. 1 cm inferior to the carina. The subcarinal space (asterisk) is bordered laterally by right and left main bronchi, anteriorly by right pulmonary artery (rpa), posteriorly by spine, superiorly by carina, and inferiorly by left atrium. aa, ascending aorta; da, descending aorta; lpa, left pulmonary artery.

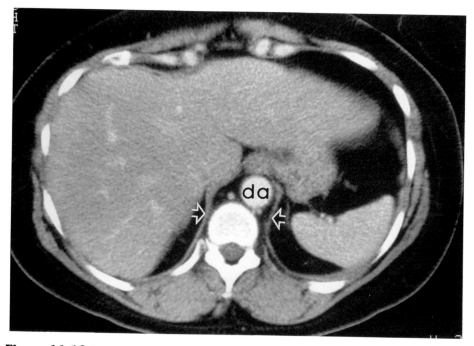

Figure 11.10 Retrocrural space. CT image at the level of the gastroesophageal junction. The descending aorta (da) and azygos and hemizygous veins are seen within the retrocrural space. This space is bordered by right and left diaphragmatic crura (open arrows) anterolaterally and by the spine posteriorly.

lymph nodes in the mediastinum provides lymphatic drainage of the lungs, mediastinal structures, portions of the upper abdomen, and the chest wall, including the breast. The regional nodal stations used in the American Thoracic Society lymph node mapping scheme include the supraclavicular nodes, upper and lower paratracheal nodes, aortopulmonary nodes, anterior mediastinal nodes, subcarinal nodes, paraesophageal nodes, pulmonary ligament nodes, tracheobronchial nodes, and intrapulmonary nodes.[10]

Small lymph nodes can normally be identified with CT in the prevascular, paratracheal, and subcarinal spaces as well as in the aortopulmonary window. Some variability in size of normal mediastinal lymph nodes has been demonstrated,[10–12] but 95% of normal mediastinal lymph nodes in these areas measure less than 1 cm in the short axis. The anterior diaphragmatic lymph nodes drain the anterior diaphragm, upper rectus abdominis muscles, and superior portion of the liver. Lymphatics draining the anterior diaphragmatic lymph nodes are contiguous with the internal mammary lymphatic trunks. The internal mammary lymph nodes drain the anterior chest wall and breast and can be involved in as many as 16% of breast cancer patients in whom axillary lymph node exploration is negative.[13] These lymph nodes, as well as those in the paracardiac, paraesophageal, and paraspinal regions are normally not visualized on CT and, if seen, should be viewed with suspicion.[14] Retrocrural lymph nodes normally are not greater than 6 mm in maximum diameter.

The superior portion of the thoracic esophagus lies behind the trachea from the thoracic inlet to the carina. Both the trachea and esophagus are enveloped by perivisceral fascia which continues into the neck.[15] The esophagus is in close contact with the left mainstem bronchus just below the carina; it then continues behind the heart anterior and to the right of the descending aorta before passing through the esophageal hiatus.[16]

The thymus is located in the anterior mediastinum anterior to the ascending aorta and arch vessels (Figure 11.11). The normal thymus reaches its largest size in adolescence and then undergoes gradual involution and fatty replacement. Thymic tissue can normally be identified on CT in all patients younger than 30 yr of age and in most patients younger than 50 yr of age. Thymic tissue is typically triangular or arrowhead in shape, but variations include separate lobes or a bilobed shape.[17]

The thoracic duct courses superiorly in the posterior mediastinum. In the lower thorax it lies along the anterior thoracic spine between the descending thoracic aorta and the azygos vein in the right hemithorax. At the level of T6, the thoracic duct crosses over to lie to the left of the esophagus in the left hemithorax and then arches laterally, frequently branching into two or three channels before entering the venous system near the junction of the left internal jugular and subclavian veins (Figure 11.12). Variations include drainage into the brachiocephalic (innominate) or external jugular veins as well as right-sided or bilateral thoracic ducts.[18]

DIAPHRAGM

The diaphragm is a thin, dome-shaped muscular sheet that divides the thoracic and abdominal cavities and allows respiration by changing intrathoracic pressure and volume. The thoracic surface of the diaphragm is invested by parietal pleura. The diaphragm has both muscular and tendinous components and its attachments are complex.[19] Anteriorly the diaphragm attaches to the xyphoid process and costal margin. Muscular slips insert into the lower ribs and their costal cartilages anterolaterally, laterally, and posterolaterally. Prominent diaphragmatic muscle slips may indent the surface of the liver and spleen and simulate lesions in these organs or mimic anterior diaphragmatic lymphadenopathy.[20]

The crura of the diaphragm are musculotendinous structures that attach along the anterolateral aspects of the first three lumbar vertebrae. They are joined anterior to the aorta

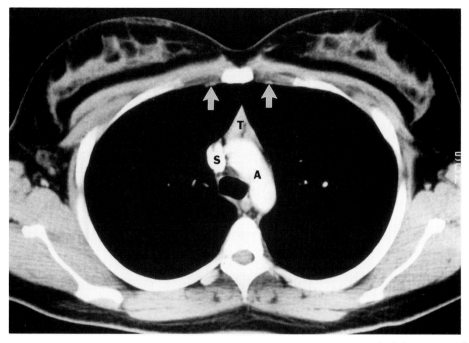

Figure 11.11 Normal thymus. Computed tomography image at the level of the aortic arch (A) in a 23-yr-old woman shows a normal arrowhead-shaped thymus (T). Note normal internal mammary vessels (arrows). S = superior vena cava.

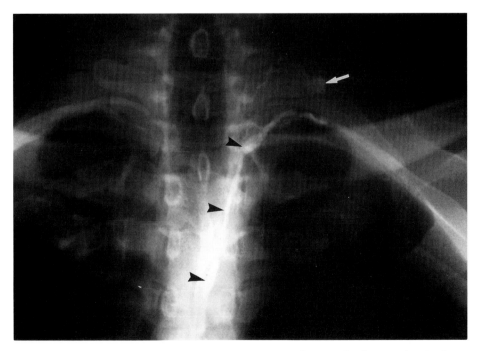

Figure 11.12 Normal thoracic duct. Lymphangiogram showing the thoracic duct in the upper chest (black arrowheads) curving to the left before emptying into the venous system. A small superior branch opacifies a normal lower cervical lymph node (white arrow).

at the T12 level by the median arcuate ligament. The aortic hiatus thus formed allows passage of the aorta, azygos and hemizygous veins, splanchnic nerves, and thoracic duct. The crura are usually asymmetric with the larger right crus often having a thickened nodular appearance anterior to the spine in the upper abdomen on cross-sectional imaging studies. The crura also appear relatively thicker on CT scans obtained during full inspiration.[21] The esophageal hiatus at the T10 levels permits passage of the esophagus and associated vessels as well as the vagus nerve. The inferior vena cava hiatus is anterior and to the right of the esophageal hiatus at the T8-T9 level. This hiatus permits passage of the inferior vena cava and branches of the right phrenic nerve.

Knowledge of normal and variant anatomy of the thorax together with basic surgical principles of respecting tissue planes will facilitate the performance of radiologic-guided percutaneous interventions and minimize the risks of procedure-related morbidity.

REFERENCES

1. Paling MR, Dwyer A: The first rib as the cause of a "pulmonary nodule" on chest computed tomography. *J Comput Assist Tomogr* 4:847–848, 1980.
2. Williams PL, Warwick R, Dyson M: *Gray's Anatomy*, ed 37. New York, Churchill Livingstone, 1989, pp 608–614.
3. Lachman E: A comparison of the posterior boundaries of lungs and pleura as demonstrated on the cadaver and on the roentgenogram of the living. *Anat Rec* 83:521–542, 1942.
4. Gamsu G, Webb WR: Computed tomography of the trachea: normal and abnormal. *Am J Roentgenol* 139:321–326, 1982.
5. Savoca CJ, Austin JHM, Goldberg HJ: Widening of the right paratracheal stripe. *Radiology* 122:295–301, 1977.
6. Naidich DP, Terry PB, Stitik FP, et al: Computed tomography of the bronchi: 1. Normal anatomy. *J Comput Assist Tomogr* 4:746–753, 1980.
7. Heitzman ER, Markarian B, Berger I, et al: The secondary pulmonary lobule: a practical concept for interpretation of chest radiographs. *Radiology* 93:507–512, 1969.
8. Godwin JD, Tarver RD: Accessory fissures of the lung. *Am J Roentgenol* 144:39–47, 1985.
9. Sone S, Hagashihara T, Morimoto S, et al: Potential spaces of the mediastinum: CT pneumomediastinography. *Am J Roentgenol* 138:1051–1057, 1982.
10. Glazer GM, Gross BH, Quint LE, et al: Normal mediastinal lymph nodes: number and size according to American Thoracic Society mapping. *Am J Roentgenol* 144:261–265, 1985.
11. Genereux GP, Howie JL: Normal mediastinal lymph node size and number: CT and anatomic study. *Am J Roentgenol* 142:1095–1100, 1984.
12. Kiyono K, Sone S, Sakai F, et al: The number and size of normal mediastinal lymph nodes: a postmortem study. *Am J Roentgenol* 150:771–776, 1988.
13. Scatarige JC, Boxen I, Smathers RL: Internal mammary lymphadenopathy: imaging of a vital lymphatic pathway in breast cancer. *RadioGraphics* 10:857–870, 1990.
14. Gamsu G: The mediastinum. In Moss AA, Gamsu G, Genant HK (eds): *Computed Tomography of the Body with Magnetic Resonance Imaging*, ed 2. Philadelphia, WB Saunders, 1994, pp 43–118.
15. Oliphant M, Wiot JF, Whalen JP: The cervicothoracic continuum. *Radiology* 120:257–262, 1976.
16. Halber MD, Daffner RH, Thompson WM: CT of the esophagus: I. Normal appearance. *Am J Roentgenol* 133:1047–1050, 1979.
17. Baron RL, Lee JKT, Sagel SS, et al: Computed tomography of the normal thymus. *Radiology* 142:121–125, 1982.
18. Kinnaert P: Anatomic variations of the cervical portion of the thoracic duct in man. *J Anat* 115:45–52, 1973.
19. Panicek DM, Benson CB, Gottlieb RH, et al: The diaphragm: anatomic, pathologic, and radiologic considerations. *RadioGraphics* 8:385–430, 1988.
20. Rosen A, Auh YH, Rubinstein WA, et al: CT appearance of diaphragmatic pseudotumors. *J Comput Assist Tomogr* 7:995–999, 1983.
21. Williamson BRJ, Gouse JC, Rohrer DJ, et al: Variation in the thickness of the diaphragmatic crura with respiration. *Radiology* 163:683–684, 1987.

CHAPTER
12

Percutaneous
Lung Biopsy

John R. Haaga
Dean A. Nakamoto
Kevin Burner

Refinements in modern imaging systems and interventional techniques have made percutaneous lung biopsy one of the most common and effective radiologic procedures.[1] We have gained valuable insights into these techniques from our experience at University Hospitals of Cleveland. This chapter will present a historical description, discuss the data from the literature, and add specific details of our own experience.

HISTORY

The concept of percutaneous aspiration of lung pathology is very old. Leyden first described its use in the diagnosis of pneumonia in 1883.[2] In 1886, Menetrier reported on the use of aspiration biopsy for the diagnosis of malignancy.[3] Unguided needle aspirations were frequent in the 1930s.[4,5] The most significant development was the use of fluoroscopy as a guide to percutaneous procedures.[6,7] Since the early reports on the use of aspiration biopsy techniques, numerous refinements and innovations in instruments, pathologic and cytologic analysis, and guidance modalities have been made.[7-13]

INDICATIONS AND CONTRAINDICATIONS

Indications

The indications for performing a percutaneous biopsy vary widely and have expanded in recent years because of the effectiveness and safety of the procedure. The most common indication for percutaneous biopsy is the need to clarify the nature of any mass or infectious process within the lung. Biopsies are used to diagnose a benign abnormality, confirm the presence of metastatic disease, or establish the nature of a primary tumor. Because of the intense, complicated, and expensive treatment required for recurrent or metastatic cancer, a definitive confirmation by tissue diagnosis is essential. Sophisticated cytologic recovery and staining methods can easily distinguish among the various tumors and permit planning of appropriate therapy.

The reason for obtaining a biopsy of suspected primary lung tumors prior to surgery is the accepted principle that treatment of small cell carcinoma of the lung is not surgical, but rather requires systemic chemotherapy. The diagnosis of and distinction among the various primary lung tumors can be consistently accomplished with percutaneous biopsy and cytopathologic techniques. As will be noted below, numerous authors have confirmed the accuracy of these methods for diagnosing adenocarcinoma, squamous and large cell carcinoma, and small cell carcinoma.

The diagnosis of benign abnormalities is difficult with aspiration biopsy samples because pathologists are unable to define benign or exclude malignant processes on the basis of cytology alone. With the recent introduction of cutting needles that obtain enough tissue for histologic analysis, progress in the diagnosis of benign lesions has been made.

With infectious diseases, a dichotomy exists between what has been reported in the literature and what actually occurs in clinical practice. Several authors have noted the benefit of percutaneous aspiration for the diagnosis of infectious processes. In our experience, determination of the etiology of a pulmonary infiltrate by aspiration methods has not been reliable. The diagnostic recovery of organisms by needle aspiration has only been effective when a discrete fluid collection exists. A small cutting needle may be helpful in assessing a dense or nodular infiltrate.

Contraindications

Absolute contraindications to a percutaneous biopsy include severe coagulopathy, the inability of the patient to cooperate, a suspected arteriovenous malformation or echinococcal lesion, or pulmonary hypertension. Once intrabronchial bleeding develops, it is very difficult to control in patients with pulmonary hypertension, and is a leading cause of death. If the operator is very experienced and familiar with the potential problems encountered in patients with pulmonary hypertension, one might consider performing an aspiration biopsy in a very rare circumstance.

The presence of restrictive lung disease, chronic obstructive pulmonary disease (COPD), emphysema, and blebs should not limit the use of percutaneous biopsy as long as the increased risk of a procedure-related pneumothorax in these patients is understood. Although the possibility of pneumothorax is worrisome, reexpansion of the lung can usually be effected by insertion of a small chest tube.

NEEDLE SELECTION AND TECHNIQUES

Needles

A variety of biopsy needles and techniques has evolved over the years. Most authors use a simple aspiration-type needle to recover cytologic samples. The choice of needle size and tip configuration has varied, but several observations seem to define the optimal device. Two authors have looked at the angle of the bevel at the end of the needle and have concluded that the best angle is about 30°.[14,15] The standard Chiba (Cook, Inc., Bloomington, IN) and the routine "spinal" needle have bevels very close to that angle. The caliber of the needles used has ranged from 18 to 25 gauge (g), but most authors support the concept that the larger the needle, the better the sample. However, the risk of postbiopsy hemoptysis is related to the size of the needle used. Khouri et al. found that the incidence of hemoptysis increases when the needle caliber is greater than 19 g.[16] Therefore, use of a 20-g Chiba needle is recommended for routine aspiration biopsies (Figure 12.1).

For optimal recovery of cells from an aspiration needle, the appropriate amount of suction on the needle should be used. It has been shown that the amount of cel-

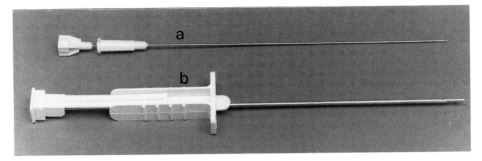

Figure 12.1 A 20-g Chiba needle **A.** for aspiration biopsies and a 14-g cutting-type needle **B.** for obtaining histologic material are shown. Small-caliber cutting needles are available.

lular return from an aspiration biopsy increases linearly with the increase in suction (vacuum) placed on the syringe attached to the needle.[17,18] The size of the syringe is not as critical as the amount of suction placed on the needle. At least 5 cc, and preferably 10 cc, of suction is required to recover the maximum amount of material. More than 10 cc of suction does not improve the diagnostic yield. Several authors have reported good results with no application of suction, but the design of these studies was poor.

It is important to handle the biopsy samples appropriately. Numerous authors have shown that recovery of diagnostic material improves if both a slide preparation and a cell-block sample are sent for pathologic evaluation.[19-21] The best slide smears are made by purging the sample from the needle directly onto the slide. The smears should be made quickly and the slide placed into a fixative to prevent drying. The needle and syringe are then irrigated with the fixative agent. The fixative containing the biopsy specimen is sent for cell block analysis. The choice of the fixative agent is usually dictated by the cytopathologist.

A cutting needle should be used when: (1) previous aspiration biopsies were negative; (2) lymphoma, mesothelioma, or a benign lesion is suspected; or the (3) anatomic approach and character of the lesion permit safe use of a cutting needle. When the lesion is based on the pleura, a 14- to 18-g needle can be used. When the lesion is within the lung parenchyma, a 20-g needle should be used.[22] If a cutting needle is used, it is prudent to evaluate the vascularity of the lesion with contrast-enhanced computed tomography (CT) beforehand. Attention to detail when performing the biopsy is important because the cutting action of the needle should be confined to the mass.

The third category of biopsy device includes small-caliber needles with special cutting tips. Small side holes in the needle tip and needles with multipointed tips are also available.[13,23,24] The Nordenstrom needle (Cook, Inc.) consists of a needle with an inner corkscrew stylet. The corkscrew stylet is longer than the outer cannula of the needle and extends into the mass. The stylet cuts a small ribbon of tissue. Generally, the specimen obtained is smaller than samples obtained with cutting needles, but the potential for complication is less.

Techniques

Three basic methods have been used for percutaneous lung biopsies: single needle, coaxial needle, and tandem or multiple needle techniques. The single needle method involves insertion of a single needle into the lesion. Multiple needle insertions are required to obtain multiple samples. The diagnostic yield and the poten-

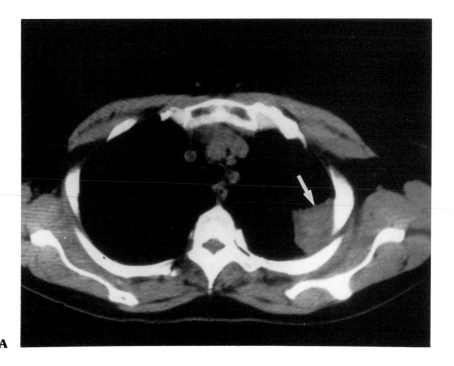

Figure 12.2 A. Pleural-based mass on the left (arrow). An oblique approach to the lesion will avoid traversing aerated lung. B. A single-needle biopsy technique is performed. The needle is advanced toward the lesion, but a rib is inadvertently impacted (arrow). Local anesthetic is infiltrated locally to reduce pain during the rest of the procedure. C and D. Following page.

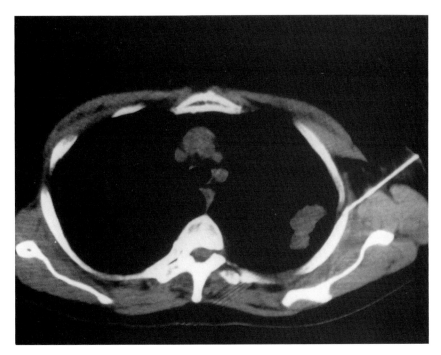

C

D

Figure 12.2 C. Adjustments are made to the needle trajectory to allow advancement of the needle over the rib to the pleural surface. Additional local anesthetic is injected to minimize discomfort during the final needle insertion. **D.** Image localizes the tip of the biopsy needle within the lesion (arrow). Typically, several needle passes are made if the lesion can be sampled without crossing lung parenchyma.

tial for complication are directly related to the number of needle passes made; the more needle passes, the greater the risk. The risk of hemoptysis is minimal when a needle 19 g or less is used. The single needle method is satisfactory for moderate or large masses that are not deep in location and when extreme accuracy is not required (Figure 12.2).

The coaxial biopsy technique employs either a long or short guiding cannula.[1,13,25] The long cannula coaxial system typically uses a larger caliber needle, such as an 18-g or 19-g needle (Greene needle; Cook, Inc.) as a guiding system. The guiding needle is positioned adjacent to or just into the abnormality. Smaller needles (i.e. 22-g) are advanced coaxially through the guiding needle into the mass. The yield depends upon the number of passes made with the smaller needles. There is minimal risk of a pneumothorax because the single larger guiding needle has only advanced across the pleural surface once. The risk of hemoptysis is somewhat greater than with the single needle technique because the size of the guiding needle is fairly large.

The short cannula, coaxial method uses a short guiding cannula that remains outside the pleural cavity. A large guiding cannula can be used since it does not penetrate the pleural surface. Therefore, a larger biopsy needle can be used and better yields obtained. We have found this to be the best method for accurately puncturing small or deep lesions, while minimizing the number of transpleural needle passes (Figure 12.3).

The tandem or multiple needle method is probably the least useful method.[25] With this technique, a single needle is placed into the mass. Additional needles are inserted adjacent to the first needle to achieve a geometric distribution within the mass. Although the diagnostic yield is good, the complication rate is higher than with the other methods.

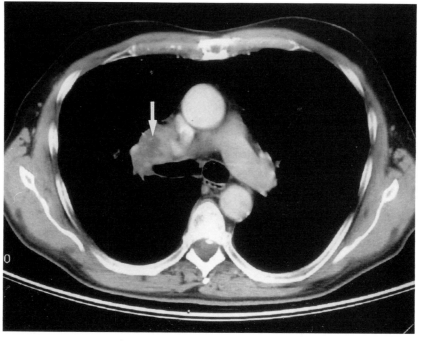

A

Figure 12.3 A. For hilar masses, a contrast-enhanced CT study is used to clearly delineate the mass (arrow) from the adjacent central vessels. **B, C, D, E,** and **F.** Following pages.

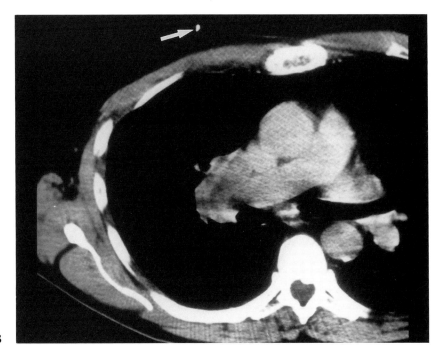

B

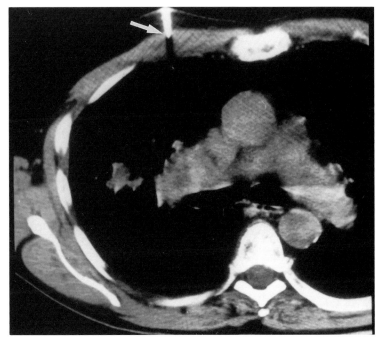

C

Figure 12.3 B. A radiopaque reference (arrow) is positioned on the overlying skin to facilitate selection of a needle entrance site. C. The short guiding cannula is inserted into the chest wall (arrow) and adjustments in cannula angulation are made until the trajectory is satisfactory. Care is taken not to penetrate the pleural surface with this cannula. D, E, and F. Following pages.

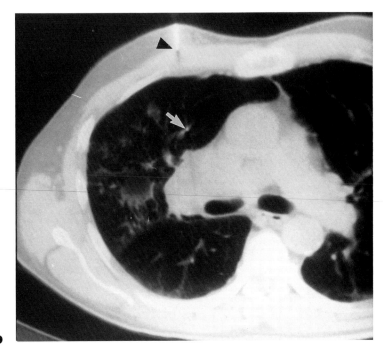

D

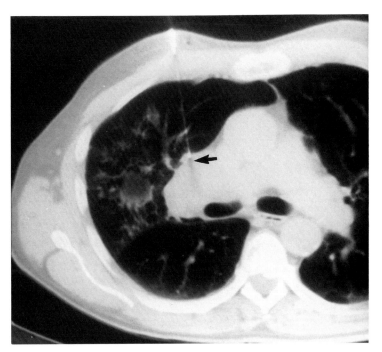

E

Figure 12.3 D. Initial passage of the biopsy needle (arrow) through the guiding cannula (arrowhead) shows the needle tip directed toward the mass. E. The needle tip is advanced into the hilar mass. The tip of the needle and its associated streak artifact are clearly delineated (arrow). F. Following page.

PREPROCEDURE EVALUATION

Prior to the procedure, information about the patient's medical history, drug history, and allergies must be acquired. A cursory evaluation of the patient's physical and men-

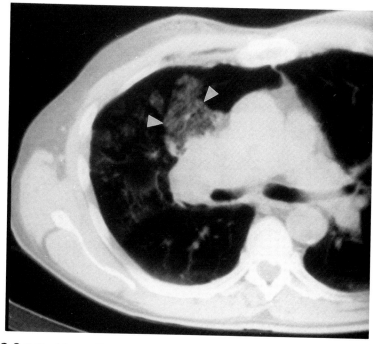

F

Figure 12.3 F. Postbiopsy CT scan shows a small amount of localized bleeding (arrowheads) in the adjacent parenchyma.

tal status should be performed. Coagulation parameters should be acceptable (prothrombin time within 3 sec of control, partial thromboplastin time within 6 sec of control, and a platelet count greater than 50,000/mm³).

The entire procedure should be clearly explained to the patient, and informed consent obtained. The purpose and advantages of performing the percutaneous procedure are detailed, and the obvious benefit of avoiding a surgical procedure is pointed out. The risks of a surgical or percutaneous procedure are discussed and compared. The risk of pneumothorax and/or hemoptysis and the management of complications are also reviewed with the patient. The remote possibility of air embolism, hemorrhage, or death must also be mentioned. The consent should be signed before any sedative is administered.

LUNG BIOPSY PROCEDURE

After the patient's vital signs are taken, intravenous access is established. Blood pressure, electrocardiogram, and oxygen saturation are monitored during the procedure. Sedation can be given, with particular care being taken not to oversedate patients who have carbon dioxide retention. The specific type of sedation depends upon the degree of anxiety of the patient, the experience of the operator, and the sedation policies of the institution. In most cases, light sedation with midazolam (Versed; Roche Lab, Nutley, NJ) is adequate, but in some cases heavier sedation may be required. For heavy sedation, it is best to have an anesthesiologist assist in the case to ensure that there is adequate monitoring of the patient while the radiologist is performing the procedure.

The risk of complication can be minimized by simply using common sense. When planning the trajectory of the needle, any obvious blebs, air cavities, or blood vessels should be avoided. The length of aerated lung crossed with the needle should be minimized, because the risk of pneumothorax is directly related to the length of lung parenchyma traversed by the needle (personal communication: John Locke, M.D., and John Haaga, M.D., Case Western Reserve University). Any skin impediment (such as the nipple) or bony structure, such as a rib or the scapula, should be avoided. The patient must be comfortable enough to stay in position (oblique, lateral, or prone) and cooperate with the radiologist. The relationship of the skin marker to the underlying deep structures can change significantly if the patient moves.

After the skin has been prepared in a sterile fashion, local anesthesia with 1% lidocaine (Xylocaine; Astra USA, Inc., Westboro, MA) is carefully administered to include the pleura. If the pleura is not anesthetized, the patient may move when the needle crosses the lung, and thereby increase the probability of a pneumothorax. If a rib or other bony structure is encountered, a large amount of local anesthetic is instilled to anesthetize the periosteum and minimize any discomfort during needle manipulation (Figures 12.2B, 12.2C, and 12.8A). The less pain the patient feels, the greater the probability he can cooperate and the procedure will go well. Mixing 10 cc of 1% lidocaine with 1 cc of 8.4% sodium bicarbonate (Abbott Laboratories, Abbott Park, IL) will lessen the stinging sensation produced by the administration of the local anesthetic.[26]

Before the procedure, the patient should practice holding his breath. This simple exercise can be reassuring, because patients realize that the duration of their breathhold will be limited. The operator can also assess potential cooperation, hearing deficiency, or comprehension problems.

The needle should only be advanced into and through lung tissue when the patient suspends his respiration. Because the lung is rather elastic and lung nodules can be firm, efficient penetration of the lesion by the needle will not be achieved unless the needle is advanced assertively. Advancing the needle slowly is more likely to deflect the mass. If the stylet of the needle is removed, the patient should suspend respiration to prevent influx of air through the needle. If the patient begins to cough when the needle is in the lung, the needle should be removed immediately; coughing may cause serious air embolism or pleural laceration.

To be absolutely certain that the specimen is diagnostic before the patient leaves, the sample can be "quick" stained and examined on site by a pathologist, or the patient can leave the biopsy suite but remain in the area until the results are known.[19,21] If the abnormality is benign, it may be difficult to know when to stop taking samples. An increase in the number of needle passes made during a biopsy procedure increases the diagnostic yield but also increases the risk of complication. Because it can be difficult to have a pathologist present for all biopsies, we perform enough needle passes to acquire the amount of material we consider adequate and then release the patient. If a nondiagnostic sample is obtained, the patient is scheduled for a repeat biopsy. If a second biopsy is necessary, the initial procedure can be reviewed to determine if a different approach or type of needle is required.

GUIDANCE MODALITIES FOR LUNG LESIONS

The three major guidance systems used for percutaneous lung biopsies are fluoroscopy, CT, and ultrasound. Fluoroscopy is best suited for well-defined, parenchymal lesions. Adjustments can be made in real time to accommodate changes in needle angle, patient respiration, or mass movement/deflection.[27] Computed tomography (CT) is the best modality for guiding biopsies of lesions located in the pleura, hila, apices, or mediastinum. Lesions that are poorly defined, cavitated, or masked by overlying structures are also best approached with CT guidance. The superiority of CT guidance for most biopsy procedures is evident in the literature.[27–36]

Ultrasound guidance can only be used for lesions based in the pleura or located in the periphery of the lung parenchyma. Small-caliber biopsy needles are usually used because even small amounts of air adjacent to the lesion can make ultrasound-guided procedures difficult. Because ultrasound guidance has such a limited role, it will not be discussed further.

Fluoroscopic Guidance

When biopsy procedures are performed under fluoroscopic guidance, there are a number of considerations that should not be overlooked.[28–35,37] If available, a movable, C-arm fluoroscopic unit should be used for the procedure. Use of a C-arm unit allows the operator to visualize the lesion in multiple planes and optimize the angle of entry into the lesion without requiring the patient to move. If the lesion is difficult to localize with C-arm fluoroscopy, CT guidance should be used. It is helpful to position the lesion at an isocentric point so that the C-arm can be rotated around the patient while keeping the lesion in the center of the fluoroscopic image (Figures 12.4 and 12.5).

There are numerous methods to confirm that placement of the needle tip is within the lesion. Use of a C-arm unit facilitates fluoroscopic triangulation. Several visual perspectives can be obtained by moving the fluoroscopic tower while the patient remains stationary. Two orthogonal views of the needle tip in the lesion are usually sufficient to confirm accurate needle placement (Figure 12.5). Slight movement of the mass when the needle penetrates the lesion or when the needle is wiggled is also useful. Most experienced operators use the tactile perception of an abrupt change in tissue texture as an indication that the needle has penetrated the mass.

When performing a fluoroscopy-guided biopsy, the operator should always be cognizant of the hazards of radiation. There are three things that can be done to minimize radiation exposure. Fluoroscopy should be used intermittently, not continuously. Second, good collimation minimizes scatter radiation to the operator and the patient. Fi-

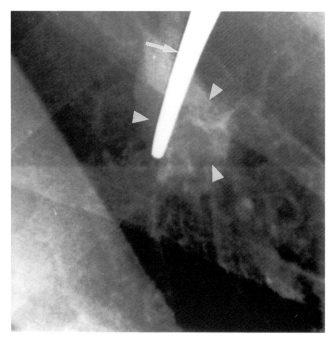

A

Figure 12.4 A. Fluoroscopy can be useful as a guidance modality for sampling well-defined parenchymal masses. Coned-down spot film shows initial localization of a mass (arrowheads) in the left lung with a metal needle holder (arrow). **B** and **C**. Following page.

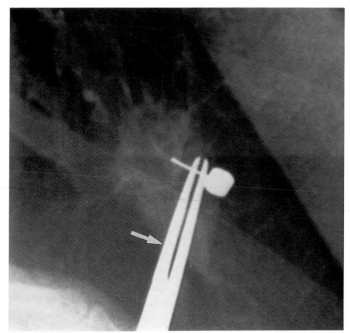

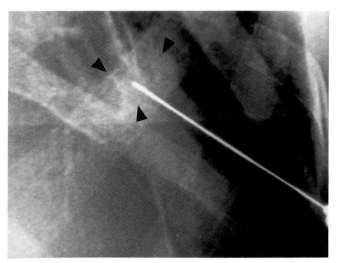

Figure 12.4 B. A needle-holding device should be used (arrow) to minimize radiation exposure to the operator's hands. C. Needle tip is seen within the mass (arrowheads).

nally, a device for holding the biopsy needle should be used whenever necessary so that direct exposure of the operator's hands to the fluoroscopic beam is avoided (Figure 12.4B). Do not lose sight of the potential hazards of radiation.

Computed Tomography Guidance

Computed tomography is well suited to a variety of biopsy procedures.[1,13] Lesions best suited for CT-guided biopsies are those in the lung apices, costophrenic and cardiophrenic angles, retrosternal area, pleura, hila, or mediastinum.[36,38–43] Biopsy of a lesion that is poorly seen on fluoroscopy because of an associated pleural effusion or overlying infiltrate can also be better performed with CT.

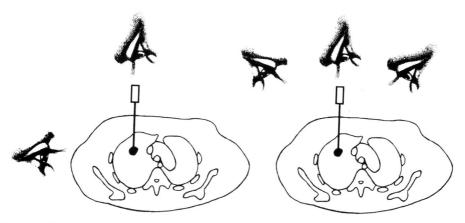

Figure 12.5 Diagram shows that right angle confirmation can be obtained by either two perpendicular views (L) or two smaller opposite angles (R). The latter approach requires less movement of the fluoroscope or the patient.

Because CT is not a real-time tool, careful selection of a needle entry site and trajectory is important. Because the ribs traverse obliquely across the anatomic area of interest on an axial CT image, the relationship of the lesion to the overlying bone is usually unreliable. Similar problems can occur with the tip of the scapula. Therefore, manual palpation for underlying bony structures at the site of planned needle entry and correlation with the CT scan prior to needle insertion are critical.

When there is an alveolar process associated with an apparent lung lesion, the spherical portions with the greatest density should be targeted for biopsy (Figure 12.6). If more than one needle pass is made, at least two different regions of the mass should be sampled. By positioning a patient with the affected lung down, a potentially mobile lung lesion can be immobilized because the weight of the ab-

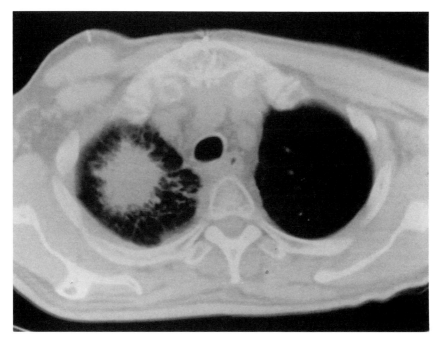

A

Figure 12.6 A. Computed tomography shows a mass with poorly defined margins due to tumor infiltration and surrounding parenchymal infiltrate. **B.** Following page.

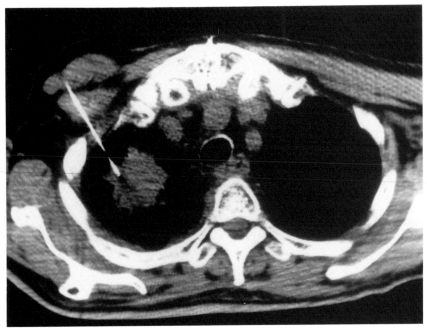

Figure 12.6 B. The needle should traverse the peripheral infiltrate and penetrate the solid component of the mass to maximize the biopsy yield.

dominal viscera will minimize movement of the ipsilateral diaphragm (Figure 12.7).

By using several important principles during a lung biopsy, the occurrence of post-procedure pneumothorax or hemoptysis can be minimized. Deliberate planning of a needle course that enters the lung through an area of pleural adhesion or avoids air cavities/blebs will reduce the risk of pneumothorax (Figure 12.8). Traversing fluid-

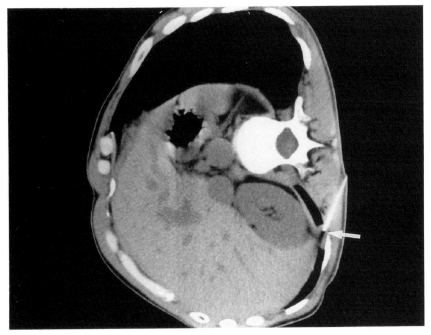

Figure 12.7 Computed tomography shows a small mass in the right posterior costophrenic angle. Placing the patient in the ipsilateral decubitus position facilitated successful needle biopsy of the mass (arrow).

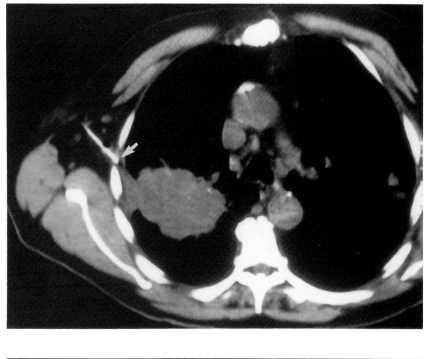

A

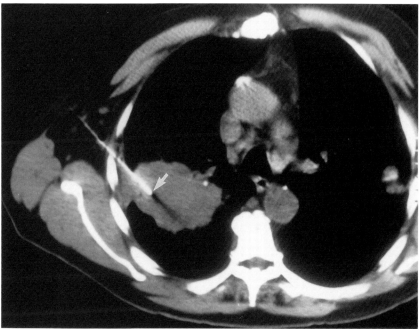

B

Figure 12.8 **A.** Preliminary CT image shows a needle trajectory that avoids penetration of aerated lung and traverses an area of pleural attachment. The needle was placed at the pleural surface (arrow) to ensure adequate local anesthesia. **B.** Placement of the needle into the mass is documented (arrow). Numerous needle aspirations or cutting needle samples can be obtained by this technique with a very low risk for a complication.

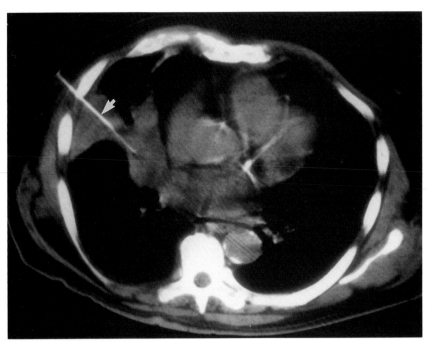

Figure 12.9 Traversing consolidated lung and avoiding aerated lung will minimize risk of a pneumothorax. This scan shows a 20-g Chiba needle (arrow) traversing a triangular infiltrate and directed toward the mass in the hilum.

filled or consolidated lung minimizes escape of air and the risk of a pneumothorax (Figure 12.9).[44] If a lesion is pleural-based, penetration of underlying air spaces can be avoided by either direct transpleural entry into the lesion (Figure 12.2A) or choosing a pathway through a pleural effusion (Figure 12.10). Severe postbiopsy hemoptysis can be minimized by avoiding major vessels, choosing the shortest needle path to the lesion, and using needles 19 g or smaller.

When performing a CT-guided lung biopsy, it is necessary to localize the lesion and then confirm accurate needle placement. The patient must be able to hold his breath consistently. Patients who are not cooperative or motivated can make lesion localization and successful biopsy quite difficult. The patient should be instructed to take gentle, comfortable breaths and stop breathing when requested. To have patients hold respiration after a full, half, or exhaled breath does not work well.

Multiple sequential, 5-mm scans in the plane of the needle will confirm placement of the needle tip. If the length of the needle is consistently seen as nontapering and cylindrical with a square end that causes a streak artifact, one can be confident that the tip is seen (Figure 12.11). With experience, the operator will be able to appreciate the change in texture between the normal lung and the firm mass during advancement of the biopsy needle.

OTHER APPLICATIONS FOR CT GUIDANCE

Mediastinal Lesions

Most mediastinal biopsies are performed under CT guidance.[1,13,27–30,36,41,42] Computed tomography provides clear visualization of the abnormality, the adjacent vascular structures, the safest path to the abnormality, and placement of the needle in the lesion. Lesions in the anterior, middle, and posterior mediastinum can also be safely and effectively sampled under CT guidance.

If an abnormality in the anterior mediastinum is large enough, it can actually ex-

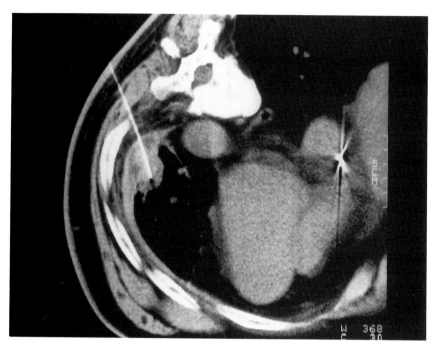

Figure 12.10 A left pleural-based lesion with an associated pleural process is biopsied without traversing aerated lung. The patient was in a decubitus position.

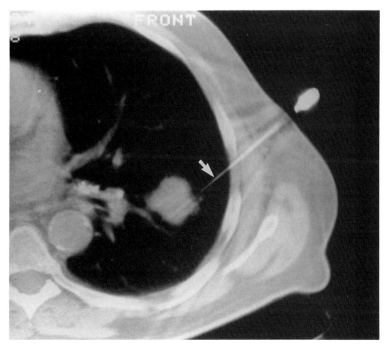

A

Figure 12.11 A. When the apparent needle tip has a "tapered" appearance on an axial CT image (arrows) and no distal streak artifact is seen, the needle tip has not been imaged. **B.** Following page.

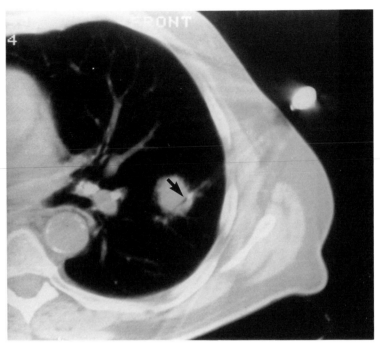

B

Figure 12.11 B. Computed tomography shows the needle tip (arrow) in the lesion. The tip has a characteristic "squared-off" appearance and also causes a distal streak artifact (also see Figures 13.3E and 13.8B).

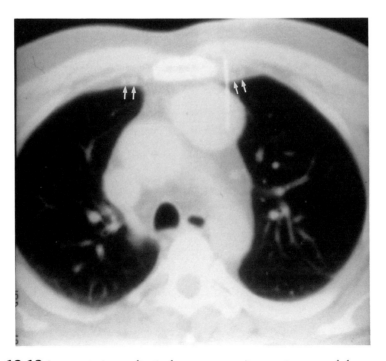

Figure 12.12 Large anterior mediastinal masses are quite easy to approach because there is no intervening aerated lung. The needle path should avoid the internal mammary vessels (arrows).

tend beyond the lateral margins of the sternum and make biopsy quite direct (Figure 12.12). When the lesion is much smaller, the biopsy device must be inserted at an acute angle under the sternum to avoid traversing aerated lung. In either case, the location of the internal mammary vessels should be noted.

Posterior mediastinal lesions are frequently adjacent to the vertebral bodies (Figures 12.13). These lesions can be targeted via the extrapleural space without travers-

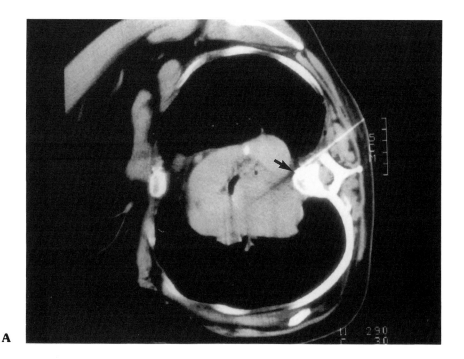

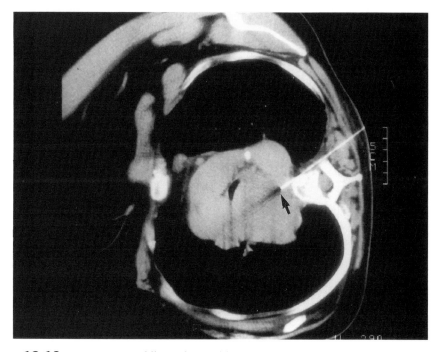

Figure 12.13 A. During a middle mediastinal biopsy, the needle is targeted to the anterior margin of the vertebral body (arrow). The patient is in a right lateral decubitus position. B. The bevel of the needle is turned so that it is toward the vertebral body. The needle is advanced slowly into the middle mediastinal mass (arrow).

ing lung parenchyma. The descending thoracic aorta and the azygos and hemizygous veins should be avoided.

Middle mediastinal lesions are very difficult to approach percutaneously. The key factor to performing a biopsy in this area is careful attention to technique. A needle path should be chosen that begins at the costovertebral junction, traverses the extrapleural space adjacent to the aorta, passes along the edge of the vertebral body, and enters the mass (Figure 12.14). To execute the maneuver, adequate local anesthetic must be given. The easiest approach is to the left of midline because the aorta "holds" the extrapleural space open for the passage of the needle. After the needle is angled appropriately at the costovertebral junction, the anterior margin of the vertebral body in the same axial plane as the lesion to be sampled is targeted. Once the needle is in contact with the periosteum of the vertebral body, a large amount of anesthetic should be administered through the needle. The bevel of the needle is then positioned against the vertebral body. The needle is advanced slowly so that it glances off the vertebral body. The most significant impediment to this maneuver is the presence of an osteophyte on the vertebral body. If an osteophyte is present and the needle cannot be advanced beyond the margin of the vertebral body, the procedure may need to be terminated. The other unusual circumstance that warrants aborting the procedure is the interposition of the aorta or hemizygous vein between the needle tip and middle mediastinal lesion. Occasionally, the hemizygous vein is interposed between the vertebral body and thoracic aorta. The biopsy should not be performed from this approach in this case. If the esophagus is traversed, a vagal reaction may occur. The major bronchi and central pulmonary vessels should also be avoided.

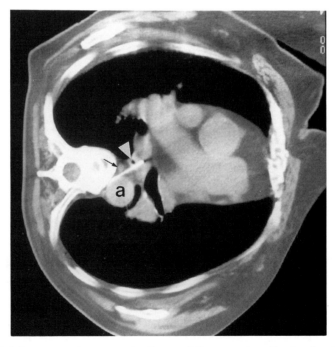

Figure 12.14 Computed tomography from a different patient (in the decubitus position) shows accurate needle placement in an abnormal-sized lymph node in the subcarinal area. Note the descending thoracic aorta (a), azygos vein (arrow), and the air-filled esophagus (arrowhead).

Apical Lung Lesions

Biopsy of an apical lung lesion is unique because of the anatomic limitations and the diverse pathologies that occur in this area.[31,38] Numerous overlying structures limit needle access to the lung apex. The brachiocephalic vessels and the clavicle limit an anterior approach. A posterior approach must be chosen carefully because of the scapula and the close apposition of the upper posterior ribs. By abducting the patient's arm, the scapula moves laterally and more space between bony structures is generated. Although the upper ribs are close together, they become concentrically smaller toward the lung apex. Therefore, a needle site slightly higher than the target lesion permits the needle to successfully traverse unimpeded over the top of the rib (Figure 12.15).

Lateral meningoceles and neurilemmomas or neurofibromas are abnormalities that can mimic a lung mass in the apex of the lung.[31] These abnormalities occur adjacent to and may enlarge the neural foramina. When unrecognized, these lesions can be inadvertently referred for biopsy. Upon puncturing a lateral meningocele, a small amount of clear, spinal fluid will be recovered. The fluid can be sent for glucose evaluation and/or the cavity can be injected with a small amount of sterile nonionic myelographic contrast material. The cavity may or may not communicate with the subarachnoid space, but the contrast will clearly define the relationship of the mass of the thecal sac. Magnetic resonance imaging (MRI) will clearly delineate its identity. Neurilemmomas are very hard, and biopsy material is difficult to obtain with needle aspiration. Larger needles are not helpful. Furthermore, the patient will complain of very intense, unremitting pain while the needle is in the lesion. No amount of local anesthetic will control the pain. Magnetic resonance imaging will usually demonstrate the relationship of the lesion to the nerve root.

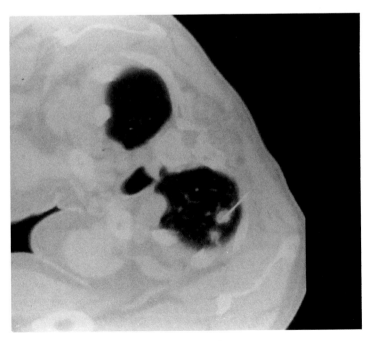

Figure 12.15 A left apical lung lesion was successfully sampled with the patient in a decubitus position, by inserting the needle with a caudal trajectory.

Hilar Lesions

Because hilar lesions are deep-seated and in close proximity to large vessels, the risk of a procedure-related complication is higher than with other thoracic biopsies.[43] Therefore, it is important to clearly define the location of the lesion relative to the central vessels (Figure 12.3). If a patient has difficulty with consistent breath-holding, a decubitus position may help stabilize the location of the lesion. For most hilar lesions, a bronchoscopy-guided biopsy should be attempted prior to any percutaneous procedure.[40,45] Hemoptysis will usually occur with percutaneous biopsy techniques, regardless of the needle size used. A patient may expectorate as much as an ounce of blood; if more bleeding occurs, careful observation is recommended (see Complications).

Pleural Lesions

Because pleural lesions are silhouetted by the pleural tissue, they are not seen well with fluoroscopy. Computed tomography is especially well suited for targeting these lesions. An aspiration biopsy procedure can be performed initially to ensure that there is sufficient local anesthetic and patient cooperation. If the pleural lesion is large with a well-defined access route, a cutting needle can be used because the risk is minimal and the diagnostic yield much improved (Figure 12.16).

DIAGNOSTIC ACCURACY

Malignant Lesions

The usefulness of percutaneous thoracic biopsies depends on the skill and expertise of the radiologist performing the biopsy and the cytopathologist interpreting the slides. Despite these uncontrollable variables, the overall success rate of percutaneous biopsy

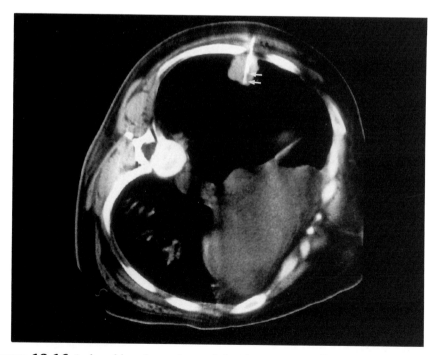

Figure 12.16 A pleural-based mass is sampled with a cutting needle. The tip of the needle is confined to the mass and the slot of the cutting blade is seen (arrows). Precise positioning of the needle tip was accomplished by careful manual adjustments. Automated biopsy devices do not afford this type of precise control.

is uniformly high, ranging between 60% and 90%.[6,12,27,35,46,47] The success rate depends on the patient population and the types of tumors included. There is a 60% to 90% correlation between the cytologic (needle) and histologic (surgical) results for primary and metastatic lung cancer. The precise correlation between cytology and histology differs with the various cell types: adenocarcinoma, 71% to 93%; squamous cell carcinoma, 81% to 100%; small cell carcinoma, poor to 90%; and metastatic disease, 60% to 80%.[48-51]

Accurate diagnosis of lymphoma, thymoma, and mesothelioma is quite difficult with aspiration biopsy techniques. Several authors have noted that the results of fine-needle aspiration can suggest the general diagnosis of lymphoma, but the results are not reliable in establishing the definitive subtype of lymphoma.[23,42,43] Establishing the specific subtype of lymphoma is critical because both the treatment and the prognosis vary greatly. Goralnik et al. have shown that large cutting needles are required to definitively diagnose most lymphomas.[22] The reported experience with thymomas and mesotheliomas is quite limited, but the literature and our experience indicate that a definitive diagnosis of these entities is difficult even with large cutting needles. Differentiation among benign thymoma, malignant thymoma, and lymphoma is very difficult.

Benign Lesions

It is difficult to use an aspiration biopsy to categorize a lesion as benign because of the problems associated with the reliability of a negative biopsy result.[12,46,52,53] In one small series, the correct diagnosis of hamartoma was obtained from cytologic material in 5 of 14 patients and in 11 of 14 cases, from histologic material.[54] Because hamartomas are very firm in texture, large needles (16-g and 20-g) and vigorous needle thrusts were necessary to obtain adequate aspiration biopsy samples. As might be expected, the authors had a higher than average complication rate.

Negative Results

Because most percutaneous biopsy procedures are performed with small-caliber needles, one must always be wary of a negative biopsy result.[51] A negative aspiration biopsy does not exclude malignancy because a negative result may be due to a technical or sampling error. Most authors agree that several repeat biopsies should be performed if there is a serious concern for malignancy. Patients should be followed carefully before a negative result is accepted. One alternative to following a patient with a negative biopsy result is to offer the patient a surgical procedure. If the patient refuses surgery after a nondiagnostic biopsy, it is our practice to monitor solitary lesions with high-resolution CT scanning at 3-month intervals for a period of 9 months. During this observation period, if the lesion completely calcifies or significantly reduces in size, our concern about malignancy lessens. Despite this, long-term follow-up is still obtained at less frequent intervals. If such a lesion grows during the observation period, a repeat biopsy and/or thoracotomy is suggested. If the lesion remains equivocal after 9 months, surgical removal is suggested.

COMPLICATIONS

Serious complications from percutaneous transthoracic lung, pleural, and mediastinal biopsies are rare as long as sound judgment and meticulous technique are used. Familiarity with factors that predispose a patient to develop a complication enables the interventional radiologist to obtain informed consent, minimize complications, and treat those that do arise. The most common complications encountered are pneumothorax and mild postbiopsy hemoptysis.[52,55-61] More serious, but less frequent, complications include tension pneumothorax, air embolism, and severe endobronchial bleeding. The most unusual complication reported is perforation of the right ventricle.[62]

Tumor Seeding

Although rare, tumor seeding along the needle track has been reported.[55-57] Such an event is unpredictable, with no definite predilection. In theory, a coaxial biopsy technique should minimize the risk.

Pneumothorax

The presence of a pneumothorax can be detected with fluoroscopy, a chest x-ray, or a CT scan. If a patient becomes acutely symptomatic, fluoroscopy can be used immediately, but this method is only useful when a large pneumothorax is present. When a patient is supine, the air in the pleural cavity is anterior in location, so that the pleural "edge" of the collapsed lung is very difficult to visualize fluoroscopically. For routine detection, a chest radiograph or CT scan will show a pneumothorax with equal accuracy.

The incidence of a postbiopsy pneumothorax is variable. The rate of asymptomatic pneumothorax ranges between 16.1% and 60%.[7-13,45,47-53] while the rate of symptomatic pneumothorax requiring chest tube insertion is 9.4% to 25%.[25,45,47-53] The distinction between a pneumothorax that is asymptomatic (not requiring treatment) and symptomatic (requiring treatment) also varies widely in the literature. In optimum circumstances, chest tube insertion can be reserved for patients who are short of breath, demonstrate an increasing pneumothorax on sequential chest radiographs, or are clinically fragile (with severe underlying lung disease, cardiac problems, advanced age, or general debilitation). Asymptomatic patients who are otherwise medically stable probably do not need a chest tube. Because of the simplicity and safety of insertion and the effectiveness of small chest tubes, strict criteria need not be established. The threshold for chest tube insertion that best suits each institution and patient can be applied.

There are numerous factors that affect development of a postbiopsy pneumothorax. One of the most significant factors affecting the occurrence of a pneumothorax is the baseline state of the patient's lung. Patients with COPD, as determined by chest radiographs and pulmonary function tests, have a postbiopsy pneumothorax rate of 46%. Patients with normal lungs have a postbiopsy pneumothorax rate of 7%.[58,59] No chest tube insertions were required in patients with normal pulmonary function, while 19% of patients with COPD required chest tube insertion after lung biopsy. In our experience, when COPD is noted on an axial CT scan, the incidences of symptomatic and asymptomatic pneumothorax were 47% and 12%, respectively.

Other factors that seem to affect the incidence of pneumothoraces include the depth and size of the lesion and the length of lung traversed by the needle. The smaller the lesion or the greater the depth of the lesion from the skin, the greater risk of a pneumothorax.[60,61] In one study, the occurrence of a pneumothorax with a CT-guided lung biopsy was directly related to the length of aerated lung crossed with the biopsy needle.[60] The risk of pneumothorax can be minimized if a needle trajectory is chosen that avoids aerated lung and traverses areas of pleural fibrosis or parenchymal consolidation (Figures 13.8–13.10).[1,44]

The development of a pneumothorax is also directly related to the number of needle passes. The caliber of the biopsy needle does not appear to affect the pneumothorax rate. The configuration of the needle tip and the mechanism of obtaining tissue have a significant effect on pneumothorax rate. If the biopsy device has a cutting tip, the pneumothorax rate is higher. For example, the Franseen needle (Cook Inc.), which has several points on its tip, is associated with a higher pneumothorax rate than a standard Chiba needle. Therefore, cutting needles should be used only if the cutting action of the needle can be confined to the mass.

Two maneuvers have been shown to be useful in reducing the pneumothorax rate. Positioning the patient with the biopsy site down for a period of 1 hr immediately after the procedure can decrease the overall pneumothorax rate from 33.6% to 17.9%, and the rate of chest tube insertion from 9.8% to 0.4%.[63,64] Because of the increased solubility of nitrogen compared with oxygen, letting the patient breathe 100% oxygen during and after the procedure has been shown to be effective in decreasing the pneumothorax rate and increasing the rate of pneumothorax resorption should one develop.[65,66] The only shortcoming of using 100% oxygen is the risk of decreasing the respiratory drive in patients with severe COPD.

Depositing collagen or blood clot along the biopsy tract to "patch" the pleura has been proposed as a means of lowering the pneumothorax rate,[45,67-71] but this technique does not appear helpful.[61,63] More recently, Engeler et al. have shown that there may be a reduction in the pneumothorax rate if collagen plugs are carefully deposited to occlude the needle pathway.[72]

Perlmutt et al. showed that if a pneumothorax develops, it occurs immediately after the biopsy in 89% of cases; an additional 9% occur at 1 hr and the remaining 2% within 4 hr after biopsy.[73] It is our practice to observe a patient for 10 to 15 min in the biopsy suite before obtaining a chest film. It is not wise to send patients for chest radiography immediately because a patient could develop a life-threatening pneumothorax in an unobserved area or during transportation. After this initial observation period, a chest film is obtained, followed by a repeat radiograph at 4 hr.

Hemoptysis

In the early years of percutaneous lung biopsies, hemoptysis occurred in as many as 21% of patients. As techniques and equipment have been refined and experience gained, the incidence of biopsy-related hemoptysis has decreased to less than 5%. Khouri et al. attributed a decrease in their hemoptysis rate primarily to a change in the size of the biopsy needle used.[16] The hemoptysis rate with an 18-g Chiba needle was 21%, whereas the rate dropped to 5% when a 20-g Chiba needle was used.

Another factor that may predispose patients to hemoptysis is the use of aspirin or other platelet inhibitors at the time of the procedure. We insist that patients discontinue medications that inhibit platelet function for at least 1 wk before the biopsy procedure. Our resolve on this issue is such that we will cancel and reschedule a procedure if any aspirin product has been taken in the preceding week. Other factors that appear to affect the rate of biopsy-related hemoptysis include the presence of congestive heart failure, lack of patient cooperation, and proximity of the lesion to large blood vessels. Berquist et al. reported a 19% hemoptysis rate with biopsies of lesions close to the hilum, compared with a 9% hemoptysis rate associated with biopsies of peripheral lesions.[60]

Endobronchial Bleeding

Severe endobronchial bleeding has been rarely reported, but its occurrence may be life-threatening.[74-78] The best method of avoiding this complication is to exclude patients who are uncooperative, have pulmonary hypertension, or are receiving anticoagulation therapy. If severe bleeding occurs, the best immediate treatment is to administer oxygen through a nasal cannula and then place the patient in a decubitus position, with the biopsy site down. This positioning maneuver will help to inhibit blood from spilling into the nonaffected lung. At the same time, an emergency code should be instituted to summon the anesthesiologist. A double-lumen endotracheal tube can be inserted so that the balloon on one lumen occludes the bronchus ipsilateral to the bleeding site, while the second lumen permits air exchange through the uninvolved lung.

Air Embolism

Air embolism is a rare but serious complication.[79-83] One possible cause is the passage of air through the open lumen of the biopsy needle. Therefore, the patient must suspend respiration when the needle lumen is open to the air (i.e., removal of the needle stylet during attachment of a syringe or vacuum device). The most plausible explanation of serious air embolism is tracking of air along the needle path from a bronchus into a pulmonary vein. This event is believed to occur when intrathoracic pressure is elevated (i.e., during a Valsalva maneuver, positive pressure ventilation, or coughing). Most reported cases of air embolism are preceded by an episode of coughing. The best method of preventing air embolism is to avoid performing the procedure on an uncooperative patient and to quickly remove the biopsy needle if any coughing occurs.

CHEST TUBE INSERTION

The indications for chest tube insertion after a biopsy differ at various institutions, but usually only symptomatic patients are treated. It is relatively easy, safe, and effective to insert a small-caliber chest tube (8- to 12-Fr nephrostomy-type catheters; Tru-Close Thoracic Vent, Uresil Corp., Skokie, IL; or Sacks One-step catheters; Elecath, Rahway, NJ) coupled to a Heimlich valve (Cook, Inc).[84-87]

The tube is inserted through the second or third anterior intercostal space on the side of the pneumothorax. The entrance site is prepared in a sterile fashion, and ample local anesthetic (down to the pleura) is instilled. After a small skin incision, the tube is advanced through the intercostal space and directed cephalad. It is preferable to position the tube in the region of the lung apex so that evacuation of air will occur whether the patient is in the supine or upright position. If the chest tube is positioned perpendicular to the chest wall, it may be quite painful because of pleural irritation, and the tube may partially trap the lung and prevent its complete reexpansion.

Chest tube function should be assessed by listening for air escaping from the Heimlich valve or by observing motion of the valve flaps. A chest radiograph should be obtained to ensure reexpansion of the lung and proper placement of the tube (Figure 12.17). In some cases, the Heimlich valve is not sufficient to allow reexpansion of the lung. In debilitated or unstable patients, in situations when the Heimlich valve is not effective, or if the lung is involved by diffuse disease, vacuum suction (Pleur-Evac; Deknatel, Fall River, MA) should be used. When there is a very large air leak, the escape of air into the pleural space can be so rapid that a large-bore chest tube attached to a Pleur-Evac will be required.

Once the lung reexpands and the air leak into the pleural space has stopped, the Pleur-Evac can be placed to water seal for 12 to 24 hr. If there is no further air leak and a repeat chest radiograph shows no recurrence of pneumothorax, the chest tube can be removed. If a Heimlich valve is used, once the lung reexpands and there is no apparent air leak, the chest tube can be capped or clamped for 6 to 12 hr while the patient is closely monitored. If the patient remains asymptomatic and a follow-up chest radiograph shows no pneumothorax, the chest tube can be removed.

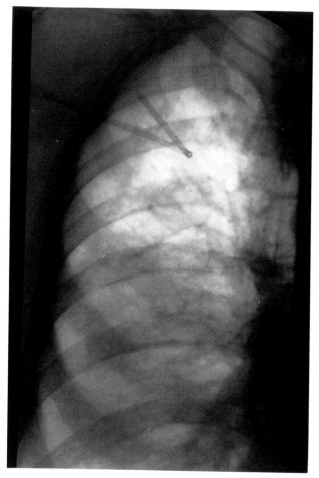

Figure 12.17 Digital radiograph shows appropriate positioning of the chest tube and complete reexpansion of the lung.

REFERENCES

1. Haaga JR: CT guided biopsy. In Haaga JR, Alfidi RJ (eds): *CT of the whole body.* St Louis, Mosby, 1988.
2. Leyden OO: Ueber infektiose pneumonie. *Dtsch Med Wochenschr* 9:52, 1883.
3. Menetrier P: Cancer primitif du poumon. *Bull Soc Anat Paris* 4:643, 1886.
4. Martin HE, Ellis EB: Biopsy by needle puncture and aspiration. *Ann Surg* 92:169–175, 1930.
5. Carver LF, Binkley JS: Aspiration biopsy of tumors of the lung. *J Thorac Surg* 8:436–463, 1939.
6. Lauby RW, Burnett WE, Rosemond GP, et al: Value and risk of biopsy of pulmonary lesions by needle aspiration: twenty-one years' experience. *J Thorac Cardiovasc Surg* 49:159–172, 1965.
7. Adamson JS, Bates JHB: Percutaneous needle biopsy of the lung. *Arch Internal Med* 119: 164–169, 1967.
8. Nordenstrom B: A new technique for transthoracic biopsy of lung changes. *Br J Radiol* 38:550–553, 1965.
9. Fontana RS, Miller WE, Beabout JW, et al: Transthoracic needle aspiration of discrete pulmonary lesions: experience in 100 cases. *Med Clin North Am* 54:961–971, 1970.
10. Meyer JE, Gandbhir LH, Milner LB, et al: Percutaneous aspiration biopsy of nodular lung lesions. *J Thorac Cardiovasc Surg* 73:787–791, 1977.

11. Turner AF, Sargent END: Percutaneous pulmonary needle biopsy: an improved needle for a simple direct method of diagnosis. *Am J Roentgenol* 104:846–850, 1968.

12. Westcott JL: Percutaneous transthoracic needle biopsy. *Radiology* 169:593–601, 1988.

13. Haaga JR, Alfidi RJ: Precise biopsy localization by computer tomography. *Radiology* 118: 603–607, 1976.

14. Andriole JG, Haaga JR, Adams RB, et al: Biopsy needle characteristics assessed in the laboratory. *Radiology* 148:659–662, 1983.

15. Dähnert WF, Hoagland MH, Hamper UM, et al: Fine-needle aspiration biopsy of abdominal lesions: diagnostic yield for different needle tip configurations. *Radiology* 185:263–268, 1992.

16. Khouri NF, Stitik FP, Erozan YS: Transthoracic needle aspiration biopsy of benign and malignant lung lesions. *Am J Roentgenol* 144:281–288, 1985.

17. Hueftle MG, Haaga JR: Effect of suction on biopsy sample size. *Am J Roentgenol* 147: 1014–1016, 1986.

18. Kreula J: Effect of sampling technique on specimen size in fine needle aspiration. *Invest Radiol* 25:1294–1299, 1990.

19. Johnsrude IS, Silverman JF, Weaver MD, et al: Rapid cytology to decrease pneumothorax incidence after percutaneous biopsy. *Am J Roentgenol* 144:793–794, 1985.

20. Greene R, Szyfelbein WM, Isler RJ, et al: Supplementary tissue-core histology from fine-needle transthoracic aspiration biopsy. *Am J Roentgenol* 144:787–792, 1985.

21. Austin JHM, Cohen MB: Value of having a cytopathologist present during percutaneous fine-needle aspiration biopsy of lung: report of 55 cancer patients and metanalysis of the literature. *Am J Roentgenol* 160:175–177, 1993.

22. Goralnik CH, O'Connell DM, El Yousef SJ, et al: CT-guided cutting-needle biopsies of selected chest lesions. *Am J Roentgenol* 151:903–907, 1988.

23. Wittich GR, Nowels KW, Korn RL, et al: Coaxial transthoracic fine-needle biopsy in patients with a history of malignant lymphoma. *Radiology* 183:175, 1992.

24. Vine HS, Kasdon EJ, Simon M: Percutaneous lung biopsy using the Lee needle and a track-obliterating technique. *Radiology* 144:921–922, 1982.

25. VanSonnenberg E, Casola G, Ho M, et al: Difficult thoracic lesions: CT-guided biopsy experience in 150 cases. *Radiology* 167:457–461, 1988.

26. Matsumoto AH, Reifsnyder AC, Hartwell GD, et al: Reducing the discomfort of lidocaine administration through pH buffering. *JVIR* 5:171–175, 1994.

27. Adler OB, Rosenberger A, Peleg H: Fine-needle aspiration biopsy of mediastinal masses: evaluation of 136 experiences. *Am J Roentgenol* 140:893–896, 1983.

28. Jereb M, Us-Krasovec M: Transthoracic needle biopsy of mediastinal and hilar lesions. *Cancer* 40:1354–1357, 1977.

29. Moinuddin SM, Lee LH, Montgomery JH: Mediastinal needle biopsy. *Am J Roentgenol* 143: 531–532, 1984.

30. Weisbrod GL, Lyons DJ, Tao LC, et al: Percutaneous fine-needle aspiration biopsy of mediastinal lesions. *Am J Roentgenol* 143:525–529, 1984.

31. Dahlgren SE, Ovenfors CO: Aspiration biopsy diagnosis of neurogenous mediastinal tumors. *Acta Radiol Diagn* 10:289–298, 1979.

32. Herman PG, Hessel SJ: The diagnostic accuracy and complications of closed lung biopsies. *Radiology* 125:11–14, 1977.

33. Sargent END, Turner AF, Gordonson J, et al: Percutaneous pulmonary needle biopsy: report of 350 patients. *Am J Roentgenol* 122:758–768, 1974.

34. Jereb M: The usefulness of needle biopsy in chest lesions of different sizes and locations. *Radiology* 134:13–15, 1980.

35. Sinner WN: Transthoracic needle biopsy of small peripheral malignant lung lesions. *Invest Radiol* 8:305–314, 1973.

36. Fink I, Gamsu G, Harter LP: CT-guided aspiration biopsy of the thorax. *J Comput Assist Tomogr* 6:958–962, 1982.

37. Stevens GM, Weigen JR, Lillington GA: Needle aspiration biopsy of localized pulmonary lesions with amplified fluoroscopic guidance. *Am J Roentgenol* 103:561–571, 1968.

38. Gatenby RA, Mulhern JR, Broder GJ, et al: Computed-tomographic-guided biopsy of small apical and peripheral upper-lobe lung masses. *Radiology* 150:591–592, 1984.

39. Gobien RP, Skucas J, Paris BS: CT-assisted fluoroscopically guided aspiration biopsy of central hilar and mediastinal masses. *Radiology* 141:443–447, 1981.

40. Sider L, Davis TM Jr: Hilar masses: evaluation with CT-guided biopsy after negative bronchoscopic examination. *Radiology* 164:107–109, 1987.

41. Kuhlman JE, Fishman EK, Wang KP, et al: Mediastinal cysts: diagnosis by CT and needle aspiration. *Am J Roentgenol* 150:75–78, 1988.

42. Rosenberger A, Adler O: Fine needle aspiration biopsy in the diagnosis of mediastinal lesions. *Am J Roentgenol* 131:239–242, 1978.

43. Westcott JL: Percutaneous needle aspiration of hilar and mediastinal masses. *Radiology* 141: 323–329, 1981.

44. Haramati LB, Austin JHM: Complications after CT-guided needle biopsy through aerated versus nonaerated lung. *Radiology* 181:778, 1991.

45. Collins CD, Breatnach E, Nath PH: Percutaneous needle biopsy of lung nodules following failed bronchoscopic biopsy. *Eur J Radiol* 15:49–53, 1992.

46. Gobien RP, Valicent JR, Paris BS, et al: Thin-needle aspiration biopsy: methods of increasing the accuracy of a negative prediction. *Radiology* 145:603–605, 1982.

47. Woolf CR: Application of aspiration lung biopsy with a review of the literature. *Dis Chest* 25:286–301, 1984.

48. Horrigan TP, Bergin KT, Snow N: Correlation between needle biopsy of lung tumors and histopathologic analysis of resected specimens. *Chest* 90:638–640, 1986.

49. Poe RH, Tobin RE: Sensitivity and specificity of needle biopsy in lung malignancy. *Am Rev Respir Dis* 122:725–729, 1980.

50. Thornbury JR, Burke DP, Naylor B: Transthoracic needle aspiration biopsy: accuracy of cytologic typing of malignant neoplasms. *Am J Roentgenol* 136:719–724, 1981.

51. Taft PD, Szyfelbein WM, Greene R: A study of variability in cytologic diagnoses based on pulmonary aspiration specimens. *Am J Clin Pathol* 73:36–40, 1980.

52. Günther RW: Percutaneous interventions in the thorax. *JVIR* 3:379–390, 1992.

53. Charig MJ, Stutley JE, Padley SPG, et al: The value of needle biopsy in suspected operable lung cancer. *Clin Radiol* 44:147–149, 1991.

54. Hamper UM, Khouri NF, Stitik EP, et al: Pulmonary hamartoma: diagnosis by transthoracic needle-aspiration biopsy. *Radiology* 155:15–18, 1985.

55. Seyfer AE, Walsh DS, Graeber GM, et al: Chest wall implantation of lung cancer after thin-needle aspiration biopsy. *Ann Thorac Surg* 48:283–286, 1989.

56. Sinner WN, Zajicek J: Implantation metastasis after percutaneous transthoracic needle aspiration biopsy. *Acta Radiol Diagn* 17:473–480, 1976.

57. Wolinsky H, Lischner MS: Needle track implantation of tumor after percutaneous lung biopsy. *Ann Intern Med* 71:359–362, 1969.

58. Miller KS, Fish GB, Stanley JH, et al: Prediction of pneumothorax rate in percutaneous needle aspiration of the lung. *Chest* 93:742–745, 1988.

59. Fish GD, Stanley JH, Miller KS, et al: Postbiopsy pneumothorax: estimating the risk by chest radiography and pulmonary function tests. *Am J Roentgenol* 150:71–74, 1988.

60. Berquist TH, Bailey PB, Cortese DA, et al: Transthoracic needle biopsy: accuracy and complications in relation to location and type of lesion. *Mayo Clin Proc* 55:475–481, 1980.

61. Locke J: University Hospitals, Cleveland, Ohio, personal communications, 1990.

62. Shevland JE: Right ventricular perforation: a rare complication of percutaneous lung biopsy. *J Thorac Imaging* 6(4):85–86, 1991.

63. Moore EH, Shepard JA, McLoud TC, et al: Positional precautions in needle aspiration lung biopsy. *Radiology* 175:733–735, 1990.

64. Cassel DM, Birnberg FA: Preventing pneumothorax after lung biopsy: the roll-over technique. *Radiology* 174:282, 1990.

65. Chadha TS, Cohn MA: Noninvasive treatment of pneumothorax with oxygen inhalation. *Respiration* 44:147–152, 1983.

66. Cormier Y, Laviolette M, Tardif A: Prevention of pneumothorax in needle lung biopsy by breathing 100% oxygen. *Thorax* 35:37–41, 1980.

67. McCartney RL, Tait D, Stilson M, et al: A technique for the prevention of pneumothorax in pulmonary aspiration biopsy. *Am J Roentgenol* 120:872–875, 1974.

68. McCartney RL: Further observations on the lung patch technique. *Am J Roentgenol* 124:397–403, 1975.

69. Herman SJ, Weisbrod GL: Usefulness of the blood patch technique after transthoracic needle aspiration biopsy. *Radiology* 176:395–397, 1990.

70. Bourgouin PM, Shepard JA, McLoud TC, et al: Transthoracic needle aspiration biopsy: evaluation of the blood patch technique. *Radiology* 166:93–95, 1988.

71. Surprenant EL: Transthoracic needle aspiration biopsy: evaluation of the blood patch technique. *Radiology* 168:285, 1988.

72. Engeler CE, Hunter DW, Castaneda-Zuniga W, et al: Pneumothorax after lung biopsy: prevention with transpleural placement of compressed collagen foam plugs. *Radiology* 184:787–789, 1992.

73. Perlmutt LM, Braun SD, Newman GE, et al: Timing of chest film follow-up after transthoracic needle aspiration. *Am J Roentgenol* 146:1049–1050, 1986.

74. McCartney RL: Hemorrhage following percutaneous lung biopsy. *Radiology* 112:305–307, 1974.

75. Milner LB, Ryan K, Guillo J: Fatal intrathoracic hemorrhage after percutaneous aspiration lung biopsy. *Am J Roentgenol* 132:280–281, 1979.

76. Norenberg R, Claxton CP, Takaro T: Percutaneous needle biopsy of the lung: report of two fatal complications. *Chest* 66:216–218, 1974.

77. Pearce JG, Patt NL: Fatal pulmonary hemorrhage after percutaneous aspiration lung biopsy. *Am Rev Respir Dis* 110:346–349, 1974.

78. Meyer JE, Ferrucci JT, Janower ML: Fatal complications of percutaneous lung biopsy: review of the literature and report of a case. *Radiology* 96:47–48, 1970.

79. Tolly TL, Feldmeier JE, Czarnecki D: Air embolism complicating percutaneous lung biopsy. *Am J Roentgenol* 150:555–556, 1988.

80. Westcott JL: Air embolism complicating percutaneous needle biopsy of the lung. *Chest* 63:108–110, 1973.

81. Aberle DR: Gamsu G. Golden JA. Fatal systemic arterial air embolism following lung needle aspiration. *Radiology* 165:351–353, 1987.

82. Baker BK, Awwad EE: Computed tomography of fatal cerebral air embolism following percutaneous aspiration biopsy of the lung. *J Comput Assist Tomogr* 12:1082–1083, 1988.

83. Cianci P, Posin JP, Shimshak RR, et al: Air embolism complicating percutaneous thin needle biopsy of lung (abstract). *Radiology* 166:290, 1988.

84. Poe RH, Kallay MC: Transthoracic needle biopsy of lung in nonhospitalized patients. *Chest* 92:676–678, 1987.

85. Casola G, vanSonnenberg E, Keightley A, et al: Pneumothorax: radiologic treatment with small catheters. *Radiology* 166:89–91, 1988.

86. Perlmutt LM, Braun SD, Newman GE, et al: Transthoracic needle aspiration: use of a small chest tube to treat pneumothorax. *Am J Roentgenol* 148:849–851, 1987.

87. Sargent END, Turner AF: Emergency treatment of pneumothorax: a simple catheter technique for use in the radiology department. *Am J Roentgenol* 109:531–535, 1970.

CHAPTER 13

Thoracic Musculoskeletal Biopsies

William N. Snearly
Phoebe A. Kaplan
Robert G. Dussault

The diagnosis and treatment of skeletal lesions is becoming increasingly complex and sophisticated. Therefore, prior to any therapeutic intervention, most skeletal lesions require a tissue diagnosis, which may be accomplished by means of an open surgical or percutaneous biopsy. The use of percutaneous biopsy in the diagnosis of skeletal neoplasms was initially reported in the early 1930s.[1] Since then, the technique has been refined and expanded to include the evaluation of osteomyelitis and other bone disorders. With the aid of computed tomographic (CT) guidance, most portions of the skeleton are accessible to percutaneous needle biopsy.

A percutaneous needle biopsy has several advantages over a surgical biopsy. Closed biopsy techniques can markedly diminish the risks and inconveniences of an open biopsy.[2] Only a small stab wound is required, which results in a smaller operative hematoma. The stab wound can easily be resected en bloc with the tumor if a surgical procedure is to be the definitive therapy. This technique also avoids creating dangerously large defects in the bone that may result in a pathologic fracture. Radiation therapy can be started earlier, as there is no concern about wound healing. Percutaneous biopsy does not require the use of a surgical suite and can be performed as an outpatient procedure at lower cost.[3] The risk of infection and tumor spillage is also reduced.[1,4–7]

Biopsy of the musculoskeletal system is not a single procedure; rather, it consists of several procedures. The type of imaging guidance, choice of needle, potential complications, and handling of the specimen all depend upon the location and appearance of the lesion.

Because of these complexities, close cooperation with the pathologist and orthopedic surgeon is needed. The pathologist should be consulted regarding the handling of the specimen and the quantity of tissue required. The pathologist should always be informed of the radiologic differential diagnosis. In cases of potential infection, material should be obtained for Gram stain and appropriate cultures as well as histologic and cytologic analysis. Consultation with the orthopedic surgeon is important to ensure that the biopsy procedure does not compromise any potential surgical resection. Skeletal lesions should be completely evaluated prior to a biopsy procedure, because the radiologic appearance, and therefore the diagnostic possibilities, may change significantly as a result of the biopsy. Biopsy of skeletal lesions is best performed at the treating institution.[8]

INDICATIONS

As a general rule, any bone lesion may be sampled by percutaneous techniques. A review of the literature indicates that almost all types of bone lesions have been diagnosed by needle biopsy.[4-6,9-15] The most frequent indication for skeletal biopsy is for tissue diagnosis of metastatic disease. Although skeletal metastases can be diagnosed with high confidence by their radiographic features, tissue diagnosis is often required to initiate or alter therapy. Percutaneous needle biopsy is often performed on the following groups of patients: (1) patients with a known primary neoplasm and a positive radionuclide bone scan; (2) patients with a known primary who develop a bone lesion which is atypical for that neoplasm; (3) patients with multiple known primary tumors who present with a bone lesion; (4) patients with a previously treated neoplasm who have been in remission and present with a new bone lesion; (5) patients with a radiographically stable metastatic lesion needing to be assessed for viable tumor cells; (6) patients with no known primary tumor who present with a bone lesion typical of metastatic disease; (7) patients who are high surgical risks; and (8) patients with osteomyelitis or infectious spondylitis in whom culture and antibiotic sensitivity results are needed to guide treatment.[5,6,14,16]

In cases of suspected primary bone tumor, the value of percutaneous biopsy has only been recently accepted. Traditionally, primary bone tumors have been subjected to open biopsy on the assumption that a large amount of tissue is needed to establish the diagnosis. This assumption was made because of the regional histologic variations within the tissue of many primary bone tumors. However, several recent reports describe successful cytologic and histologic diagnosis of selected primary bone tumors from percutaneous biopsy specimens.[17-20] Moreover, the increased use of neoadjuvant chemotherapy for bone tumors has increased the need for tissue diagnosis prior to operative resection. Percutaneous needle biopsies are indicated in patients with suspected primary bone tumors when: (1) patients with round cell tumors (myeloma, lymphoma, or Ewing sarcoma) will be treated by radiation or chemotherapy without surgical resection; (2) patients with eosinophilic granuloma or unicameral bone cysts will be treated with intralesional injection of methylprednisolone; (3) patients with osteosarcomas will be treated by limb salvage; and (4) a round cell lesion must be differentiated from osteomyelitis. An open biopsy is recommended after two unsuccessful needle biopsy attempts. Percutaneous biopsy is not recommended for patients with suspected cartilaginous tumors because they are often difficult to grade even with surgical specimens.[7]

CONTRAINDICATIONS

There are no absolute contraindications to percutaneous skeletal biopsy. A relative contraindication is a high risk of hemorrhage due to an uncorrectable bleeding diathesis. Platelet counts below 50,000 should be corrected prior to the biopsy.[5,21] Partial thromboplastin time (PTT), prothrombin time (PT), and platelet count should be evaluated before the procedure.[21]

A patient with a lesion that will be treated surgically should not be subjected to percutaneous biopsy unless the result will significantly alter the surgical approach. As with any other procedure, the risks of the biopsy must be weighed against the risks of initiating treatment without a specific diagnosis.

LOCALIZATION OF THE LESION

Before the biopsy is performed, a complete radiographic evaluation of the lesion should be performed. Generally, this will include plain films and a whole body nuclear medicine bone scan. Most patients will also be studied with CT or magnetic resonance imaging (MRI) to assist in staging the lesion. All of the available studies must be reviewed to help plan the biopsy. The lesion selected for biopsy should be the most accessible lesion. The approach should take into consideration the local anatomy and any potential surgical resection. As with any biopsy, special attention must be paid to the location of blood vessels, nerves, lung, or other vital structures to minimize the risk of complication.

Many imaging modalities are available to guide needle placement. Excellent results have been reported with fluoroscopy, CT, ultrasonography, and bone scintigraphy. Selection of the guiding modality is based upon the location of the lesion and the experience of the radiologist. Fluoroscopy is well suited for use in the extremities or ribs.[4,9,10,13,15,22,23] Computed tomography has been recommended for vertebral biopsies due to the complex anatomy.[24–28] Ultrasound and scintigraphic guidance have also been successfully used to guide biopsies of rib lesions.[29–34]

INSTRUMENTATION

There are a wide variety of biopsy needles available. In general, the types of needles available for percutaneous bone biopsies can be divided into four groups: spinal-type, cutting, trephine, and combination-type needles that combine features of a few types of needles.

Spinal-type Needles

Spinal-type needles are most commonly used for aspiration bone biopsy. Useful sizes range from 16 to 22 gauge with a variety of angled bevels. The bevel angle has a significant effect on the specimen size and quality, particularly when small-bore needles are used. In a laboratory evaluation of a variety of 22-gauge needles, the best samples were obtained with a 25° beveled needle (Chiba; Becton Dickinson, Franklin Lakes, NJ)[35] (Figure 13.1). The small caliber needles are especially useful for biopsing deeply located lesions or those that are adjacent to neurovascular structures. In addition, a small, spinal-type needle with a removable hub (e.g., van Sonnenberg or CoANS; Cook Inc., Bloomington, IN) can be used as a guide for the introduction of a larger needle, thereby increasing the safety of the procedure.[36] Once this type of needle is inserted into the lesion, negative pressure is applied on the needle with a syringe while it is rapidly inserted in and out of the lesion. Material obtained is suitable for cytologic analysis.

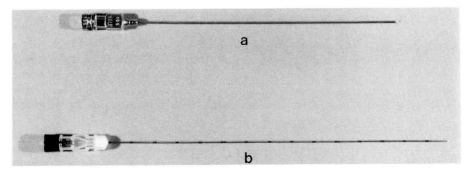

Figure 13.1 A conventional 22-gauge spinal needle (a) and a 22-gauge Chiba needle (b). The 25° bevel on the Chiba needle is highly effective in obtaining an adequate sample. Centimeter markings on the Chiba needle aid in its positioning.

Cutting Needles

The cutting needles are most useful for obtaining a core of soft tissue material for histologic analysis without significant crush artifacts.[37] This type of needle consists of an inner component that catches and holds a small amount of tissue in a recessed notch. A sharp cutting cannula is then advanced, cutting the tissue and retaining it for retrieval. Important variables with cutting needles are the length of the channel in which the sample is obtained and the distance the needle tip advances when the sample is obtained. Needle selection will therefore vary with lesion location and size. The lightweight and compact Temno needle (Bauer Medical Inc., Clearwater FL) is available in a number of combinations of channel and needle lengths and with a coaxial guiding needle through which multiple tissue samples can be obtained (Figure 13.2). Cutting needles are well suited for soft-tissue masses or osteolytic bone lesions.

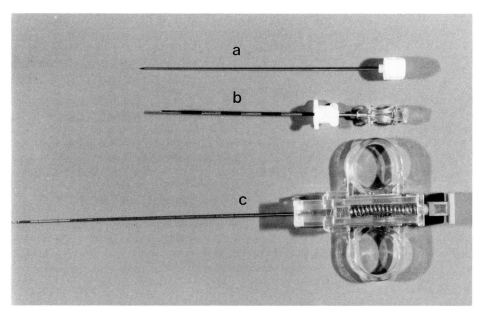

A

B

Figure 13.2 A. The coaxial Temno system. The sharp obturator (a) is placed inside the 17-gauge coaxial needle (b) as it is inserted into the lesion. A small locking stopper on the coaxial needle guards against insertion beyond the required depth. Then the obturator is removed and the spring-loaded 18-gauge biopsy needle (c) is inserted up to its hub. The needle is armed by pulling back on the plunger until a click is felt. The plunger is depressed to advance the specimen notch and advanced further to trigger the cannula to close over the notch, trapping the specimen. **B.** Magnified view: detail of the specimen notch.

Trephine Needles

The basic trephine needle consists of a large outer cannula fitted with a sharp obturator. Trephine needles are generally larger than spinal and cutting needles and are used to obtain cores of bone for histologic analysis. With smaller trephine needles, such as the 18- to 22-gauge Franseen (Cook Inc.), the outer cannula has a number of cutting teeth that can drill into the bone. With larger trephines such as the Craig (10-gauge, Becton Dickinson Co.) or Ackerman (12-gauge, Slanco, Becton Dickinson Co) needle, the obturator is replaced by an inner cannula containing the cutting teeth (Figure 13.3). The tip of the outer cannula is beveled, thus acting as a wedge that can be secured into the bone. This type of needle is most useful for obtaining large samples and for lesions that are osteoblastic or located beneath intact cortical bone. Percutaneous penetration of extremely thick cortex or very osteoblastic lesions may require the use of a hand drill or one of several motor-driven biopsy devices.[38–40]

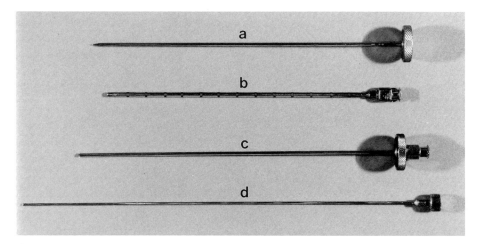

A

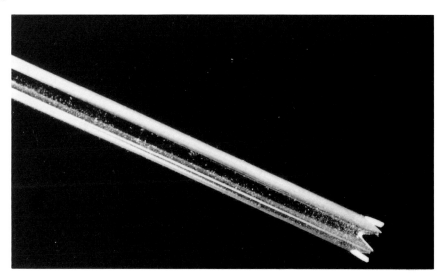

B

Figure 13.3 A. The Ackerman trephine needle biopsy set. The sharp obturator (a) is placed within the outer cannula (b) which is advanced until it is wedged into the bone. The obturator is then removed and replaced by the trephine needle (c). The trephine needle is advanced by a combination of axial and rotational forces. A blunt obturator (d) aids in removal of the specimen from the trephine. B. Magnification view of the cutting tip.

Combination Needles

Two other needles are available that combine features of the cutting and trephine needles. The Jamshidi needle (Manan Medical Products Inc., Northbrook, IL), initially devised for bone marrow aspiration, consists of a sharp beveled tip with an inner obturator (Figure 13.4). It is available in either 11 or 12 gauge and is equipped with a fixed handle to facilitate use in hard bone. The beveled tip can be used to cut out a core of cancellous bone. As there is no outer cannula to secure the specimen, negative pressure should be applied to the hub with a syringe during needle withdrawal.

The second combination needle is the Ostycut (C.R. Bard, Covington, GA) which consists of an outer beveled cutting needle with a threaded tip and a sharp inner obturator (Figure 13.5). The outer needle can be fitted with a handle to facilitate use in very hard bone.

Combinations of needles can be used effectively in a coaxial fashion for obtaining material for cytology and histology. For example, a Jamshidi needle may be used as a guiding cannula through which specimens can be obtained with a small spinal-type needle for cytology, or a cutting or trephine needle for histology. Several specimens can be obtained without additional imaging because the Jamshidi ensures a consistent location within the lesion. The Jamshidi needle itself can be used to obtain an additional histologic specimen if needed. We generally obtain material for cytology with three different needle passes and for histology with two core specimens.

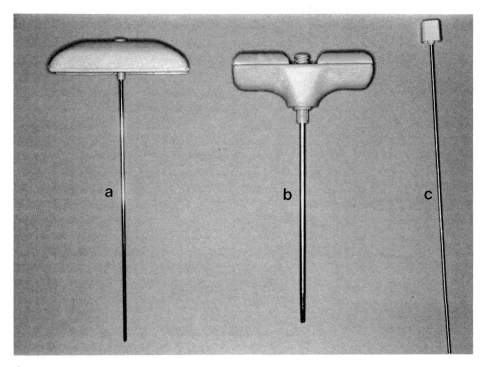

A

Figure 13.4 A. Disposable Jamshidi biopsy needle. The sharp obturator (a) and the cutting needle (b) fit together to form a T-shaped handle. A Luer-Lok hub on the cutting needle is used for aspiration biopsy and to apply suction as the needle is withdrawn. The blunt obturator (c) is used to dislodge the specimen from the cutting needle. **B.** Following page.

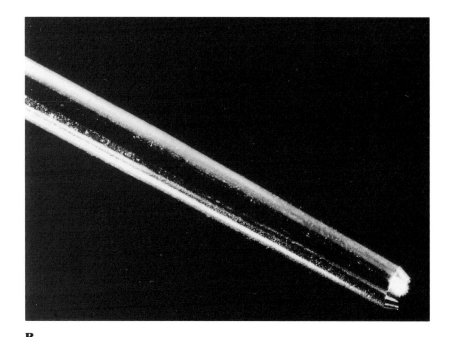

B

Figure 13.4 B. Magnification view of the cutting needle.

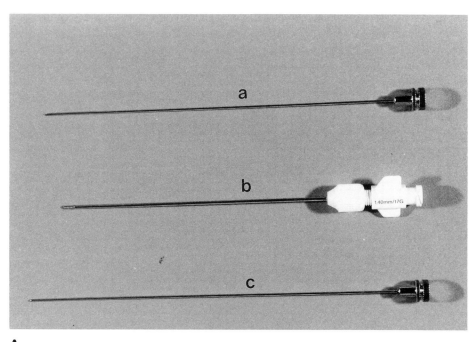

A

Figure 13.5 A. The Ostycut biopsy needle. A sharp obturator (a) and the cutting needle (b) are combined as the tip is anchored in the bone. The obturator is removed and the needle advanced by clockwise rotation. The threaded tip cuts a core as it is screwed into the bone. A slight change in direction while advancing the final 1–2 mm will sever the specimen. A syringe is attached to the hub during specimen withdrawal. The blunt obturator (c) aids in specimen extraction. B. Following page.

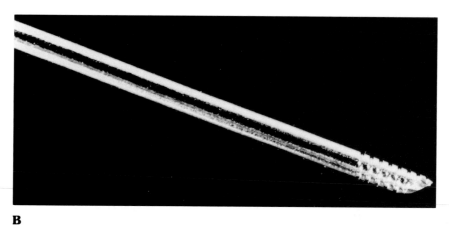

B

Figure 13.5 B. Magnified view of threaded tip of the cutting needle.

PREBIOPSY PREPARATION

Once all of the available imaging studies have been reviewed and the most accessible lesion identified, the route of approach is chosen. Consideration should be given to the anatomic relationships of adjacent structures and the shortest route from the skin to the lesion. The type of imaging guidance is determined in advance and the types, sizes, and lengths of needles are selected and their availability confirmed. In cases of primary skeletal neoplasms, it is essential that the procedure be discussed with the treating surgeon.

The patient should be asked to void before the procedure. When use of intravenous (IV) sedation is anticipated, the patient is instructed to begin a clear liquid diet at 8:00 am and IV access should be established. Although there are many options available for sedation, we generally use midazolam and fentanyl. Midazolam is a short-acting benzodiazepine that also impairs memory of periprocedural events. The dosage should be titrated slowly in 1 mg increments IV over at least 2 min to avoid acute respiratory depression. Sedative effects are evident in 3 to 5 min. The respiratory depressant effects of midazolam can be reversed with flumazenil (0.2 mg IV over 15 sec, repeated at 60-sec intervals to a total dose of 1.0 mg). Fentanyl is a narcotic analgesic with a 30- to 60-min duration of action. The dosage should be titrated slowly to the level of analgesia desired. The IV dosage range is 2 to 20 μg/kg. Maintenance doses of 25 to 100 μg can be given as needed. The effects can be reversed with naloxone 0.4 mg IV, repeated at 2- to 3-min intervals as required, to a total of 2.0 mg. In all cases requiring sedation, the blood pressure, pulse, and oxygen saturation should be monitored (Marquette Electronics, Milwaukee, WI). A physician or a nurse should be present whose only responsibility is to administer the IV medications and monitor the patient.

FLUOROSCOPY GUIDANCE MODALITIES

The patient is placed on the fluoroscopic table in the most comfortable position that affords accessibility to the lesion. A C-arm or biplane fluoroscopic unit can be quite useful. The entry site is marked on the skin with an indelible marker. The area is then prepared and draped in a sterile fashion. One percent lidocaine with epinephrine (1:100,000 to reduce capillary bleeding) is injected to anesthetize the skin and subcutaneous tissues. The periosteum is richly innervated and should be anesthetized with adequate amounts of local anesthetic. With the exception of vertebral body biopsies or pediatric cases, IV sedation is usually not required. A small dermatotomy is made to facilitate needle entry. The biopsy needle is then advanced under intermittent fluoroscopic guidance until it is in contact with the lesion (Figure 13.6). When a spinal-type

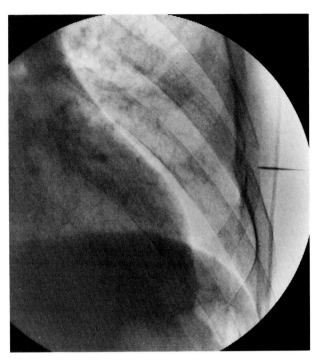

Figure 13.6 Fluoroscopically guided biopsy. Destructive lesion in the left fifth rib of a patient with squamous cell carcinoma of the lung. A spinal needle was inserted into the lesion under fluoroscopic guidance and aspiration biopsy performed. Pathologic examination demonstrated a metastatic lesion.

needle is used, it is advanced into the lesion and the stylet removed. The aspiration is performed by applying negative pressure with a syringe and moving the needle back and forth a few millimeters. When a cutting needle is used to obtain tissue from a soft-tissue mass or an osteolytic bone lesion, it is inserted in the closed position. Once proper placement in confirmed, the inner cannula is advanced. The outer cannula is then used to detach a small core of tissue. The needle is removed in the closed position to retain the specimen.

For a trephine biopsy, once the obturator and outer cannula are firmly anchored into the cortical bone, the obturator is removed. The trephine needle is advanced through the outer cannula with a rotating movement so that its teeth cut out a core of tissue. The needle is then moved from side to side to detach the specimen. Negative pressure should be applied to the back of the needle with a syringe to assure retention of the specimen as the trephine is removed. To increase the diagnostic yield, specimens should be obtained from several areas of the lesion, including any soft-tissue component. The histologic specimen can be stored and submitted if cytologic analysis is negative or if histologic evaluation is required.

Computed Tomography

Although many authors have reported successful use of fluoroscopy for vertebral body biopsies.[5,9,13,23,27] we prefer to use CT guidance because of the proximity of the vertebrae to vital structures.[24,25] The patient is placed in the CT scanner in the prone position. Before the biopsy, contiguous 5-mm axial images are obtained through the region of interest. A radiopaque skin marker is positioned. One of the commercially available radiopaque grids (e.g., Fast Find Grid; E-Z-EM, Inc., Westbury, NY), barium dots, hypodermic needles, or any other readily available marked can be used. From these initial images, the CT couch is then positioned at the location most likely to provide safe access to the lesion. The laser-positioning light on the CT scanner and the marker grid are used to localize and mark the site of skin puncture. The skin is then prepared and draped in a sterile manner.

The distance from the skin and the angle of needle insertion to the lesion are determined (Figure 13.7). The needle is then slowly advanced toward the lesion. Although many needle-guiding devices have been developed, we find the free-hand technique the most rapid and versatile. Computed tomographic images are obtained as needed to confirm proper needle position. Once the needle is within the lesion, aspiration or trephine biopsy can be performed.

Nuclear Medicine

Bone scintigraphy is the most commonly used modality in the detection of skeletal metastatic lesions. However, abnormal uptake on the bone scan is associated with a normal radiograph in approximately 50% of cases.[31] In such cases, fluoroscopic guidance cannot be used. Several authors have described techniques using the bone scan to localize skeletal lesions for biopsy.[29,31,34] In addition to less radiation exposure to the patient and physician, nuclear medicine guidance provides a more physiologic imaging technique for location of skeletal abnormalities. This technique is most useful with rib lesions, which can be successfully biopsied without further imaging.

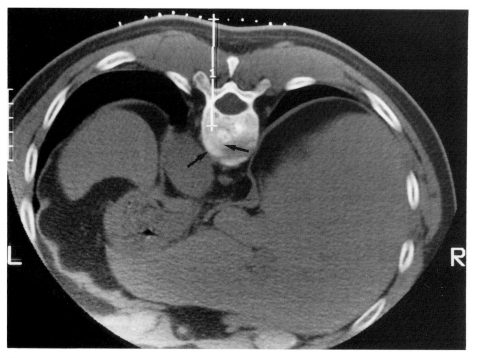

A

Figure 13.7 Computed tomography guided vertebral biopsy using a transpedicular approach. Patient with prostate carcinoma and a low signal lesion in the T11 vertebral body with MRI (not shown). **A.** CT image with radiopaque grid placed reveals an ill-defined region of increased attenuation within the T11 body that corresponded to the MRI abnormality (arrows). Electronic calipers are used to plan the needle depth and path. **B** and **C.** Following page.

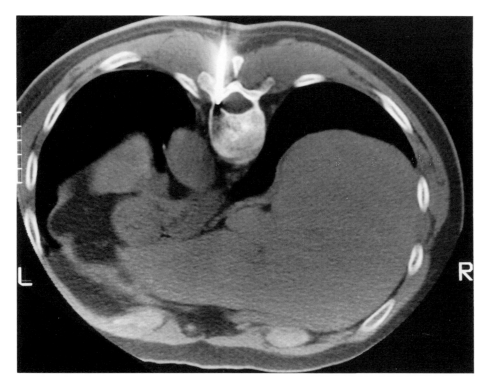

B

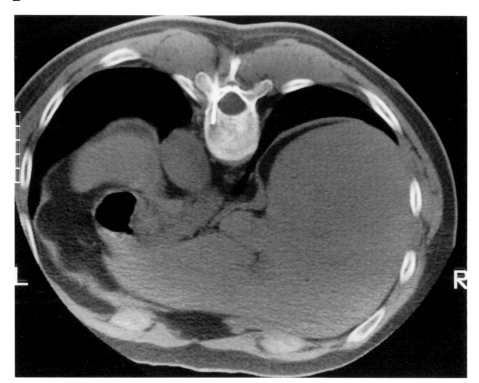

C

Figure 13.7 B. After placement of a Jamshidi needle, a repeat scan shows the needle tip within the left pedicle. The streak artifact is seen at the needle tip. C. A repeat scan shows an Ostycut needle that was inserted coaxially through the Jamshidi needle to obtain core specimens for histology. Chiba needles were also used coaxially to obtain cytologic material. Specimen analysis revealed normal bone and marrow elements.

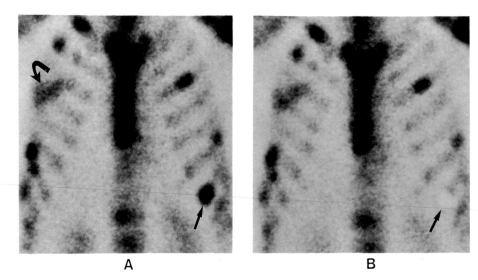

Figure 13.8 Scintigraphically guided biopsy. **A.** Anterior image of the chest following intravenous injection of Tc-99m MDP demonstrates multiple metastatic rib lesions (left image). Uptake is also seen in the peripheral lung mass (curved arrow). **B.** A lead disc (arrow) was positioned over the lesion in the right seventh rib and the lesion was marked for aspiration biopsy. Metastatic adenocarcinoma was detected.

The technique is typically performed following an initial bone scan on which skeletal metastases are suggested. If no plain film abnormality is present to guide biopsy, another bone scan can be used for localization. On the day of the biopsy, the patient is injected with 20 mCi of technetium (Tc) 99m-labeled methylenediphosphonate (MDP). Approximately 2 hr later, a gamma camera image is obtained with the patient in the position in which the biopsy will be performed. A small photon-attenuating marker (a coin or lead disc) is used to localize the specific lesion to be biopsied (Figure 13.8). The percutaneous biopsy can be accomplished with a spinal-type needle. This technique can also be used to mark the skin and the periosteum of a rib with methylene blue for subsequent surgical biopsy.

Ultrasound

Ultrasound has been successfully used to detect destructive rib lesions and to guide percutaneous biopsy in cases of suspected metastatic disease.[30,32,33] Ultrasound energy is poorly transmitted by normal cortical bone. However, rib lesions can be detected by ultrasound, often before plain films demonstrate an abnormality.[33] In all reported cases, ultrasound demonstrates interruption of the cortical bone in the areas of abnormality. There is a heterogeneous decrease in the echogenicity of the abnormal rib, and extraosseous tumor extension is often visible. A biopsy guide can be used, or the biopsy needle can be inserted into the lesion under direct ultrasound visualization. Complications are extremely uncommon with either method as the needle is always seen and the underlying pleura can be avoided. Results are comparable to those obtained with other imaging guidance.[30,32,33]

BIOPSY OF SPECIFIC REGIONS

The basic techniques described above apply to the majority of bone biopsies. However, some modifications are necessary in certain anatomic regions.

Ribs

In rib lesions, the adjacent neurovascular bundle and the underlying lung should be avoided. Therefore, the lower rib margin should be avoided because the neurovascular bundle runs in a groove along the posterior margin of the inferior aspect of the rib. The perpendicular approach should also be avoided since it yields only a small amount of material and any undue pressure might push the needle through the rib with the attendant risk of pneumothorax. A tangential biopsy approach is safer and will yield a larger specimen.[5]

Sternum

The sternum is another flat bone with important structures (heart, great vessels, lung) immediately beneath it. As with rib lesions, a tangential approach will avoid inadvertent sternal penetration and provide a greater specimen volume. Although the sternum can be easily biopsied using fluoroscopic guidance, CT better delineates the anatomy and may provide a greater margin of safety.

Thoracic Vertebral Body

Biopsies of the thoracic vertebral bodies also require care to avoid the lungs, aorta, and dural sac. Although techniques have been described to safely biopsy the thoracic spine fluoroscopically, we prefer CT guidance.[5,12,23] Whenever the situation allows, an approach from the right side of the vertebral body is preferable because the aorta is not as close to the needle path. There are two different approaches to thoracic spine lesions that avoid the dural sac, lungs, and other adjacent structures: transpedicular (Figure 13.7) and transcostovertebral.[24,25,27] The transcostovertebral approach utilizes the interval between the medial end of the rib and the transverse process of the vertebral body.[24] This approach avoids the intercostal neurovascular bundle, exiting nerve roots, lungs, and aorta.

While most patients will require some degree of IV sedation for vertebral body biopsies, the patient should not be so heavily sedated as to be unable to immediately inform the radiologist of any neurologic symptoms. If such symptoms are reported, the course of the needle should be altered.

LABORATORY EXAMINATION OF THE SPECIMEN

Once the histologic and cytologic specimens have been obtained, it is important that they be handled properly. The pathologic evaluation of bone lesions has become increasingly sophisticated; techniques such as imprints, immunostains, and electron microscopy are often critical in establishing a diagnosis. Specialized staining methods require the use of specific fixatives for the biopsy specimen. Therefore, it is critical that the pathologist be consulted before the procedure so that the differential diagnosis can be discussed and adequate biopsy material obtained for any specialized evaluation. It is also very helpful to have a cytotechnologist in attendance during the biopsy to prepare slides for cytology and supervise handling of the specimen.

Because intracellular organelles dissipate quickly, samples for electron microscopy should be immediately placed in glutaraldehyde. After any imprints or touch-preps are made, the remainder of the histologic specimen should be placed in an appropriate fixative. In most cases, tissue can be placed in a formalin solution. For cases in which gout is suspected and for all tumors in which Ewing's sarcoma enters into the differential diagnosis, samples should be placed in absolute alcohol. In cases of known or suspected lymphoma, specimens should be placed in glutaraldehyde for electron microscopy, in 80% alcohol for glycogen stains, and in saline for other stains. If frozen-section analysis is desired, the tissue should be taken to the pathology department in a sterile manner without the use of any fixatives. Any cytologic aspirates, including intraosseous blood, should be placed in an appropriate preservative such as Mucolex and sent to the laboratory. Finally, it is important to collect some material for culture and Gram stain when an infection is suspected.[5,7]

RESULTS

In most of the recent large series, the accuracy of percutaneous bone biopsy reported ranges from 72% to 97%.[2,4–6,9–11,13,15] The diagnostic accuracy varies depending on the clinical setting, although the reported rates of accuracy for metastatic neoplasm, primary neoplasm, and infection are similar. Adequate material for diagnosis is obtained in as many as 95% of patients and accuracy is increased when aspiration biopsy is combined with trephine biopsy.[5,28] Nondiagnostic specimens are most often obtained when the lesion is cystic or densely osteoblastic. In such cases, an attempt should be made to biopsy any soft-tissue or lytic component or the least sclerotic region of bone.[4,9] Due to difficulties with histologic grading of cartilaginous neoplasms, percutaneous biopsy is not recommended when a cartilage matrix is identified.[7,9]

COMPLICATIONS

Percutaneous biopsy of the musculoskeletal system is associated with few complications. A review of over 9,500 procedures reported a serious complication rate of 0.2%.[13] Complications included bleeding, infection, pneumothorax, and neurologic damage.[5,6,13,22]

Pain is the most common side effect and is often related to application of negative pressure within the marrow cavity. Penetration of the periosteum is painful, and care should be taken to use adequate amounts of local anesthesia. Intravenous sedation is rarely necessary except for vertebral body biopsy, deep-seated lesions, or pediatric cases. Infection has been reported in 0.3% of cases, making adherence to aseptic technique essential.[22] Significant bleeding is another potential complication that can be avoided by proper planning of the needle path and correction of any clotting abnormalities before the procedure.[21] Pneumothorax has been reported in association with rib and vertebral biopsies in as many as 4% of cases and can often be managed conservatively.[22]

Neurologic damage is the most serious complication that has been reported, with an estimated incidence of 0.08%.[22] However, surgical exploration and postmortem examinations have demonstrated that cord damage was often caused by tumor invasion or bleeding within a tumor and was not a direct result of the biopsy procedure.[5]

The possibility of tumor spread along the needle track is another unlikely, but potential, complication.[2,8,41] However, there have been no documented cases of this complication in more than 15,000 biopsies, and it has not been possible to produce spread of tumor along needle tracks in experimental animals.[5,22]

POSTPROCEDURE CARE

A short period of observation following the procedure will aid in detecting immediate complications. Generally, we observe the patient for 20–30 min after completion of the biopsy or 45 min after the last IV sedation. The biopsy site and the patient's vital signs are monitored every 15 min. In cases of rib or sternal biopsies, an upright expiratory chest radiograph is obtained to assess for pneumothorax. Any discharge instructions or follow-up appointments are reviewed with the patient. Upon discharge, the patient may resume a normal diet and activity level.

SUMMARY

Percutaneous needle biopsy of the thoracic skeleton is a safe, accurate, and economical method of obtaining tissue for cytologic, histologic, or bacteriologic analysis. The procedure can be easily repeated when needed and does not preclude subsequent surgical biopsy or treatment. It should be emphasized that the procedure is a team effort that includes the patient, the radiologist, the referring physician, the orthopedic surgeon, and an experienced pathologist.

REFERENCES

1. Coley BL, Sharp GS, Ellis EB: Diagnosis of bone tumors by aspiration. *Am J Surg* 13: 215–224, 1931.
2. Moore TM, Meyers MH, Patzakis MJ, et al: Closed biopsy of musculoskeletal lesions. *J Bone Joint Surg* 61-A:375–380, 1979.
3. Fraser-Hill MA, Renfrew DL, Hilsenrath PE: Percutaneous needle biopsy of musculoskeletal lesions. II. Cost-effectiveness. *Am J Roentgenol* 158:813–818, 1992.
4. Carrasco CH, Wallace S, Richli WR: Percutaneous skeletal biopsy. *Cardiovasc Intervent Radiol* 14:69–72, 1991.
5. deSantos LA, Lukeman JM, Wallace S, et al: Percutaneous needle biopsy of bone in the cancer patient. *Am J Roentgenol* 130:641–649, 1978.
6. deSantos LA, Murray JA, Ayala AG: The value of percutaneous needle biopsy in the management of primary bone tumors. *Cancer* 43:735–744, 1979.
7. Mirra JM: *Bone Tumors: Clinical, Radiologic, and Pathologic Correlations.* Philadelphia, Lea & Febiger, 1989.
8. Mankin HJ, Lange TA, Spanier SS: The hazards of biopsy in patients with malignant primary bone and soft-tissue tumors. *J Bone Joint Surg* 64-A:1121–1127, 1982.
9. Ayala AG, Zornosa J: Primary bone tumors: percutaneous needle biopsy. *Radiology* 149: 675–679, 1983.
10. El-Khoury GY, Terpeka RH, Mickelson MR, et al: Fine-needle aspiration biopsy of bone. *J Bone Joint Surg* 65-A:522–525, 1983.
11. Fraser-Hill MA, Renfrew DL: Percutaneous needle biopsy of musculoskeletal lesions. I. Effective accuracy and diagnostic utility. *Am J Roentgenol* 158:809–812, 1992.
12. Kattapuram SV, Rosenthal DI: Percutaneous biopsy of skeletal lesions. *Am J Roentgenol* 157:935–942, 1991.
13. Murphy WA, Destouet JM, Gilula LA: Percutaneous skeletal biopsy 1981: a procedure for radiologists—results, review, and recommendations. *Radiology* 139:545–549, 1981.
14. Onik G, Shang Y, Maroon J, et al: Percutaneous automated biopsy in the diagnosis of primary infectious spondylitis. *Neurosurgery* 26(2):234–237, 1990.
15. Tehranzadeh J, Freiberger RH, Ghelman B: Closed skeletal needle biopsy: review of 120 cases. *Am J Roentgenol* 140:113–115, 1983.
16. Mondal A: Cytologic diagnosis of vertebral tuberculosis with fine-needle aspiration biopsy. *J Bone Joint Surg* 76-A:181–184, 1994.
17. Fanning CV, Sneige NS, Carrasco CH, et al: Fine needle aspiration cytology of chondroblastoma of bone. *Cancer* 65(8):1847–1863, 1990.
18. Kumar RV, Rao CR, Hazarika D, et al: Aspiration biopsy cytology of primary bone lesions. *Acta Cytol* 37(1):83–89, 1993.
19. Nauert C, Zornoza J, Ayala A, et al: Eosinophilic granuloma of bone: diagnosis and management. *Skeletal Radiol* 10:227–235, 1983.
20. Vetrani A, Fulciniti F, Boschi R, et al: Fine needle aspiration biopsy diagnosis of giant-cell tumor of bone. *Acta Cytol* 34(6):863–867, 1990.

21. Silverman SG, Mueller PR, Pfister RC: Hemostatic evaluation before abdominal interventions: an overview and proposal. *Am J Roentgenol* 154:233–238, 1990.

22. Griffiths HJ: Interventional radiology: the musculoskeletal system. *Radiol Clin North Am* 17(3):475–484, 1979.

23. Larédo JD, Bard M: Thoracic spine: percutaneous trephine biopsy. *Radiology* 160:485–489, 1986.

24. Brugieres P, Gaston A, Heran F, et al: Percutaneous biopsies of the thoracic spine under CT guidance: transcostovertebral approach. *J Comput Assist Tomogr* 14(3):446–448, 1990.

25. Ghelman B, Lospinuso MF, Levine DB, et al: Percutaneous computed tomography-guided biopsy of the thoracic and lumbar spine. *Spine* 16(7):736–739, 1991.

26. Klose KC, Mertens R, Alzen G, et al: CT-guided percutaneous large-bore biopsies in benign and malignant pediatric lesions. *Cardiovasc Intervent Radiol* 14:78–83, 1990.

27. Mick CA, Zinreich J: Percutaneous trephine bone biopsy of the thoracic spine. *Spine* 10(8): 737–740, 1985.

28. Tikkakoski T, Lähde S, Puranen J, et al: Combined CT-guided biopsy and cytology in diagnosis of bony lesions. *Acta Radiol* 33:225–229, 1992.

29. Collins JD, Bassett L, Main GD, et al: Percutaneous biopsy following positive bone scans. *Radiology* 132:439–442, 1979.

30. Hsu WH, Chiang CD, Hsu JY, et al: Impalpable thoracic bony lesions diagnosed by sonographically guided needle aspiration biopsy. *J Ultrasound Med* 11:105–109, 1992.

31. Moores DWO, Line B, Dziuban SW JR, et al: Nuclear scan-guided rib biopsy. *J Thorac Cardiovasc Surg* 99:620–621, 1990.

32. Targhetta R, Balmes P, Marty-Double C, et al: Ultrasonically guided aspiration biopsy in osteolytic bone lesions of the chest wall. *Chest* 103:1403–1408, 1993.

33. Vogel B: Ultrasonographic detection and guided biopsy of thoracic osteolysis. *Chest* 104: 1003–1005, 1993.

34. Zegel HG, Turner M, Velchik MG, et al: Percutaneous osseous needle biopsy with nuclear medicine guidance. *Clin Nucl Med* 9:89–91, 1984.

35. Andriole JG, Haaga JR, Adams RB, et al: Biopsy needle characteristics assessed in the laboratory. *Radiology* 148:659–662, 1983.

36. Geremia GK, Charletta DA, Granato DB, et al: Biopsy of vertebral and paravertebral structures with a new coaxial needle system. *AJNR* 13:169–171, 1992.

37. Schweitzer ME, Deely DM: Percutaneous biopsy of osteolytic lesions: use of a biopsy gun. *Radiology* 189:615–616, 1993.

38. Ahlström KH, Åström KGO: CT-guided bone biopsy performed by means of a coaxial biopsy system with an eccentric drill. *Radiology* 188:549–552, 1993.

39. Cohen MA, Zornosa J, Finkelstein JB: Percutaneous needle biopsy of long-bone lesions facilitated by the use of a hand drill. *Radiology* 139:750–751, 1981.

40. Vorwerk D, Klose KC, Günther RW, et al: A new motor-driven percutaneous bone biopsy system: technical note. *Cardiovasc Intervent Radiol* 12:232–235, 1989.

41. Simon MA, Biermann JS: Biopsy of bone and soft-tissue lesions. *J Bone Joint Surg* 75-A: 616–621, 1993.

C H A P T E R
14

Management of Intrathoracic Fluid Collections

Dean A. Nakamoto
John R. Haaga

Improvements in imaging technology, refinements in catheter construction, and the success of percutaneous interventions in the abdomen have led to a larger and more important role for percutaneous intervention in the management of patients with intrathoracic fluid collections. Imaging-guided techniques are associated with less morbidity than surgery, and some patients may be stabilized by a percutaneous drainage procedure so that needed surgery can be performed more safely. Many disease processes originally considered amenable only to surgical management can now be effectively treated by interventional radiologists. However, it is still important for interventional radiologists to work closely with their surgical colleagues, since some diseases may not be cured with percutaneous techniques alone.

In the thorax, abnormal fluid can accumulate in the pleural space, lung parenchyma, or mediastinum. Etiologies that can lead to the accumulation of complicated pleural fluid collections include infection, malignancy, surgery, and trauma. Percutaneous diagnostic aspiration can be performed safely and accurately, and drainage catheters can be placed for treatment of infected or otherwise symptomatic collections.

Although there are few contraindications to most imaging-guided fluid aspirations and drainages, one important contraindication is an uncooperative patient. Relative contraindications include patients with abnormal clotting parameters: an elevated prothrombin time 3 sec or more above control, a partial thromboplastin time 6 sec or more above control, or a platelet count less than 50,000/mm³. These abnormalities can usually be corrected with appropriate blood products. If a patient is febrile and an infected collection is suspected, we prefer that the patient have at least one dose of broad-spectrum antibiotics intravenously prior to the procedure. One dose of antibiotics usually does not alter the results of the specimen culture.

PLEURAL FLUID COLLECTIONS

Abnormal fluid in the pleural space is easily accessible by percutaneous methods. The four percutaneous procedures most commonly performed are diagnostic thoracentesis, therapeutic thoracentesis, pleural sclerosis, and empyema drainage.

Diagnostic Thoracentesis

Diagnostic thoracentesis is usually performed to evaluate for empyema or malignancy. Other indications for the procedure include evaluation for chylous or bloody fluid. Patients are usually referred on the basis of findings from chest radiographs or a computed tomographic (CT) study of the chest.

Technique

Almost all diagnostic thoracenteses can be performed with ultrasound guidance. Sonography is quick and accurate and delineates even small amounts of fluid in the pleural space. When pleural collections are difficult to visualize with ultrasound due to the patient's body habitus or the presence of air within the collection, CT guidance may be used.

The patient is comfortably seated on a chair or stretcher with his back to the interventionalist. Patients who cannot tolerate this position are placed in a lateral decubitus position with the affected side up. The fluid is localized with either a sector or linear array ultrasound transducer. It is important to identify the position of the diaphragm to avoid inadvertent puncture of the liver or spleen. The skin should be marked over the largest component of the pleural collection. Standard aseptic technique should be used. Local anesthesia usually provides sufficient analgesia as long as particular attention is paid to the parietal pleural surface. The needle should be advanced over the superior surface of the rib to avoid the neurovascular bundle located along the inferior aspect of the rib.

Most pleural fluid collections can be aspirated with a 20-gauge (g) spinal needle. The needle is connected to plastic tubing, which is directly connected to a syringe. This "closed" system minimizes the chance for inadvertent introduction of air into the pleural space. If fluid cannot be aspirated through the 20-g spinal needle, and 18-g angiocatheter can be used. When using an angiocatheter, it is important to have the patient suspend respirations before attaching the catheter to the connecting tubing, in order to prevent air from entering the pleural space. If fluid still cannot be obtained, the effusion may actually represent pleural thickening or may be too viscous to be aspirated with small catheters. Further evaluation with CT is then usually helpful.

A postprocedure upright chest radiograph should be obtained to evaluate for a pneumothorax. The pneumothorax rate following diagnostic thoracocentesis is 2–3%, and the rate of those requiring treatment is even lower.[1,2] If there is a small asymptomatic pneumothorax that remains stable, no intervention is needed. However, if the pneumothorax increases in size over a 4-hr period of observation, the patient should be watched carefully because a chest tube may be needed. If the pneumothorax causes dyspnea, a small-bore chest tube attached to a Heimlich valve can be easily placed under fluoroscopic guidance.

Therapeutic Thoracentesis

The most common indication for a therapeutic pleural drainage procedure is the need to remove large volumes of fluid for relief of respiratory symptoms. Such effusions may be transudative secondary to congestive heart failure or liver failure, or may be exudative secondary to a malignancy. Therapeutic thoracentesis may also be performed in patients with large simple parapneumonic effusions to prevent empyema formation and improve respiratory function.

Technique

The collection is localized by ultrasound. A diagnostic thoracentesis should be performed prior to catheter placement. The fluid should be sent for appropriate laboratory studies. If the collection is large, a single-step catheter with a trocar can be used. For smaller collections, a 19-g needle with an 18-g Teflon sheath (Longdwel catheter; Becton-Dickinson Co., Rutherford, NJ) can be used to enter the collection. The needle is removed and a standard 0.035-inch guidewire is placed through the Teflon sheath into the fluid collection. A pigtail catheter of appropriate size can be introduced over the guidewire under ultrasound or fluoroscopic guidance, although in experienced hands, imaging guidance may not be necessary for this step. Care should be exercised to prevent inadvertent introduction of air into the pleural space.

Once the catheter is within the fluid collection, it is connected to plastic tubing and a three-way stopcock. The fluid can then be withdrawn by a syringe or connected to a vacuum bottle. Rapid withdrawal of more than 1 liter of pleural fluid at a time is not recommended. Reexpansion pulmonary edema can result from pleural space evacuation, and rapid shifts in intravascular fluid volumes can cause hypotension.[3] If the patient has any chest discomfort, dyspnea, or excessive coughing, a chest film should be obtained to evaluate for a pneumothorax. After the fluid has been removed, the catheter is withdrawn and a chest radiograph is obtained. The pneumothorax rate is similar to the rate seen with diagnostic thoracocenteses. Small, asymptomatic pneumothoraces can be left to resorb spontaneously. Symptomatic pneumothoraces require chest tube placement.

Pleural Sclerosis

Some pleural effusions do not respond to simple thoracentesis. Recurrent effusions are often secondary to pleural involvement or central lymphatic obstruction by malignancy. Cirrhosis, congestive heart failure, nephrotic syndrome, and systemic lupus erythematosus can also cause recurrent benign effusions. Treatment options for recurrent symptomatic pleural effusions include pleurectomy, mechanical pleurodesis, talc poudrage, or percutaneous tube thoracostomy with chemical sclerosis. The pleural space should be adequately drained so that the lung can fully reexpand prior to any treatment. Pleural sclerosis should only be performed if the pleural effusion is symptomatic and recurrent despite appropriate medical therapy and/or drainage, and if the underlying lung is able to fully reexpand.

Surgical Techniques

Although surgical pleurectomy may be effective, it is a relatively major procedure and may be complicated by bleeding from pleural metastases.[4] Thoracoscopy and talc poudrage have recently been advocated as both safe and effective in the treatment of malignant and nonmalignant effusions.[4,5] With video-assisted thoracoscopy, the pleural fluid can be drained, adhesions lysed, and talc insufflated into the pleural space. The talc is asbestos-free and nonpyrogenic, and is insufflated dry by use of an atomizer.[4] LoCicero had nearly 100% success in treating recurrent effusions in 40 patients using this technique.[4] However, he recommends this procedure only for those patients with moderate to good performance status; patients with severe debility are better managed with tube thoracostomy and sclerosis.

Percutaneous Techniques

Percutaneous chest tubes have been used to instill various agents into the pleural space for pleurodesis. Tetracycline is usually effective, easy to use, and inexpensive as an intrapleural sclerosant.[2,6,7] However, it has recently been discontinued as a parenteral agent and is no longer available for use. Doxycycline has been suggested as an alternative agent, but there is insufficient data to recommend its intrapleural use. Bleomycin has also been used as a pleural sclerosant; however, it is expensive and must be prepared in a protective hood.[7,8]

Talc suspensions can be instilled via chest tubes. As described for thorascopic insufflation, the talc should be asbestos-free and sterile. It is important to mix the talc suspension (5 gm of talc in 100 cc of saline) well so that the talc does not clump and all of it can be instilled through the tube into the pleural space.[4] The tube is clamped for 6 hr while the patient undergoes positional maneuvers to ensure distribution of the talc over all pleural surfaces. The chest tube is then opened to drainage. Webb et al. reported good short-term results with the talc pleurodesis.[9]

Drainage of loculated, malignant pleural effusions can be difficult because the septations within the collection can prevent adequate drainage by a single catheter. Intrapleural administration of urokinase can dissolve the septations, allowing the loculated collections to flow freely through a single chest tube (see pages 323–326). Once the collection is drained, the cavity can be sclerosed.

Chylothorax

Chylothorax is the accumulation of lymphatic fluid in the pleural space. It occurs in a variety of conditions, particularly in malignancies that obstruct the main lymphatic ducts such as lymphomas. Chylothorax may also occur in association with chylous ascites, systemic lupus erythematosis, intestinal lymphangiectasia, and chest trauma.

Post-traumatic chylothoraces will usually resolve with conservative management including parenteral nutrition and bowel rest. Thoracic duct ligation is usually performed if conservative management fails. Pleurodesis with talc and fibrin glue has been described in refractory cases.[10,11] Pleurodesis may be particularly desirable for infants or severely debilitated patients.

Empyema

Empyema thoracis refers to the accumulation of purulent material within the pleural space. Despite the development of new antibiotics, empyema remains a common problem and is associated with mortality rates as high as 40%.[12]

Pathogenesis and Etiologies

There are three stages in the evolution of an empyema.[13,14] The stage determines the management of the empyema. The first stage is the exudative stage, in which there is accumulation of sterile, free-flowing pleural fluid. The pleural fluid at this time contains rare polymorphonuclear leukocytes (PMNs), a normal glucose level, and a normal pH. The second stage is the fibropurulent stage in which the sterile pleural fluid has become infected with bacteria, and the cellularity and protein content in the pleural fluid increase. Fibrin is deposited on the visceral and parietal pleura. As this stage progresses, loculations form. The pleural fluid pH and glucose decrease, and the lactic dehydrogenase (LDH) level and the number of PMNs increase. In the third or organization stage, fibroblasts and capillaries grow into the exudate and form a pleural peel. If untreated, this stage may result in entrapment of adjacent lung or drainage of fluid through the chest wall (empyema necessitatis) or into the lung (bronchopleural fistula). Although the best method of managing an empyema is controversial, early intervention is the key to preventing pleural peel formation and the development of an entrapped lung. Once a peel forms, decortication is almost always necessary, although there is evidence that some pleural peels can resolve spontaneously if the underlying empyema is treated satisfactorily.[15]

Infected pleural fluid has developed in association with pulmonary infections, surgery, trauma, foreign bodies, esophageal perforation, or inflammatory processes below the diaphragm. Pulmonary infection (pneumonia) is the associated etiology in

65% of empyemas.[14] An empyema due to pneumonia appears to have a better response rate than either a postsurgical or post-traumatic empyema.[5,12,16]

Anaerobic bacteria have replaced Gram-positive organisms as the most common cause of infected pleural fluid collections in adults.[14] More than one anaerobic organism is usually cultured from an empyema. Because anaerobes are fastidious and so common, culture specimens should be handled appropriately to ensure positive culture results. The specimens should be cultured quickly, and they should be exposed to as little air as possible, because air may kill the organisms. Although there has been a recognizable change in the organisms associated with empyema, management and clinical outcome with treatment have not been altered.[17,18] *Staphylococcus aureus* remains the most common organism found in empyemas in children.

Diagnosis

Analysis of the pleural fluid by routine thoracentesis determines the stage of the empyema and the most appropriate management. If there is aspiration of gross pus or if the Gram stain is positive, the pleural space should be drained immediately. A positive Gram stain, even if nonpurulent fluid is obtained, is indicative of advanced disease, and drainage is recommended.[13] If the pleural fluid is not grossly purulent and does not have microorganisms on the Gram stain, then assessment of the fluid composition can be used to direct management. The most important pleural fluid components to measure are pH, glucose, and LDH levels. When the pleural space becomes infected, the pleural fluid glucose level decreases due to glycolysis from PMN phagocytosis and bacterial metabolism. This increase in glucose metabolism results in accumulation of lactic acid and CO_2, which decreases the pleural fluid pH. The pleural fluid LDH level rises due to cell lysis. Of these three components, the pleural fluid pH will usually decrease before the glucose level decreases and the LDH level increases.[14] These three parameters are important predictors of whether an effusion will resolve with or without drainage.[14] Many authors use criteria based on the combined pleural fluid data of Sahn[13] and Light.[14] For pleural fluid with a pH< 7.10, glucose<40 mg/dl, and LDH >1,000 U/L, early drainage is recommended to avoid subsequent development of a complicated, multilocated effusion or a pleural peel. For free-flowing fluid with a pH >7.30, glucose >60 mg/dl, and LDH< 1,000 U/L, the fluid will probably resolve spontaneously if appropriate antibiotics are given. For fluid with a pH between 7.10 and 7.30, it is recommended that antibiotics be given and the patient be observed closely. If needed, repeat thoracentesis can be performed.

Indications for Chest Tube

As stated above, the primary indication for chest tube placement is to drain an empyema and prevent progression of the pleural process to the organized stage. Although recent radiologic series have demonstrated fairly high success rates with percutaneous drainage, there is still controversy as to whether radiologic or surgical tubes should be used.[19-28] Indications for imaging-guided pleural catheter placement include failure of surgically placed chest tubes, collections too small for safe surgical tube placement, debilitated patients who are too ill to undergo an operative procedure, and multiple, loculated fluid collections.

Percutaneous Technique

Prior to the procedure, patients should receive appropriate antibiotics. If the pleural fluid is free-flowing, a diagnostic thoracentesis can be performed with ultrasound guidance. If there is gross pus or a positive Gram stain, a drain can then be placed. However, many pleural fluid collections are already loculated when the patients are referred for percutaneous drainage. We prefer to use CT guidance both to perform diagnostic aspirations and for placement of drainage catheters in loculated collections. Computed tomography provides optimal visualization of all loculations, differentiates between collapsed lung and pleural fluid, and allows visualization of the needle, guidewire, and catheter during the drainage procedure.

Once the loculated collection is localized, the patient is placed in a position that allows optimal access. A diagnostic thoracocentesis is performed. Because CT provides complete visualization of the collection, the trajectory of the needle can be planned such that the entire collection can be traversed. We prefer an anterolateral approach when possible, especially for posteriorly located collections (Figure 14.1). Using this approach for drainage of a posteriorly located empyema allows the patient to lie supine without kinking the catheter. A direct posterior approach can be used, but the catheter may become kinked when the patient lies down. Drainages performed with ultrasound are usually limited to a posterior approach for posteriorly located collections.

For CT-guided drainages, we prefer a 19-g needle with an 18-g Teflon sheath (Longdwel catheter). Using the Teflon sheath, even very thick purulent fluid can be aspirated with little difficulty. If drainage is desired, a standard 0.035-inch guidewire can be placed through the 18-g sheath into the empyema for subsequent catheter placement.

We generally use the Seldinger technique to introduce the catheter into the pleural space. Single-step catheters with trocars can be used, but the Seldinger technique provides better control and reduces the chance of injury to the underlying lung. Inadvertent entry of air during dilatation of the tract is not a problem because the collections are usually loculated. The viscosity of the fluid determines the size of the catheter.

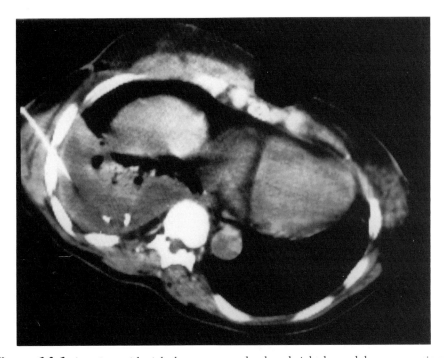

Figure 14.1 A patient with right breast cancer developed right lower lobe pneumonia and secondary empyema and was treated with an 8-Fr pigtail catheter. Drainage during the first 2 days was minimal due to multiple thin septations. She was then treated with 4 days of intrapleural urokinase, 125,000 IU twice daily. The empyema resolved 7 days later and the catheter was removed. Note the lateral approach for this posteriorly located effusion. This trajectory allows the patient to lie down without kinking the catheter.

Most collections can be drained with 8- to 10-Fr self-retaining nephrostomy-type catheters (Percuflex nephrostomy; Boston Scientific Corp., Natick, MA). It is sometimes technically difficult to introduce a catheter into the pleural space because the catheter or the guidewire may buckle. Adequate dissection of the subcutaneous tissues along the needle tract and use of a stiffer guidewire (Rosen guidewire; Cook Inc., Bloomington, IN), help to prevent this buckling. Occasionally, a 12-Fr catheter will be needed to drain the viscous fluid. Insertion of a large catheter can be difficult without fluoroscopic guidance. If needed, catheter upsizing can be performed 1 to 2 days later under fluoroscopic guidance. We rarely use a catheter larger than 12-Fr; instead we instill urokinase into the pleural space (see discussion below).

Apparent unilocular collections frequently contain multiple, thin septations that cannot be visualized on CT images. These septations become apparent only when small amounts of fluid can be aspirated from a catheter positioned in the middle of the collection. Despite being fine and delicate, these thin septations are probably just as responsible for the failure of percutaneous drainage as the viscosity of the fluid.[13,26] If multiple thin septations are present within a fluid collection, it is helpful to have the needle traverse as much of the collection as possible before removing the sharp stylet. The sharp needle point punctures the septations, subsequently allowing a single catheter to drain many of the loculations. Although additional mechanical disruption of the septations can be performed, we prefer to instill urokinase to dissolve these septations.

To achieve optimal drainage, it is helpful to have the pigtail portion of the catheter in a dependent position within the fluid. Nephrostomy-type catheters with sideholes in the distal pigtail are the type of drainage catheters most frequently used. Catheters with additional sideholes more proximal to the pigtail (biliary-type) can be used, however, care must be taken to ensure that all of the sideholes remain within the pleural collection.

Once the catheter is placed, it can be sutured to the skin or attached with adhesive fixation devices (Percufix Catheter Cuff Kit, Boston Scientific Corp.). The adhesive devices reduce infections at the skin entrance site and the skin irritation caused by suture material. Once the patient returns to the hospital ward, the drain is placed to a standard water seal (Pleur-Evac; Deknatel, Fall River, MA) and wall suction at -20 cm of water. The patient is continued on antibiotics tailored to the culture and sensitivity results of the fluid sample. The pleural fluid output is monitored daily. Assuming there is good drainage, the tube position can be checked every 2–4 days with chest radiographs. If there are any problems, a repeat CT can be performed to check tube position. Additional drainage tubes can be placed as needed for any separate collections not being drained.

Once the fluid has become serous, the tube output has decreased to less than 20 cc per 24 hr, the patient has defervesced, and the white blood cell count is normal, the tube may be removed. A repeat CT should be performed prior to tube removal to ensure that there are no undrained collections.

When empyema drainage is performed, it is important to work closely with the thoracic surgeon. Not all collections are amenable to percutaneous drainage. Patients who develop a pleural peel (Figure 14.2) or who have persistent fevers and elevated white blood cell counts despite 48–72 hr of adequate drainage and appropriate antibiotics may require surgical drainage and decortication. Surgical treatment for such patients should not be delayed.

Fibrinolytic Agents

Recognizing the need to break down loculations in an empyema, investigators have long tried to use intrapleural fibrinolytic agents. As early as 1949, Tillet et al. instilled streptokinase and streptococcal deoxyribonuclease into empyemas.[29] However, allergic reactions to the streptokinase were not well tolerated by some patients. Even with the advent of purified streptokinase, allergic reactions still occurred.[20] In 1988, Haaga introduced the use of urokinase for lysing loculations in abscess collections.[30] Moulton

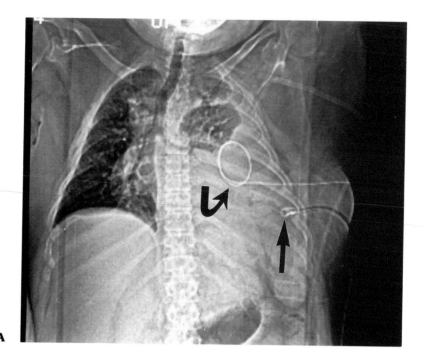

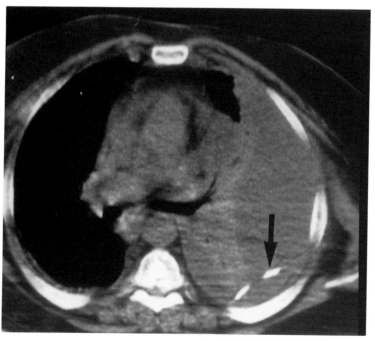

Figure 14.2 A. A 42-yr-old patient had a community-acquired left lower lobe pneumonia complicated by a large loculated empyema. He was initially treated with a surgically placed chest tube (straight arrow) which only drained a minimal amount of purulent material. An 8-Fr pigtail catheter was placed using a lateral approach (curved arrow). B. Note how the guidewire and catheter (arrow) remained coiled within a thin septation. The initial overnight drainage was minimal, so the patient was treated with 4 days of intrapleural urokinase, 125,000 IU twice daily. More than 1 L of fluid was removed in 4 days. C. Following page.

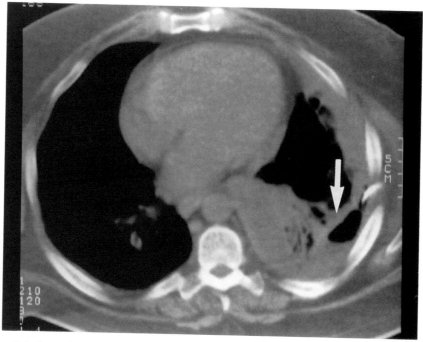

C

Figure 14.2 C. Although there was significant improvement in the empyema, the patient developed a pleural peel (arrow) and a decortication was performed semielectively.

et al.[20] successfully drained 12 of 13 loculated pleural collections by using adjunctive intrapleural urokinase. Lee et al.[19] treated 10 patients with multiloculated pleural effusions with a single 8-Fr catheter and intrapleural urokinase. They instilled 100,000 IU of urokinase per session, the total amount of urokinase ranging from 100,000 to 700,000 IU. They cured nine patients and one patient had a recurrence that was subsequently successfully treated percutaneously. More recently, Moulton et al. reported on 118 patients with complicated pleural fluid collections treated with image-guided drainage.[31] Surgical thoracostomy drainage had failed in 41 of these patients. Adjunctive intrapleural urokinase was used in 98 patients. Drainage was successful in 94% (111 of 118), although 45% (53 of 118) required placement of more than one drainage catheter. The mean duration of drainage was 6.3 days, and the mean total dose of urokinase per case was 466,000 IU. There were no reported complications.

Because the safety and efficacy of intracavitary urokinase for abdominal abscesses has been well demonstrated, we are now using urokinase liberally to treat empyemas. The decision to proceed with the use of urokinase is based on the amount of fluid remaining after satisfactory catheter placement. If pleural fluid is difficult to aspirate, loculations are visible on CT, or any significant fluid collection is present on follow-up imaging, instillation of urokinase into the pleural space is instituted. Our current protocol uses 125,000 IU of intrapleural urokinase every 12 hr for 4 days. Prior to the instillation of urokinase, the drainage catheter is aspirated as much as possible with a syringe and the amount of aspirate recorded. The urokinase is then instilled into the chest tube, followed by a 5-cc saline flush. Whenever possible, patients are instructed to change positions to facilitate distribution of the urokinase throughout the pleural space. The catheter is clamped for 30 min and then restored to wall suction. After 4 days or until complete resolution of the fluid collection, the urokinase is discontinued and the catheter is irrigated with 10 cc of saline twice daily until the tube is ready to be removed, as previously discussed. To reduce cost, a 250,000 IU vial of urokinase is reconstituted in the morning, so that 125,000 IU is used in the morning and the remainder is used at night. Relative contraindications include bronchopleural fistulae, a coagulopathy with prothrombin time 3 sec or more above control, pregnancy, or known central nervous system metastases. Bleeding complications related to intrapleural instillation of urokinase are extremely rare and allergic reactions have not been reported.[19,20,31] Although lytic agents are active in the pleural space, they have been shown to have no measurable effect on systemic coagulation parameters.[19,20,32]

Results

The success rate of imaging-guided percutaneous empyema drainage ranges from 70% to 94%, with a cumulative success rate of approximately 85%.[19–27,31] This rate compares favorably with success rates of 35–75% for surgically placed chest tubes.[16–18] It is difficult to compare the radiologic and surgical series directly, because the patient populations were so variable in these studies. However, some general principles are apparent from the literature. Most authors agree that early drainage is important. A high percentage of early stage empyemas with free-flowing fluid can be treated with either surgically or percutaneously placed chest tubes. Failure of chest tube drainage is usually due to thick, viscous fluid and loculations. Such collections resist even large-bore chest tubes, but it appears that greater success can be achieved with the adjunctive use of intrapleural urokinase (Figure 14.3). Once a pleural peel develops, decortication is usually required, although there are some authors who suggest that some pleural peels may resolve spontaneously after treatment of the underlying empyema.[14,15] In debilitated patients who develop pleural peels, conservative management can be tried, and in some of these patients decortication may be avoided. However, for otherwise healthy patients, the surgical literature suggests that decortication should not be delayed when there is persistent pleural sepsis in the presence of a pleural peel.[33,34]

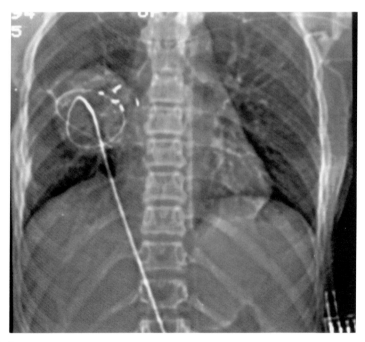

A

Figure 14.3 An 11-yr-old female developed a postoperative empyema after a right middle lobectomy for bronchiectasis. **A.** The CT topogram demonstrates the wire and catheter coiled within the empyema. **B.** Following page.

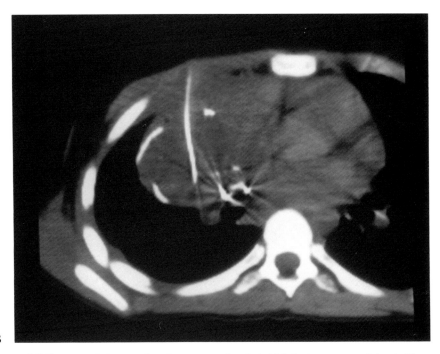

B

Figure 14.3 B. An 8-Fr pigtail catheter was placed. Initial drainage was minimal. She was started on intrapleural urokinase, 50,000 IU three times daily for 4 days. The empyema resolved with percutaneous drainage only.

In the surgical literature, rib resection, limited thoracotomy, and thorascopic debridement have all been advocated as the treatment of choice for empyema.[16,18,35] Currently, there is a trend toward early decortication.[12,33] Ashbaugh reviewed the effects of delayed surgical treatment and the choice of operation on the morbidity rate in patients with empyema.[33] He concluded that decortication is the procedure of choice when tube drainage fails. Decortication had the lowest morbidity and mortality rates when compared to tube or open surgical drainage.

The timing of decortication is important.[12] The fibroblastic pleural peel usually organizes by 8 wk, at which time a decortication can be performed. There is also an early window during the first 2–3 wk before the fibroblastic reaction begins when decortication can be performed easily. However, between 3–6 wk, the fibroblastic membrane is poorly developed and adherent to the lung. Attempts to perform decortication at this time can lead to tearing of lung tissue and the development of a bronchopleural fistula.

Complications

Serious complications from "blind" insertion of surgical chest tubes have been reported. These include lung laceration, diaphragmatic and intra-abdominal organ injury, and neurovascular injury.[36,37] None of these complications has occurred in the radiologic series. The only two complications reported in the radiologic series were an episode of transient bacteremia and a cardiopulmonary arrest from which the patient was successfully resuscitated.

Conclusions

Early drainage is very important in the management of an empyema. Imaging-guided chest tube placement is becoming the method of choice because of its accuracy, safety, and patient acceptance. It can also be used as an adjunct to surgically placed chest tubes to treat any undrained loculated collections. Even if an empyema does not completely resolve after percutaneous placement of a drainage catheter, a critically ill patient may be stabilized enough to permit a more elective surgical procedure. Because not all empyemas are amenable to percutaneous drainage, it is important to work closely with the thoracic surgeons. Intrapleural urokinase is a promising therapeutic agent to facilitate drainage of complicated or multiloculated pleural fluid collections. Formation of a pleural peel, persistent sepsis, and lack of response to catheter drainage are indications for prompt surgical intervention.

LUNG ABSCESSES

Although empyemas usually require some form of drainage to resolve, 80–90% of lung abscesses will heal with conventional antibiotic therapy.[38–40] Despite this, the reported mortality rate associated with a lung abscess is as high as 28%.[39]

Etiology

Primary lung abscesses are most commonly caused by oropharyngeal aspiration due to alcoholic stupor, general anesthesia, seizure disorders, or cerebrovascular accidents.[38,41,42] Other predisposing factors for aspiration include a hiatal hernia, esophageal dysmotility, and gastroesophageal reflux. Poor oral hygiene, although not a direct cause of aspiration, is a major factor in the development of a lung abscess because it provides the inoculum when a patient aspirates.[41]

Pneumonia is the other common cause of a primary lung abscess. Nosocomial pneumonias tend to be mixed with anaerobic bacteria and aerobic Gram-negative bacteria and frequently develop in debilitated patients. These pneumonias also have higher morbidity and mortality rates compared with community-acquired pneumonias.[41] While lung abscess formation is more commonly associated with anaerobic pneumonias, there are some aerobic organisms that can cause lung necrosis. These organisms include *Klebsiella pneumoniae, Staphylococcus aureus,* and various *Pseudomonas* species.[38]

Secondary lung abscesses result from a variety of conditions: malignancy, septic emboli and infarction, obstructing lesions or foreign bodies, and structural defects such as bronchiectasis, abnormal mucociliary mechanisms, or lung cysts.[38,41] Carcinoma of the lung is one of the more common causes of a secondary lung abscess.

Regardless of the etiology, lung abscesses often arise within the periphery of the lung.[43] The inflammatory process surrounding an abscess frequently extends to the visceral pleura and then to the parietal pleura, where it can cause a focal pleurodesis and a lesion-pleural symphysis.[43] This pleural symphysis is free of aerated lung and permits percutaneous access to a lung abscess, with minimal risk of pneumothorax or contamination of the pleural cavity.[43–46]

Diagnosis

Imaging plays an important role in the diagnosis and management of a lung abscess. Chest radiographs can be used to monitor areas of consolidation for possible cavity formation. Computed tomography is the imaging procedure of choice once a cavity is identified or if there is strong suspicion for the presence of small, subtle cavities. Computed tomography accurately delineates the lung parenchyma and pleura, thus differentiating between empyema and lung abscess. This difference is vital to directing subsequent management. Although early drainage is important for treating empyemas, medical management is preferred for treating lung abscesses.

Appropriate samples from lung abscesses are required to obtain accurate culture results and to determine the correct antibiotic regimen. Deep sputum expectoration can be used, but transtracheal aspirates have been shown to be more accurate.[41,47] Some authors recommend bronchoscopy to obtain a diagnostic sample and evaluate for an unsuspected endobronchial lesion or anatomic abnormality.[42,45,48] Bronchoscopy may be particularly helpful in young children who may be unable to cough up sputum due to the presence of bronchial stenosis or a foreign body.[45] However, the usefulness of bronchoscopy in adults is limited because the samples obtained may still be contaminated.[47] Contamination can be a problem in patients with chronic bronchitis, bronchiectasis, or bronchial neoplasms. These patients can have relatively large numbers of bacteria in the lower respiratory tract although they are not clinically infected.[41,47] Percutaneous transthoracic aspiration has the advantage of obtaining culture samples with almost no risk of specimen contamination.[45]

Medical Management

Lung abscesses and aspiration pneumonias will usually resolve when treated with appropriate antibiotics and postural drainage. Antibiotics commonly used include penicillin and clindamycin or a combination of penicillin and metronidazole.[41] Additional antibiotics may be necessary to treat certain aerobic infections. Although lung abscesses generally respond to antibiotics, resolution may be prolonged, with an average of 65 days to cavity closure.[41] In Bartlett's experience with 193 patients, infection was the cause of death in eight patients (4%) and a factor in lethal outcome in 14 (7%).[41] All patients with community-acquired pneumonia survived, but there was a 20% mortality rate in patients with nosocomial infections.

In addition to antibiotics, drainage of an abscess via the airways by deep sputum expectoration is important for cure, particularly in children. Kosloske et al.[45] recommended that lung abscesses be treated with appropriate antibiotics and drained by chest physiotherapy in those children who are able to cough up deep sputum. In those patients unable to cough sufficiently (usually children younger than 7 yr) or in those patients who are deteriorating, percutaneous drainage or surgical resection is recommended.

Although bronchoscopy may have a role in making an initial diagnosis, particularly in young children unable to cough, it has a more limited role in adults.[39,41] Because it can open occluded bronchi, bronchoscopy may be most helpful for those patients who cannot expectorate sputum or in patients with an infected cavitary neoplasm.[39] Some lung abscesses have been successfully drained by placement of coronary artery catheters into the involved bronchi transtracheally or through a bronchoscope.[42] Otherwise, bronchoscopy offers few therapeutic benefits.[41]

Surgical Management

Surgical alternatives include lobectomy, pneumonectomy, and surgically placed chest tubes. In the preantibiotic era, lung abscesses were drained by thoracotomy or percutaneous chest tubes.[44] With the use of modern antibiotics, most lung abscesses are now successfully treated medically. Surgical methods are required only in the 10–20% of patients in whom medical therapy has failed.[39–41] Lobectomy is the standard surgical treatment.[39,41] Indications for lobectomy include significant hemoptysis, suspected underlying malignancy, massive necrosis, and delayed closure of an abscess, (i.e., more than 6–8 wk of adequate antibiotic therapy).[42,44] A more limited segmentectomy may be performed; however, this may violate the infected lung parenchyma, thus increasing the chance of pleural contamination.[42] Other possible complications of lobectomy include hemorrhage, bronchopleural fistula, and contamination of the contralateral lung.

Percutaneous Management

While surgery is a treatment alternative for lung abscesses, there is a trend toward managing lung abscesses with percutaneous chest tube drainage.[40,44,49] The success of percutaneous chest tubes in the treatment of critically ill patients with lung abscesses unresponsive to antibiotics has been the catalyst for this trend.[40,44] Weissberg cured 7 of 7 patients in critical condition with percutaneous tube drainage.[44] The chest tubes were inserted through the abscess–pleural symphysis under general anesthesia. If the pleural symphysis was not present, stay sutures were placed in the lung to prevent leakage of pus into the pleural space. Rice et al. used either chest radiographs, fluoroscopy, or CT to guide chest tube placement, and cured 11 of 14 patients.

Although critics of percutaneous chest tube drainage cite the possible complications of pleural cavity contamination and bronchopleural fistula formation,[39,42] these complications have been fairly rare, ranging from 0% to 4% in most series.[38,44–46,49] In Rice's series, all 11 patients developed bronchopleural fistulas but these fistulas did not interfere with ventilation, and eight closed spontaneously.[40] The use of the abscess–pleural symphysis for access is not mentioned by these authors. They also had two episodes of hemorrhage requiring treatment.[40] Weissberg, using surgical techniques, did not have any patients develop bronchopleural fistulas, significant hemorrhage, or empyemas.[44] The absence of such complications in this series is probably due to the use of the abscess–pleural symphysis or stay sutures in the lung to minimize leakage of abscess fluid into the pleural space.

Imaging-guided Intervention

Cross-sectional imaging defines the presence, location, and size of an abscess. In addition, the abscess–pleural symphysis can usually be well delineated, identifying a percutaneous access site into the abscess. Use of imaging guidance also facilitates drainage of small abscesses, even in pediatric patients. The indications for placement of a drainage tube into a lung abscess under imaging guidance are essentially the same as for surgical resection: persistent sepsis after 5–7 days of appropriate antibiotic therapy, abscesses 4 cm or greater in diameter, which are under tension or enlarging; or failure to wean from a ventilator due to a large abscess.[40] Other indications include the need for obtaining a specimen in infants and children who are either too young or too debilitated to produce adequate sputum.[50,51] Relative contraindications include the inability of a patient to cooperate, the lack of an abscess–pleural symphysis, and a coagulopathy. Most patients with intact cough mechanisms and patent bronchi should be cured with conservative medical management.[46] As with an empyema, it is important to work closely with the thoracic surgeons.

Technique

We prefer to use CT guidance for all lung abscess drainages. The abscess is first localized and measured, and then the abscess–pleural symphysis is delineated (Figure 14.4). If no pleural symphysis is visualized, it is preferable to defer percutaneous drainage. Central abscesses are usually best managed surgically. Some authors have recommended positioning the patient such that the contralateral, noninfected lung is in a nondependent location in order to avoid endobronchial spread of purulent material to the uninfected lung during the drainage procedure.[46] However, lung abscesses requiring percutaneous drainage often do not have adequate drainage through the bronchial tree, which is why the medical therapy failed. Therefore, the normal lung can occasionally be placed in a dependent position as long as the patient is not coughing up sputum, since the chance of soiling the normal lung through the bronchial tree is small (Figure 14.5).

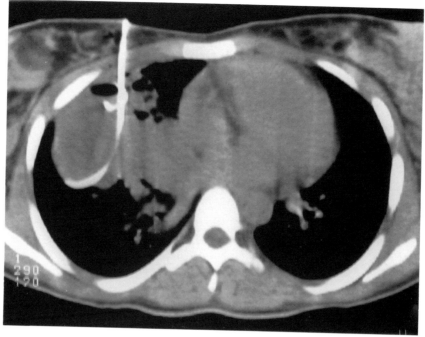

A

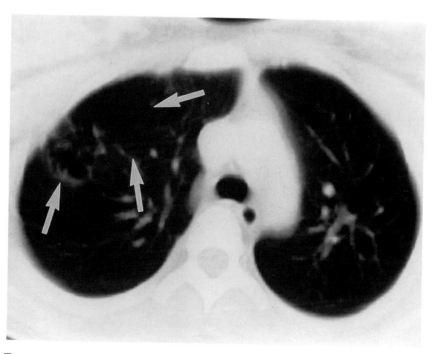

B

Figure 14.4 A. A previously asymptomatic 17-yr-old female presented with fever and a right upper lobe lung abscess, which was drained with an 8-Fr catheter. B. Emphysematous changes were noted in the noninfected superior portions of the right upper lobe (arrows). This suggested that the patient had a congenital lung lesion which was secondarily infected, not a primary lung abscess. C and D. Following page.

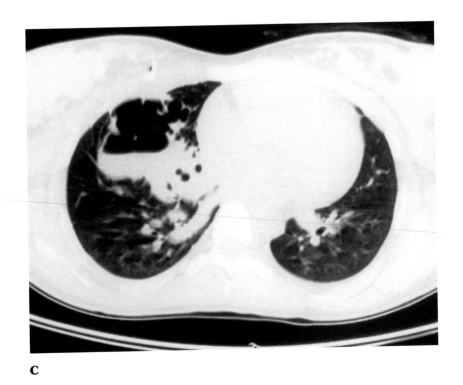

C

D

Figure 14.4 C. Axial image at lung window settings shows a decrease in abscess size after 1 wk of drainage. D. After 10 days of percutaneous drainage, the abscess continued to decrease in size and the peripheral blood leukocyte count returned to normal. The patient subsequently underwent a semielective right middle and upper lobectomy. This proved to be a cystic adenomatoid malformation.

Once the trajectory of the needle is determined, the patient is prepared and draped in a standard fashion. An 18-g Longdwel catheter is used to obtain a specimen sample for appropriate laboratory studies. A standard 0.035-inch guidewire can then be inserted through the Teflon sheath into the abscess cavity. The tract is then dilated and an 8- to 10-Fr nephrostomy-type pigtail catheter introduced. This dilatation can be performed on the CT table if the interventionalist is experienced. Alternatively, after the guidewire is placed in the abscess cavity, the patient can be carefully moved to the fluoroscopy suite for catheter placement. For very large abscesses, a single-step catheter on a trocar can be used, but we prefer the control of the Seldinger technique for smaller abscesses or for abscesses located near vital organs. One should not be too vigorous with catheter or guidewire manipulations within the abscess cavity while performing catheter insertions or exchanges since lung abscesses may have fine strands of residual normal parenchyma which can bleed.[40]

Ultrasound and fluoroscopy can also be used to guide aspiration and drainage of lung abscesses.[40,43,47,50,51] Yang et al. used ultrasound to guide aspiration of lung abscesses in 31 of 33 patients.[43] The abscess–pleural symphysis was visualized in 25 patients, and only two small pneumothoraces developed. Nonvisualization of some abscesses due to gas and the inability to image an entire abscess and the surrounding structures are limitations of ultrasound. Fluoroscopy is limited in its ability to visualize the abscess–pleural symphysis. However, a combination of ultrasound-guided aspiration followed by guidewire insertion and tract dilatation under fluoroscopy can be performed.

Once the catheter is within an abscess, it can be placed to gravity drainage or to a Pleur-Evac and wall suction at −20 cm of water. Follow-up should be performed with chest radiographs either daily or every other day during the first week, and less frequently thereafter, until the cavity is closed.

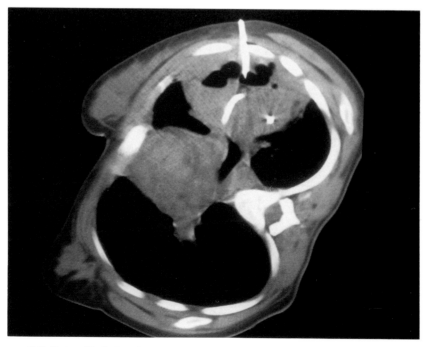

Figure 14.5 An elderly female patient with a lung abscess and a nonproductive cough could not lie supine. Because she was not producing sputum, the abscess could be drained with the uninvolved lung in a relatively dependent position, with little risk of endobronchial contamination from the abscess.

The catheters can be removed either blindly or under fluoroscopic visualization when the output decreases to less than 20 cc per day, the fluid becomes serous, the cavity appears closed, and the patient remains afebrile with normalization of the white blood cell count. Failures may occur with multiloculated abscesses, infected tumor cavities, or chronic, thick-walled abscesses.[45,46]

For infants and small children, percutaneous aspiration of lung abscesses has been advocated as both diagnostic and therapeutic.[50,51] In children younger than 8 yr old, early intervention is recommended because the airway may be too small to adequately drain the abscess, even with an intact cough mechanism.[45,50] In two separate reports, lung abscesses were successfully aspirated in three premature infants and one 17-month-old infant.[50,51] Complications include bacteremia, which resolved after reaspiration of the abscess, a small pneumothorax, and partial collapse of one lobe. The last two complications were not clinically significant.

Fibrinolytic Agents

We have been instilling urokinase into selected lung abscesses. The protocol is similar to the regimen used for intra-abdominal abscesses. It is based on the size of the abscess, assuming the abscess has a spherical shape. The following amounts of urokinase are instilled into the abscess cavity every 8 hr for 4 days. For abscesses 0–3 cm in diameter, 10,000 IU urokinase; 3–5 cm diameter, 25,000 IU urokinase; and 5–10 cm diameter, 50,000 IU urokinase. The catheter is flushed with 5 cc of saline after instillation of the urokinase, and the catheter is clamped. After 15 min, the catheter is unclamped and returned to suction. Relative contraindications for intra-abscess administration of urokinase include prolonged coagulation times (prothrombin time [PT] 3 sec or more above control), known brain metastases, pregnancy, nursing mother, or allergy to urokinase. If needed, the urokinase can be instilled for longer than 4 days, however we have found that 4 days is usually sufficient.

Success rates for imaging-guided percutaneous lung abscess drainage range from 67% to 100%.[38,46,52–55] Reported complications include spillage of infected material into the adjacent lung, hemothorax, one episode of increased intracranial pressure when the catheter traversed normal lung, and clogged catheters. Other possible complications include bronchopleural fistula, empyema, and pneumothorax.

Conclusions

Despite current medical management techniques, lung abscesses are associated with mortality rates of 5–28%.[39,41] Surgical resection has been the standard treatment. However, percutaneous transthoracic tube drainage may soon become the intervention of choice for lung abscesses in which medical therapy fails. The use of imaging guidance to direct drainage tube insertion minimizes complications such as bronchopleural fistula, pneumothorax, and contamination of the pleural space.

PERICARDIAL FLUID COLLECTIONS

Pericardial effusions may accumulate due to malignancy, infections and/or autoimmune pericarditis, or as a sequela of cardiac surgery. The effusions may be acute, subacute, or chronic. Aspiration of the fluid may be needed to determine the etiology of the collection. Indications for drainage include large effusions that cause clinical deterioration, hemodynamic compromise, and cardiac tamponade.[56,57]

Prior to the use of imaging-guided methods, pericardiocentesis was associated with significant complications, including perforation of the heart, laceration of the coronary vessels, arrhythmias, bleeding, and death.[58,59] Fluoroscopic and/or sonographic guidance for pericardiocentesis have been recently advocated.[56,57,59–62] Those authors using sonography or a combination of sonography and fluoroscopy have had fewer complications and no procedure-related deaths.[56,59,62,63] We have found CT to be an effective modality to guide aspiration and drainage of pericardial effusions. Computed tomography allows visualization of an effusion and its relationship to the heart, lungs, and other vital structures such as the liver and internal mammary arteries. It may be particularly helpful in visualizing infected collections containing air bubbles and loculated effusions.[64]

Surgical pericardial window formation is usually performed in patients whose effusions do not respond to percutaneous drainage. Indications for surgical intervention include cytologic confirmation of suspected malignancy in recurrent effusions, management of malignant effusions that do not respond to routine therapy in patients with otherwise limited tumor extent and favorable survival time, and benign effusions that recur rapidly following needle drainage.[65] In patients who undergo surgery, success can be expected in more than 90% of cases; however, postoperative complications may also occur in as many as 65% of these patients.[65,66] Some surgeons prefer to perform a total pericardiectomy, particularly when the estimated survival time of the patient is greater than 1 yr.[67]

Percutaneous Drainage Technique

The patient is positioned in the CT gantry so that the trajectory of the needle avoids the lung, internal mammary arteries, and heart. An intercostal approach, similar to that used in sonographically guided pericardiocentesis is preferred.[56,59,63] An approach perpendicular to the pericardial effusion increases the chances of the needle point striking the heart, especially if the effusion is small (Figure 14.6). Therefore, an obtuse angle of

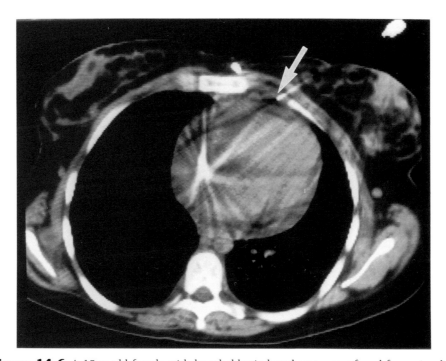

Figure 14.6 A 15-yr-old female with lymphoblastic lymphoma was referred for pericardial aspiration to evaluate for possible malignant pericardial effusion. A left anterior approach, avoiding the internal mammary arteries, heart, and pleural space, was used. Note the obtuse angle of the needle (arrow) relative to the anterior pericardium. This is important if the pericardial effusion is small. The risk of puncturing the heart is increased if a more perpendicular approach is used. This effusion was nonmalignant. If drainage had been desired, a catheter could have been placed by using the Seldinger technique.

approach to the fluid is safer. An 18-g Longdwel catheter is used to aspirate the fluid. If drainage is desired, a 0.035-inch guidewire is advanced into the effusion, and subsequent dilatations can be performed either on the CT gantry or in a fluoroscopy suite. During the procedure, it is important to monitor the patient appropriately and to have intensive care unit (ICU) support staff present if the patient is unstable. The patient should have good intravenous access in case pharmacologic intervention is required. If the effusion is large, the initial drainage should be limited to 200–400 cc during the first 20 min to decrease the risk of compromising cardiac hemodynamics.[62] The remainder of the fluid can be removed gradually by gravity drainage.

Results

Pericardiocentesis has been successful in almost all cases of sonographic guidance.[55,59,61–63] The only reported failure was in a patient with a very small effusion.[59] Placement of drainage catheters has also been very successful; however, as many as 24% of these patients eventually require a surgical procedure.[56] Some critically ill patients cannot undergo surgery. In such patients, successful percutaneous pericardial window formation with a valvuloplasty balloon under fluoroscopic guidance has been described.[67, 68]

Complications

Despite imaging guidance, there are significant risks to pericardiocentesis. Most of the complications are due to the needle touching or penetrating the heart. Cardiac penetration may occur, however, this is usually not a major complication as long as small-caliber needles are used and only a ventricle is penetrated.[59,60,62] The thick, highly contractile walls of the ventricles presumably cause the needle tract to seal. However, penetration into an atrium or laceration of a coronary artery may cause very serious bleeding.[60] Fluoroscopically guided pericardiocentesis has a 5–10% incidence of cardiac penetration leading to significant morbidity.[57,58,60] The reported incidence of cardiac penetration with sonographic guidance is 0–2%, with minimal associated morbidity.[56,59–63] Other complications encountered during pericardial drainages include arrhythmias, bleeding, pneumopericardium, and injury to the diaphragm or liver. Surgical techniques can have high success and low morbidity and mortality rates, but significant complications have also been reported.[65,66]

Conclusions

Imaging-guided pericardiocentesis and drainage have proved to be relatively safe, reliable, and effective. In critically ill patients who eventually will require a surgical procedure, an imaging-guided drainage may allow the patient's condition to be stabilized until surgery can be performed.

MEDIASTINAL ABSCESSES

Mediastinal abscesses may result from penetrating trauma, iatrogenic etiologies, esophageal perforation, or the spread of infection from adjacent tissue spaces. Patients with mediastinal abscesses are often critically ill, so that surgery may be difficult and risky. Imaging-guided drainage is ideal in such patients because a catheter can be placed within the abscess to stabilize and possibly cure critically ill patients.

Percutaneous Drainage Technique

Computed tomography is the guiding modality of choice. The approach should avoid the lung and all major cardiovascular and tracheobronchial structures. The needle and catheter should remain extrapleural. Posterior mediastinal abscesses can usually be drained from a direct posterior approach without crossing the pleura or other vital structures. Anterior mediastinal abscesses can be drained from an anterolateral approach. It is important to avoid the internal mammary artery and all of the mediastinal great vessels.

Middle mediastinal abscesses are more difficult to drain. A posterolateral approach is usually required, either through the right or left paraspinal space (Figure 14.7). It is easier to remain extrapleural and avoid the lung by using the left paraspinal approach. It is also important to use adequate local anesthesia. The needle should enter the skin at the level of the costotransverse process junction. Once the needle reaches the vertebral body, the needle bevel is turned toward the vertebral body and the needle is advanced slowly. The needle path must be carefully planned before the mediastinum is entered, because once the needle is against the vertebral body it is difficult to change its trajectory. Once the needle passes medial to the descending aorta, the bevel can be adjusted to facilitate entry into the abscess. If the abscess is paratracheal or subcarinal, it is important to avoid the esophagus, trachea, and main bronchi. An anterior approach can be used for a middle mediastinal abscess; however, it may be difficult to avoid the lung or major vessels unless there is a large amount of mediastinal fat.

While single-step catheters on trocars may be used for large abscesses in the anterior or posterior mediastinum, we always use an 18-g Longdwel catheter and the Seldinger technique to enter and drain middle mediastinal abscesses. Once the needle enters the collection, a small amount of fluid is aspirated and visually inspected. If the fluid is grossly purulent, a 0.035-inch guidewire is coiled into the collection. The tract is dilated and an 8- to 10-Fr self-retaining catheter is placed. If the aspirated fluid is

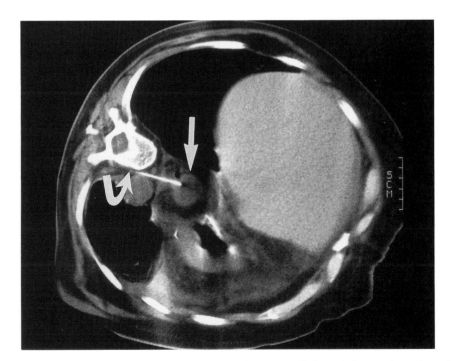

Figure 14.7 A patient, after esophagectomy and gastric pull-through for esophageal cancer, developed a postoperative fever, elevated white blood cell count, and a small middle mediastinal fluid collection (straight arrow). The collection was aspirated from a left paraspinal approach, with the needle (curved arrow) passing between the aorta and spine. The aspirated fluid was clear yellow, so only a small sample was sent for culture. This was subsequently shown to be sterile and resolved spontaneously. If purulent material had been obtained, or if the cultures were positive, a catheter could have been placed from the same trajectory.

clear, only a small fluid sample is sent for Gram stain and culture and sensitivity. If the culture result is positive, the collection can then be reaspirated and drained. Initial aspiration of the entire collection is not recommended because the "target" will be too small to easily drain if the specimen culture is positive. For those collections in which the initial aspirate appears questionably infected or when the collection is in a difficult location, a 5-Fr angiographic pigtail catheter can be placed into the collection. If the 24-hr culture result is positive, the patient can be returned to the angiographic suite, and a larger self-retaining catheter can be placed. If the culture result is negative, the 5-Fr catheter can be easily removed.

Results

Because mediastinal abscesses are not common, there are not many reports of percutaneous drainage. Gobien et al. cured 5 of 6 patients with mediastinal abscesses, and stabilized the sixth patient for later elective surgery.[69] They also excluded the diagnosis of infection in three patients by proving that the mediastinal fluid collections were sterile. Wittich et al. reported successful CT-guided catheter drainage of 24 of 26 (92%) mediastinal abscesses. Failures were secondary to phlegmonous collections. No significant complications occurred.[70]

Complications

The major complications associated with this procedure include inadvertent puncture of cardiovascular or tracheobronchial structures, esophagus, or the pleura and lung. If vascular structures are punctured, the bleeding should stop quickly unless the vessel is lacerated. Although erosion into vessels or other structures by an indwelling catheter is a possible risk, this has not yet been reported.[69]

Conclusions

Infected mediastinal fluid collections that are accessible by percutaneous techniques should respond to catheter drainage as well as empyemas and intra-abdominal abscesses as long as meticulous technique is used.

REFERENCES

1. O'Moore PV, Mueller PR, Simone JF et al: Sonographic guidance in diagnostic and therapeutic interventions in the pleural space. *Am J Roentgenol* 153:941, 1989.
2. Lee MJ, Saini S, Brink JA, et al: Interventional radiology of the pleural space: diagnostic thoracentesis, therapeutic thoracentesis, pleural biopsy, and pleural sclerosis. *Semin Intervent Radiol* 8:23–28, 1991.
3. Trapnell DH, Thurston JGB: Unilateral pulmonary edema after pleural aspiration. *Lancet* 1:1367, 1970.
4. LoCicero J: Thoracoscopic management of malignant pleural effusion. *Ann Thorac Surg* 56:641–643, 1993.
5. Bresticker MA, Oba J, LoCicero J, et al: Optimal pleurodesis: a comparison study. *Ann Thorac Surg* 55:364–367, 1993.
6. Zaloznik AJ, Oswald SG, Langin M: Intrapleural tetracycline in malignant pleural effusions: a randomized study. *Cancer* 51:752–755, 1983.
7. Ruckdeschel JC, Moores D, Lee JY, et al: Intrapleural therapy for malignant pleural effusions: randomized comparison of bleomycin and tetracycline. *Chest* 100:1528–1535, 1991.
8. Morrison MC, Mueller PR, Lee MJ, et al: Sclerotherapy of malignant pleural effusion through sonographically placed small-bore catheters. *Am J Roentgenol* 158:41–43, 1992.
9. Webb WR, Ozmen V, Moulder PV, et al: Iodized talc pleurodesis for the treatment of pleural effusions. *J Thorac Cardiovasc Surg* 103:881–886, 1992.
10. Adler RH, Levinsky L: Persistent chylothorax: treatment by talc pleurodesis. *J Thorac Cardiovasc Surg* 76:859–864, 1978.

11. Akaogi E, Mitsui K, Sohara Y, et al: Treatment of postoperative chylothorax with intrapleural fibrin glue. *Ann Thorac Surg* 48:116–118, 1989.

12. Mandal AK, Thadepalli H: Treatment of spontaneous bacterial empyema thoracis. *J Thorac Cardiovasc Surg* 94:414–418, 1987.

13. Sahn SA: Management of complicated parapneumonic effusions. *Am Rev Respir Dis* 148:813, 1993.

14. Light RW: Parapneumonic effusions and empyema. *Clin Chest Med* 6:55–61, 1985.

15. Neff CC, vanSonnenberg E, Lawson DW, et al: CT follow-up of empyemas: pleural peels resolve after percutaneous drainage. *Radiology* 176:195–197, 1992.

16. Lemmer JH, Botham MJ, Orringer MB: Modern management of adult thoracic empyema. *J Thorac Cardiovasc Surg* 90:849–855, 1985.

17. Mavroudis C, Symmonds JB, Minagi H, et al: Improved survival in management of empyema thoracis. *J Thorac Cardiovasc Surg* 82:49–55, 1981.

18. Van Way C, Narrod J, Hopeman A: The role of early limited thoracotomy in the treatment of empyema. *J Thorac Cardiovasc Surg* 96:436–439, 1988.

19. Lee KS, Im J, Kim YH, et al: Treatment of thoracic multiloculated empyemas with intracavitary urokinase: a prospective study. *Radiology* 179:771–775, 1991.

20. Moulton JS, Moore PT, Mencini RA: Treatment of loculated pleural effusions with transcatheter intracavitary urokinase. *Am J Roentgenol* 153:941–945, 1989.

21. Silverman SG, Mueller PR, Saini S, et al: Thoracic emyema: management with image-guided catheter drainage. *Radiology* 169:5–9, 1988.

22. Hunnan GR, Flower CDR: Radiologically guided percutaneous catheter drainage of empyemas. *Clin Radiol* 39:121–126, 1988.

23. Merriam MA, Cronan JJ, Dorfman GS, et al: Radiographically guided percutaneous catheter drainage of pleural fluid collections. *Am J Roentgenol* 151:1113–1116, 1988.

24. Westcott JL: Percutaneous catheter drainage of pleural effusion and empyema. *Am J Roentgenol* 144:1189–1193, 1985.

25. vanSonnenberg E, Nakamoto SK, Mueller PR, et al: CT and ultrasound guided catheter drainage of empyemas after chest-tube failure. *Radiology* 154:349–353, 1984.

26. Lee MJ, Saini S, Brink JA, et al: Interventional radiology of the pleural space: management of thoracic empyema with image-guided catheter drainage. *Semin Intervent Radiol* 8:29–35, 1991.

27. Lambiase RE, Deyoe L, Cronan JJ, et al: Percutaneous drainage of 335 consecutive abscesses: results of primary drainage with 1-year follow-up. *Radiology* 184:167–179, 1992.

28. Tarver RD, Dewey DJ: Interventional chest radiology. *Radiol Clin North Am* 32:689–709, 1994.

29. Tillet WS, Sherry S, Reed CT: The use of streptodornase in the treatment of chronic empyema. *J Thorac Surg* 21:325–341, 1951.

30. Haaga JR: CT-guided procedures. In Haaga JR, Alfidi RJ: *Computed Tomography of the Whole Body,* ed 2. St Louis, CV Mosby, 1988, pp 1200–1320.

31. Moulton JS, Benkert RE, Weisinger KH, et al: Treatment of complicated pleural fluid collections with image-guided drainage and intracavitary urokinase. *Chest* 108:1252–59, 1995.

32. Lahorra JM, Haaga JR, Stellato T, et al: Safety of intracavitary urokinase with percutaneous abscess drainage. *Am J Roentgenol* 160:171–174, 1993.

33. Ashbaugh DG: Empyema thoracis: factors influencing morbidity and mortality. *Chest* 99:1162–1165, 1991.

34. Morin JE, Munro DD, Maclean LD: Early thoracotomy for empyema. *J Thorac Cardiovasc Surg* 64:530–536, 1972.

35. Ridley PD, Brainbridge MV: Thorascopic debridement and pleural irrigation in the management of empyema thoracis. *Ann Thorac Surg* 51:461–464, 1991.

36. Miller KS, Sahn SA: Chest tubes: indications, technique, management and complications. *Chest* 91:258–264, 1987.

37. Millikan JJ, Moore EE, Steiner E, et al: Complications of tube thoracostomy for acute trauma. *Am J Surg* 140:738–741, 1980.

38. Moore AV, Zuger JH, Kelley MJ: Lung abscess: an interventional radiology perspective. *Semin Intervent Radiol* 8(1):36–43, 1991.

39. Hagan JL, Hardy JD: Lung abscess revisited. *Ann Surg* 197:755–761, 1983.

40. Rice TW, Ginsberg RJ, Tomas RJ, et al: Tube drainage of lung abscesses. *Ann Thorac Surg* 44:356–359, 1987.

41. Bartlett JG: Anaerobic bacterial infections of the lung. *Chest* 91:901–909, 1987.
42. Estrera AS, Platt MR, Mills LJ, et al: Primary lung abscess. *J Thorac Cardiovasc Surg* 79: 275–282, 1980.
43. Yang P, Luh K, Lee Y, et al: Lung abscesses: US examination and US-guided transthoracic aspiration. *Radiology* 180:171–175, 1991.
44. Weissberg D: Percutaneous drainage of lung abscess. *J Thorac Cardiovasc Surg* 87:308–312, 1984.
45. Kosloske AM, Ball WS, Butler C, et al: Drainage of pediatric lung abscess by cough, catheter, or complete resection. *J Pediatr Surg* 21:596–600, 1986.
46. vanSonnenberg E, D'Agostino HB, Casola G, et al: Lung abscess: CT-guided drainage. *Radiology* 178:347–351, 1991.
47. Grinan NP, Lucena FM, Romero JV, et al: Yield of percutaneous needle lung aspiration in lung abscess. *Chest* 97:69–74, 1990.
48. Pohlson EC, McNamara JJ, Char C, et al: Lung abscess: a changing pattern of the disease. *Am J Surg* 150:97–101, 1985.
49. Yellin A, Yellin EO, Liebermann Y: Percutaneous tube drainage: the treatment of choice for refractory lung abscess. *Ann Thorac Surg* 39:266–270, 1985.
50. Lorenzo RL, Bradford BF, Black J: Lung abscesses in children: diagnostic and therapeutic needle aspiration. *Radiology* 157:79–80, 1985.
51. Lee SK, Morris RF, Cramer B: Percutaneous needle aspiration of neonatal lung abscesses. *Pediatr Radiol* 21:254–257, 1991.
52. Ha HK, Kang MW, Park JM, et al. Lung abscess: percutaneous catheter therapy. *Acta Radiol Scand* 34:362–365, 1993.
53. Parker LA, Melton JW, Delaney DJ, et al: Percutaneous small bore catheter drainage in the management of lung abscesses. *Chest* 92:213–218, 1987.
54. Ball WS, Bisset GS, Towbin RB: Percutaneous drainage of chest abscesses in children. *Radiology* 171:431–434, 1989.
55. Cuestas RA, Kienzle GE, Armstrong JD: Percutaneous drainage of lung abscesses in infants. *Pediatr Infect Dis J* 8:390–392, 1989.
56. Kopecky SL, Callahan HA, Tajik AJ, et al: Percutaneous pericardial catheter drainage, report of 42 consecutive cases. *Am J Cardiol* 58:633–635, 1986.
57. Zahn EM, Houde C, Benson L, et al: Percutaneous pericardial catheter drainage in childhood. *Am J Cardiol* 70:678–680, 1992.
58. Wong B, Murphy J, Chang C, et al: The risk of pericardiocentesis. *Am J Cardiol* 44:1110, 1970.
59. Callahan JA, Seward JB, Nishimura RA, et al: Two-dimensional echocardiography guided pericardiocentesis, experience in 117 consecutive patients. *Am J Cardiol* 58:633–635, 1986.
60. Duvernoy O, Borowiec J, Helmius G, et al: Complications of percutaneous pericardiocentesis under fluoroscopic guidance. *Acta Radiol* 12:147, 1991.
61. Taavitsainen M, Bondestam S, Mankinen P, et al: Ultrasound guidance for pericardiocentesis. *Acta Radiol* 32:9, 1991.
62. Gatenby RA, Hartz WH, Kesslar HB, et al: Percutaneous catheter drainage for malignant pericardial effusion. *JVIR* 2:151, 1991.
63. Clarke DP, Cosgrove DO: Real-time ultrasound scanning in the planning and guidance of pericardiocenteses. *Clin Radiol* 38:119, 1987.
64. Higgins CB, Mattery RF, Shea P: CT localization and aspiration of postoperative pericardial fluid collection. *J Comput Assist Tomogr* 7:734, 1983.
65. Gregory JR, McMurtry MJ, Mountain CF: A surgical approach to the treatment of pericardial effusion in cancer patients. *Am J Clin Oncol* 8:319–323, 1985.
66. Fredriksen RT, Cohen LS, Mullins CB: Pericardial windows or pericardiocentesis for pericardial effusion. *Am Heart J* 82:158–162, 1971.
67. Selig MB: Percutaneous transcatheter pericardial interventions: aspiration, biopsy, and pericardioplasty. *Am Heart J* 125:269–271, 1993.
68. Palacios IF, Tuzcu M, Ziskind A, et al: Percutaneous balloon pericardial window for patients with malignant pericardial effusion and tamponade. *Cathet Cardiovasc Diagn* 22:244–249, 1991.
69. Gobien RP, Stanley JH, Gobien BS: Percutaneous catheter aspiration and drainage of suspected mediastinal abscesses. *Radiology* 151:69–71, 1984.
70. Wittich GR, vanSonnenberg E. Percutaneous drainage of mediastinal fluid collections. *Radiology* 189(P):156, 1993.

C H A P T E R
15

Management of Tracheobronchial Stenoses with Metal Stents

Alan H. Matsumoto
J. Fritz Angle
Charles J. Tegtmeyer

INTRODUCTION

Progressive narrowing of the tracheobronchial airways can be very distressing for the patient and is potentially life-threatening. Signs and symptoms include breathlessness, wheezing, stridor, and recurrent infections. Treatment for airways obstruction varies, depending upon the length of the lesion, the etiology of the obstruction, and the age and overall prognosis for the patient.

Malignancy is the most frequent cause of tracheobronchial obstruction in the adult population and is rarely amenable to reconstructive surgery. External beam irradiation, intraluminal brachytherapy, or endoscopic resection using diathermy, laser, or cryotherapy have been used in this setting.[1-5] Most of these treatment options provide only temporary relief of symptoms because of the rapid regrowth of residual tumor.

The majority of benign strictures of the trachea and major bronchi are due to iatrogenic causes, but prior infections, sarcoidosis, amyloid disease, vascular rings, trauma, or disease processes which affect the integrity of the cartilaginous rings of the trachea can also lead to airway stenosis. Short, circumscribed, benign lesions of the cervical trachea are usually best treated by surgical resection.[6-8] Long strictures are more difficult to treat but can occasionally be treated by very complex surgical procedures which incorporate the use of free or pedunculated grafts of different types of tissues.[9,10] Unfortunately, resection of long segments of the airway (greater than 6 cm) frequently results in respiratory problems secondary to collapse of the graft or recurrent anastomotic strictures.[7]

Benign lesions have been treated with a variety of endoscopic techniques. These therapeutic modalities usually produce immediate improvement and occasional long-term successes, but recurrences are the general rule.[4,5] Dilatations of benign tracheobronchial stenoses using balloons and bougies have also been performed.[11-15] Limited follow-up is available in these reports, and repeat dilatations have been required in most instances. In one case, balloon dilatation was repeated six times over a 5-month interval. The frequent need to supplement dilatation techniques with adjunctive endoscopic therapy or stents suggests that balloon or bougie dilatation alone is not effective in providing long-term palliation for benign tracheobronchial stenoses.[16,17] Despite this, balloon dilatation may have a role in neonates and infants as a temporizing measure to allow growth of the child until a more definitive procedure can be performed.

Long-term tracheostomy has occasionally been employed to manage chronic upper airways obstruction. The disadvantage of a tracheostomy is the inability to maintain peroral and pernasal breathing, speech, and adequate clearance of secretions.

PLASTIC STENTS

In 1965, Montgomery described the use of a T-shaped silicone tube designed to be used both as a tracheal stent and as a tracheostomy tube.[18] The tube is positioned in the trachea, with the sidearm of the T projecting through the tracheostomy. The sidearm prevents tube migration and provides access for clearance of secretions. In 1982, Westaby and Shepherd described a silastic tracheobronchial stent with the lower end forming a reverse Y configuration. This stent is designed to rest on the carina and has a sidearm that extends out of the tracheostomy site.[19] The Westaby tube design prevents distal and proximal migration and allows the entire length of the trachea and both mainstem bronchi to be stented. The silicone stent that is most widely used at this time is the Dumon endoprosthesis.[20] It is designed with no external components and can be inserted using a rigid bronchoscope. The outside surface of this stent has rounded studs that protrude from its surface. The studs are designed to prevent the stent from sliding or turning. The Dumon stent is available in several sizes for both tracheal and bronchial applications.

Plastic stents are fairly well tolerated. They have been shown to be effective in relieving respiratory symptoms in patients with large airway obstruction secondary to extrinsic compression or long-segment disease of the cartilaginous rings of the trachea and in some patients with large, bulky, intrinsic tumors.[21,22] Silastic stents have also been used for definitive treatment of benign disease or as an adjunct to or in preparation for definitive surgical reconstruction.[23] These stents have provided palliation of symptoms for 5 to 10 years in patients with benign disease.[23,24]

The most frequent problems associated with the use of plastic stents are stent migration and mucous plugging.[24–27] Migration is most likely to occur in short, conical stenoses with intact, smooth mucosa or in the presence of tracheobronchial malacia. In both situations, the underlying anatomy does not permit firm anchorage of the stent. The mucosa under most plastic stents undergoes a metaplastic alteration with impediment of mucous clearance.[28] The presence of the plastic stent also appears to reduce the effectiveness of the mucociliary clearance mechanism, leading to recurrent plugging of the stent. In most instances, migration or mucous plugging of the stent can be managed by endoscopic repositioning or replacement of the silastic stent.

The large profile of the plastic stent relative to its intraluminal diameter remains a problem and may further predispose the stent to plugging. The large size of the stent also makes insertion and replacement somewhat difficult. Although there is one report on the use of a fenestrated silicone chest tube as an endobronchial stent, most of the plastic tracheobronchial stents do not have sideholes.[29] Therefore, placement of a nonfenestrated stent peripheral to a major bronchus will lead to obstruction of segmental bronchi.

METAL STENTS

Metal tracheobronchial devices have been in use since the early 1950s.[30–32] There are several potential advantages of metal stents compared to plastic stents. Metal stents have a relatively low profile on insertion. The thickness of the wall of the metal stent relative to its intraluminal diameter is negligible. Following placement of a metal stent, the normal respiratory epithelium protrudes through the open lattice, and metaplastic squamous epithelium overgrows and incorporates the stent into the wall of the airway.[28] The neoepithelium overlying the stent also appears to maintain some rudimentary ciliary function (Figure 15.1). Potential problems associated with the use of a metal stent in the tracheobronchial system include ingrowth of granulation or tumor tissue through the open lattice of the metal stent, leading to recurrent airways obstruction.[24,28] Because metal stents become incorporated into the wall of the airway within 4 to 6 weeks, they are also very difficult to remove without surgery.

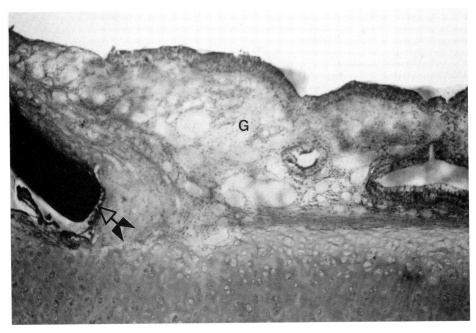

A

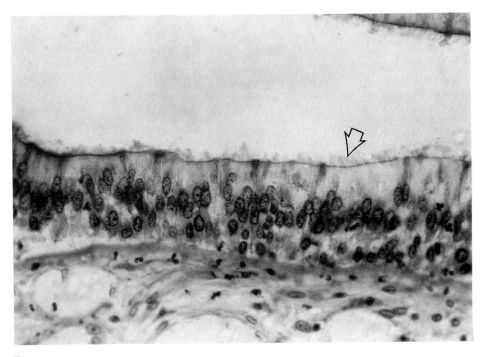

B

Figure 15.1 A. A microscopic section of an autopsy specimen from a patient with an endo-bronchial Palmaz stent in place for 27 months shows the stent strut (arrow). Overlying the stent strut is granulation tissue (G). B. Further magnification of the specimen reveals ciliated neoep-ithelium (arrow) along the luminal surface of the airway.

There are two basic designs to metal stents: balloon-expandable and self-expanding. At the time of this writing, there are only two types of metal stents that are approved by the Food and Drug Administration (FDA) for application in the tracheobronchial system: the Gianturco tracheobronchial stent (Cook, Inc., Bloomington, IN) and the Wallstent tracheobronchial endoprosthesis (Schneider, Inc., Minneapolis, MN). Both of these stents are self-expanding. The Wallstent is also available in a silicone-covered model (Permalume covering).

Gianturco Stent

The Gianturco tracheobronchial stent is a self-expanding device that is constructed in a zigzag configuration from a rigid stainless steel wire. It is available in diameters of 15, 20, 25, 30, and 35 mm and in one length, 5 cm.[33] The stent is designed to be introduced through a 14.5 F or 16.5 F introducer sheath. The sheath is positioned in the obstructing lesion, and the stent is advanced to the tip of the sheath using a pusher rod. While maintaining pressure against the stent with the pusher rod, the introducer sheath is then retracted. The stent is uncovered and self-expands. The fixation hooks on the stent help to minimize migration of the stent once it is deployed (Figure 15.2). Further expansion of the stent several days after its deployment has been observed.[34]

Gianturco stents have been used to treat airway compression caused by extrinsic malignancy and intraluminal obstruction secondary to intrinsic tumors of the airway. In one report, 17 of 21 (81%) patients who underwent stent placement for treatment of tracheobronchial obstructions secondary to malignancy had improvement in their clinical symptoms.[34] Following stent placement, the clinical benefit persisted for a mean survival period of 134 days (range, 2 to 799 days). The only early complication observed in this series was stent migration, which required stent removal. Late complications included the development of a tracheal-pharyngeal fistula and separation of two consecutive stents, requiring the placement of additional stents. Recurrent obstruction was seen in two patients. In both of these cases, tumor growth occurred distal to the stents. The large gap between the metal wires of the Gianturco stent also allows ingrowth of tumor through the stent. This can lead to recurrent airway obstruction. Therefore, if Gianturco stents are used in the presence of intraluminal malignancy, adjunctive radiation or endoscopic therapy should be considered.[34–36]

The Gianturco stent has been used in the management of tracheobronchial malacia, postinflammatory and postintubation strictures, and anastomotic stenoses.[36–40] Most of these series reporting on the use of the Gianturco stent in patients with benign disease are small, yet it appears that almost 70% of patients with tracheobronchial malacia have long-term improvement in their cough efficiency and expiratory volumes.[39,40] Some ingrowth of granulation tissue through the stent can be seen in up to 80% of patients with long-term follow-up. In most instances, this granulation tissue can be managed with endoscopic therapy.[37,40] In patients with benign fibroinflammatory stenoses, the formation of granulation tissue can be recurrent and refractory to endoscopic treatment. In one series, it was necessary to remove the stents in three patients because of exuberant granulation tissue formation.[40] Displacement of the stent during suctioning, stent migration, disruption of the stent, and erosion of the stent into an adjacent artery causing massive bleeding have also been reported with the use of the Gianturco stent.[39,41,42]

Recurrent infections related to the presence of a Gianturco stent have not been a clinical problem. Stent struts have been seen to traverse upper lobe bronchi without causing upper lobe atelectasis or recurrent pneumonias. Coughing has been seen immediately following stent placement, but this problem usually resolves with time.

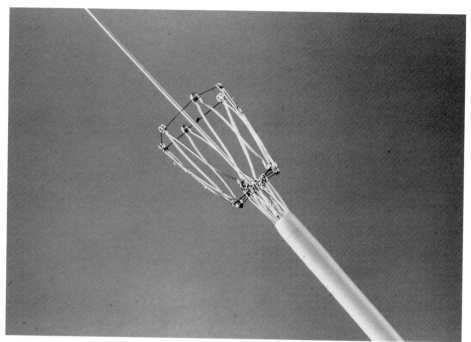

A

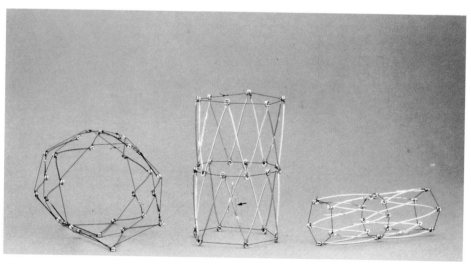

B

Figure 15.2 A. A partially deployed Gianturco tracheobronchial stent is demonstrated. B. Fully deployed Gianturco tracheobronchial stents with retention hooks (arrow) are shown.

Wallstent Tracheobronchial Endoprosthesis

The Wallstent tracheobronchial endoprosthesis is a flexible, self-expanding metal stent. It is woven into a cylindrical tube from 20 monofilaments of a stainless steel alloy. The delivery system has a sleeve which constrains the metal endoprosthesis, thereby minimizing the profile of the metal stent during its insertion. When the sleeve on the delivery catheter is retracted, the metal stent self-expands and foreshortens in length (Figure 15.3). The diameter of the stent is selected to be larger than the target

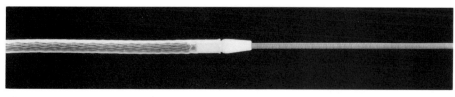

A

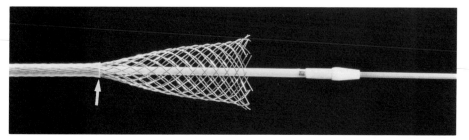

B

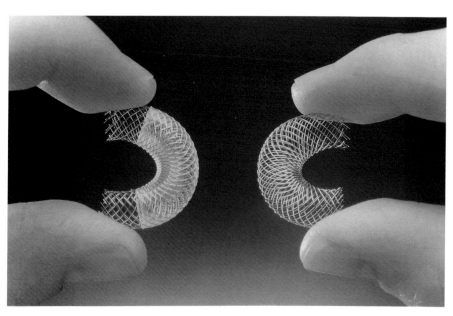

C

Figure 15.3 A. The delivery device with a constrained Wallstent tracheobronchial endoprosthesis is shown. B. The constraining sleeve (arrow) has been withdrawn, allowing partial expansion of the Wallstent. During the expansion process, the Wallstent has foreshortened. C. Silicone-covered and uncovered Wallstents are demonstrated.

airway. Upon deployment, the stent expands to the diameter of the airway and is held in place by the radial force generated by the stent (Figure 15.4). Because the stent is flexible, it will attempt to conform to the underlying anatomy. Wallstents are currently available in diameters of 5 to 24 mm and in lengths from 20 to 94 mm.

The Wallstent endoprosthesis has been used in the treatment of both benign and malignant strictures[24,39,43–45] (Figure 15.4). The Wallstent appears to be useful in relieving symptoms caused by extrinsic compression of the airways.[24,39,43,44] Intrinsic tu-

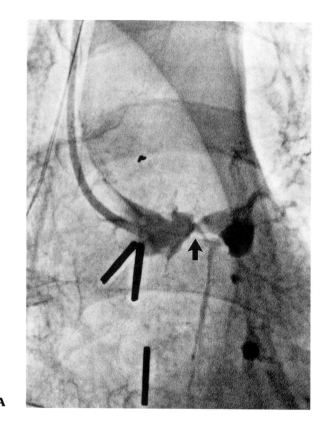

A

B

Figure 15.4 A. A bronchogram using nonionic contrast reveals a significant stricture (arrow) at the left lung transplant anastomosis. B. A Wallstent endoprosthesis is shown positioned across the region of the anastomotic stricture (arrow). Two Wallstents are present. The initially deployed stent retracted proximal to the stricture; therefore, a second Wallstent was advanced coaxially through the first stent to bridge the stricture. **C** and **D**. Following page.

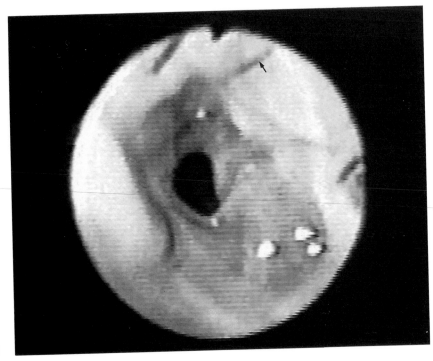

C

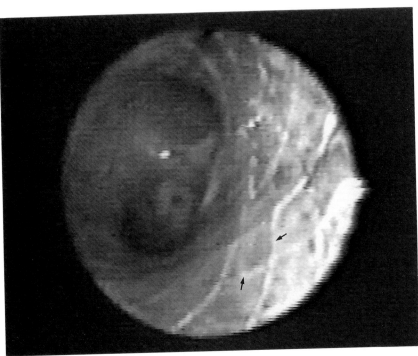

D

Figure 15.4 C. Bronchoscopic exam reveals a very narrow bronchial anastomosis prior to stent placement. Suture material is visualized (arrow). D. Following deployment of the Wall-stent, bronchoscopic evaluation reveals a widely patent airway with visualization of the distal bronchi. The stent filaments are seen (arrows).

mors of the airway can grow through the open wire-mesh of the Wallstent. Therefore, in the presence of an intraluminal tumor, placement of an uncovered Wallstent frequently requires adjunctive radiation or endoscopic therapy to maintain airway patency.[24,39,43]

The Wallstent has also been used to treat benign postsurgical anastomotic stenoses, postintubation stenoses, tracheal amyloid, severe scoliosis, postinfectious lesions, Wegener's granulomatosis, and tracheobronchial malacia.[24,39,45] Following Wallstent implantation, immediate symptomatic improvement has occurred in almost all patients with benign lesions. The mean follow-up period in most series is 8 to 10 months, with the longest follow-up being 27 months.[39,45] Formation of granulation tissue within the stent occurs in approximately 20% of the patients and can usually be managed with repeat balloon dilatation, additional stent placement, or endoscopic resection techniques (cryotherapy, laser photoblation, or bipolar electrocautery). The ingrowth of granulation tissue appears to become self-limiting 18 to 24 months after stent implantation, although this has not been completely defined.[24,39,45]

In rare instances, ingrowth of granulation tissue may be recurrent and refractory to therapy, especially in lesions with ongoing, active inflammation. Therefore, if there is endoscopic evidence of inflammation in a benign tracheobronchial lesion, initial use of a plastic stent may be beneficial until the inflammatory tissue matures. The resultant fibrous stricture can then be treated with a metal stent once the need for long-term stenting has been demonstrated.[46]

Other complications associated with the use of the Wallstent have been relatively rare. Coughing and hemoptysis have been observed in a case in which the stent diameter was too small and did not approximate the bronchial wall in all areas.[39] Recurrent pneumonia, stent fracture and migration, mucous plugging, and excessive secretions have not been a problem. The stent has also been positioned so that the wire mesh covered lobar bronchi. Although this did not result in recurrent pneumonia or lobar atelectasis,[43] some authors advocate removing the stent filaments that cross a bronchial orifice with the use of an endoscopic laser.[39]

Palmaz Stent

The Palmaz stent is a rigid, balloon-expandable stent made from 316-L stainless steel. It is FDA approved for use in the biliary and vascular systems. The primary advantages of the Palmaz stent are that it can be precisely placed and it has excellent radial hoop strength. The disadvantage is that it is rigid. In addition, once the Palmaz stent is deformed, it remains deformed.

We have placed 18 Palmaz stents for the treatment of 11 benign stenoses involving the main bronchi in 10 patients. The age range of these patients was 13–69 years. All diagnoses were made using bronchoscopic and clinical evaluation. The lesions treated included 10 transplant strictures and 1 stenosis secondary to compression of the left mainstem bronchus by extensive mediastinal histoplasmosis. The indications for stent placement were failure to wean from a ventilator in five patients and lifestyle-limiting shortness of breath in the remaining five patients.

Preprocedural evaluation included pulmonary function tests with flow-volume loops of the patients not on ventilators and bronchoscopic evaluation of all 10 patients. A computed tomography (CT) scan of the chest was not routinely obtained, but if a CT scan was available, it was reviewed prior to the procedure. All stents were placed using fluoroscopic guidance with the assistance of general anesthesia. Bronchoscopy was also performed immediately following stent deployment (Figure 15.5). Prophylactic antibodies were given for 24 hours.

The technical success rate was 100% (10/10). Immediate clinical success was achieved in 80% (8/10) of the patients: 5 of 5 treated for shortness of breath and 3 of 5 treated for inability to wean from a ventilator. The two clinical failures were in patients

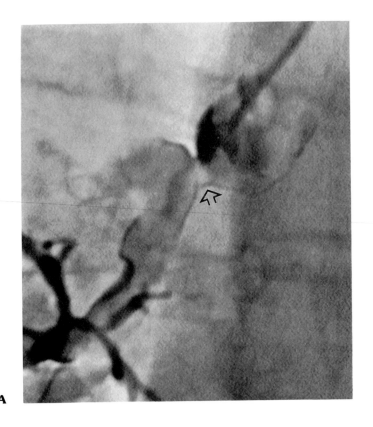

A

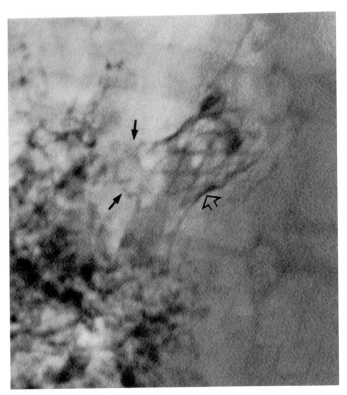

B

Figure 15.5 A. A right lung bronchogram reveals a stricture (arrow) at the anastomotic site of a right lung transplant. B. Following placement of a 12-mm-long Palmaz stent (open arrow), the airway is widely patent. The Palmaz stent was dilated to 9 mm in diameter. The upper lobe bronchus (straight closed arrows) was not traversed by the stent. C, D, and E. Following pages.

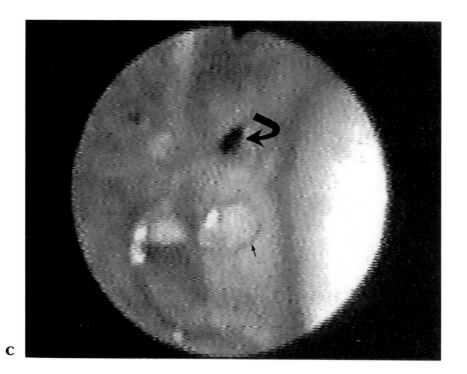

C

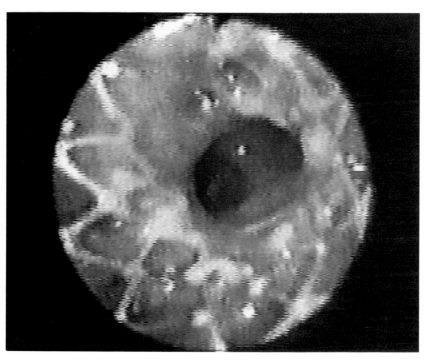

D

Figure 15.5 C. Bronchoscopic evaluation reveals the markedly narrowed right lung transplant anastomosis (curved arrow). Suture material is seen (small arrow). **D.** Following deployment of the Palmaz stent, the airway is patent, with visualization of distal bronchi. **E.** Following page.

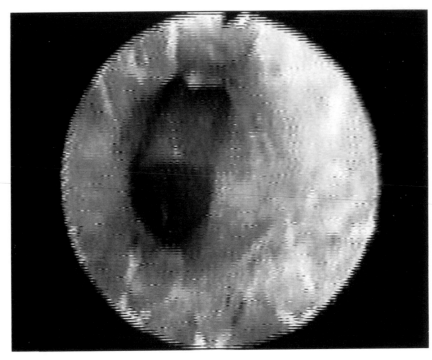

E

Figure 15.5 E. Follow-up bronchoscopy at 6 months reveals continued airway patency. The struts of the stent are partially covered by neoepithelium.

with lung transplants. One of these patients had a stent placed 1 day following lung transplantation and died despite a widely patent bronchus. Autopsy revealed diffuse infection involving the transplanted lung, with findings most consistent with preservation injury. The second clinical failure was in a patient who underwent right lung transplantation for pulmonary lymphangiomatosis. Following lung transplantation, the patient was unable to be weaned from the ventilator. At the time of placement of the bronchial stent, the patient had been ventilator dependent for 7 months. Following stent placement, there was no improvement in the pulmonary status and the patient died several months later.

Pulmonary function tests, bronchoscopy, and clinical follow-up were obtained in all patients. Of the eight patients who derived clinical benefit, three died at 7, 12, and 14 months, respectively, after stent placement. All three patients had bronchoscopic evidence of a widely patent stent immediately prior to their death. None of the deaths were felt to be related to the presence of the bronchial stent. Two more patients developed symptomatic narrowing 2 months and 4 months, respectively, after stent placement secondary to ingrowth of granulation tissue. Both of these patients underwent successful endoscopic bipolar electrocautery and balloon dilatation of the stent (Figure 15.6). The stents in both of these patients remained widely patent until their death at 18 and 27 months, respectively. All seven patients who died were lung transplant recipients. None of the deaths were believed to be related to the presence of the stent.

Three patients are currently alive and well 38, 56, and 57 months, respectively, after stent placement. All three of these patients have developed granulation tissue within the stent. In one patient, the development of granulation tissue and partial collapse of the stent 18 months after stent placement resulted in recurrent symptoms (Figure 15.7). This problem was successfully treated with endoscopic bipolar electrocautery, balloon dilatation, and placement of a second stent. This patient has done well for an additional 38 months (56 months assisted patency). One patient required bipolar electrocautery and balloon dilatation at 10 months and 24 months. This patient is cur-

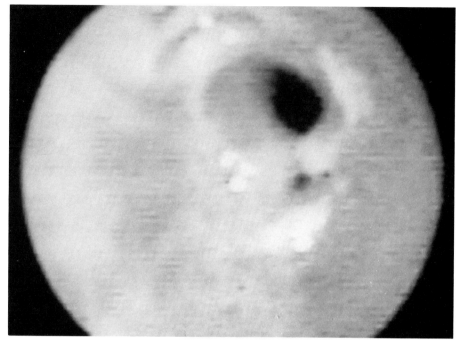

A

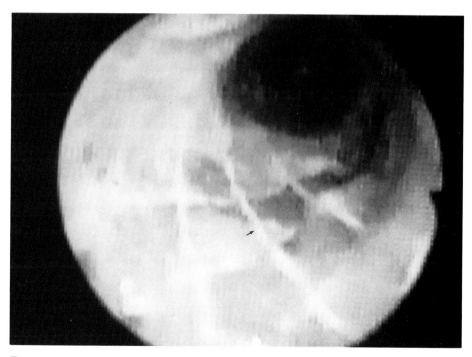

B

Figure 15.6 A. Bronchoscopic evaluation of a left lung transplant reveals a stricture at the anastomotic site. B. Following dilatation of a 30-mm-long Palmaz stent to 10 mm in diameter, the anastomotic stricture is open. The struts of the Palmaz stent are seen (arrow). C. Following page.

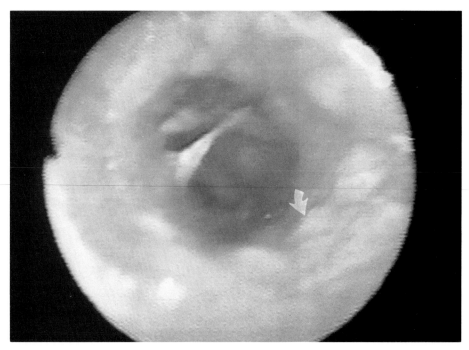

C

Figure 15.6 C. Follow-up bronchoscopy for recurrent shortness of breath at 4 months reveals complete covering of the stent by exuberant granulation tissue (arrow). Bipolar electrocautery and balloon dilatation were successful in reestablishing airway patency.

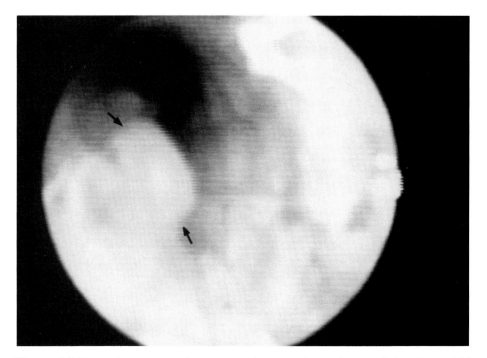

Figure 15.7 Bronchoscopy reveals narrowing the airway lumen by granulation tissue within the stent (arrows).

rently doing well 14 months (38 months assisted patency) after the last intervention. The last patient is a 32-year-old female with histoplasmosis. This patient has developed exuberant granulation tissue formation within the stent requiring repeat bronchoscopy and bipolar electrocautery at 3- to 6-month intervals.

To summarize, three of eight patients had primary patency of their stent until their death. An additional three patients required only one reintervention to maintain stent patency. The remaining two patients have required multiple sessions of endoscopic bipolar electrocautery and balloon dilatation. The mean follow-up for the eight patients was 28 months (range, 7 to 57 months).

Of the eight patients who benefited from placement of the Palmaz stent, some component of stent collapse was present in four of the patients who developed ingrowth of granulation tissue. In each instance, stent collapse was easily addressed with balloon dilatation. There were no stent fractures, stent migrations, clinically significant episodes of hemoptysis, or coughing. There were no stent-related infections. There was partial covering of the right upper lobe bronchus in two patients without clinical sequelae. Histologic examination was performed in one patient with a stent in place for 27 months (Figure 15.1).

In one other small report, Palmaz stents were used to treat neonatal tracheomalacia in three patients.[47] Two of these patients had ongoing sepsis at the time of the procedure and died within 3 weeks of stent implantation. The remaining patient has done well, but follow-up has been limited.

Nitinol Stents

Nitinol is a binary alloy of nickel and titanium. This metal alloy has thermal-memory characteristics. At lower temperatures, it is very malleable. At higher temperatures, the metal will assume a predetermined shape. Nitinol is also very kink resistant. Stents constructed from nitinol have included coil, knitted, Z, and diamond-shaped lattice configurations. Nitinol stents are self-expanding, and most of the designs demonstrate food flexibility. Nitinol has been demonstrated to be well tolerated in the tracheobronchial systems of animals.[48]

Several European centers have clinical experience with the use of nitinol-based stents in the tracheobronchial system.[27,49,50] These reports suggest that after implantation of a nitinol tracheobronchial stent for either malignant or benign etiologies, 90% of patients demonstrate a significant improvement in their respiratory status. In about 20% of the patients, ingrowth of granulation tissue occurs. As with all uncovered metal stents, ingrowth of intraluminal malignancy remains problematic.[50] Complications and long-term patency rates with nitinol stents are not well defined at this time.

Covered Metal Stents

As previously noted, management of airway obstruction secondary to intraluminal malignancy is quite challenging. Although metal stents may provide immediate palliation, rapid tumor ingrowth can lead to recurrent symptoms of airway obstruction. Gianturco stents covered with a Dacron mesh or polyester sleeve have been fashioned to address this problem.[51,52] Unfortunately, covered Gianturco stents are not widely available.

More recently, a silicone-covered Wallstent (Permalume covering) has been FDA approved for use in the tracheobronchial system (Figure 15.3C). The covered Wallstent is currently available in diameters of 8 to 14 mm and in lengths of 20 to 80 mm. The introducer device is similar to the original biliary Wallstent design and incorporates a rolling membrane deployment mechanism. The delivery system is 11F for the 14-mm stent and 7.5F for the smaller prosthesis. The primary indication for the use of a covered stent in the tracheobronchial system is for treating airway obstruction secondary to intraluminal tumor and for treating fistulas.

There is no available literature on the use of the covered Wallstent, although we have placed one in a patient with metastatic renal cell carcinoma with multiple intraluminal metastatic deposits to the left mainstem bronchus and extensive mediastinal disease causing compression of the left mainstem bronchus (Figure 15.8). The patient's respiratory symptoms improved following covered-stent placement. Follow-up bronchoscopy at 1 month and clinical follow-up for 6 months revealed continued symptomatic improvement.

IMPLANTATION TECHNIQUE AND FOLLOW-UP

Prior to stent insertion, it is extremely important to define the proximal and distal extent of the lesion, the relationship of the lesion to the main and segmental bronchi and the vocal chords, and the nature of the lesion (extrinsic compression, bulky intraluminal tumor, or malacia). Some investigators also believe that it is important to define whether there is an active inflammatory or granulomatous component to the lesion prior to placement of a metal stent. These authors have found that in the presence of active inflammation, ingrowth of granulation tissue can become quite problematic.[24,39,45] Stents placed within 2 cm of the vocal cords can cause recurrent aspiration and problems with phonation (Bryan D. Peterson, MD, SCVIR Meeting, Washington, DC, 1997).

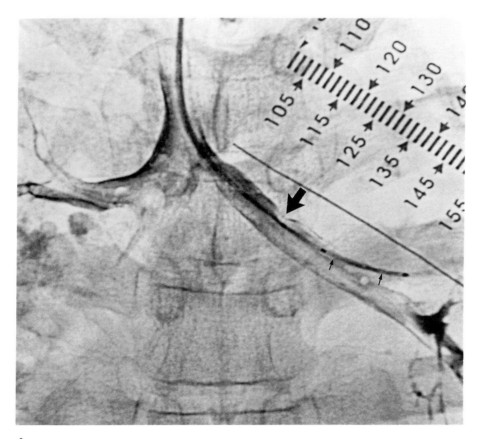

A

Figure 15.8 A. A bronchogram reveals diffuse narrowing of the left mainstem bronchus, with bronchographic findings of an intraluminal deposit of renal cell carcinoma (arrow). A radiopaque reference (LeMaitre Stent Guide, Vascutech, Inc., Burlington, MA) has been taped to the patient's anterior chest wall. The guide facilitates accurate placement of the stent. A guidewire with radiopaque markers (Magic Torque guidewire, Boston Scientific Corp., Natick, MA.) is also present (small arrows). This helps to determine the length and diameter of the lesion. **B** and **C**. Following page.

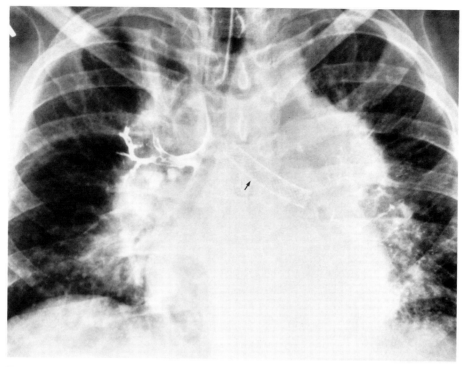

B

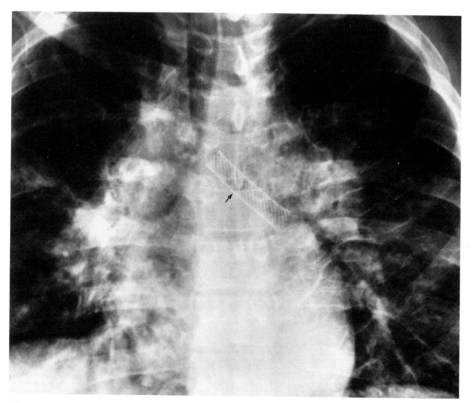

C

Figure 15.8 B. A chest X-ray following the procedure demonstrates satisfactory positioning of the covered Wallstent (arrow). Extensive mediastinal and hilar adenopathy and mild compression of the distal trachea are seen. C. A follow-up chest X-ray several months later demonstrates further expansion of the covered Wallstent.

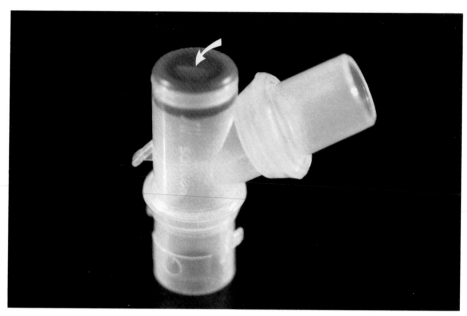

Figure 15.9 The adapter for the endotracheal tube as a slit-like valve (arrow), which permits insertion of a bronchoscope or introducer sheath while simultaneously ventilating the patient.

Several methods have been used to define the anatomy of upper airway obstructions: rigid and flexible bronchoscopy, bronchography with fluoroscopy, and CT. At our institution, an interdisciplinary team of pulmonologists, thoracic surgeons, and interventional radiologists is involved in the initial evaluation, treatment, and follow-up of these patients.

Patients are selected for stent placement based upon the presence of clearly defined respiratory symptoms, bronchoscopic findings of an obstructing airway lesion, and pulmonary function tests with flow loops suggestive of large airway obstruction. In most instances, the patient has also had a CT scan of the chest and mediastinum, but this is not a necessity. Although a number of authors implant metal tracheobronchial stents using only neuroleptic analgesia, all bronchial stent implantations at our institution have been performed while the patient was under general anesthesia. Whenever possible, a No. 8 endotracheal tube is used in combination with a Y adapter (Swivel Elbow, Diemolding Healthcare Div., Canastota, NY) (Figure 15.9). The Y adapter allows flexible bronchoscopy or stent insertion to be performed while continually ventilating the patient. An endotracheal tube smaller than a No. 8 will not permit simultaneous ventilation during flexible bronchoscopy. Unless bronchoscopic evaluation has been performed within 2 weeks of the planned procedure, bronchoscopy is repeated to ensure that there has been no significant change in the underlying obstructive anatomy.

A 10F, short hemostatic sheath (Cook, Inc.) is then introduced through the "slit" on the Y adapter on the endotracheal tube. This minimizes air leakage during the procedure. A flexible J wire (Tapered J, Cook, Inc.) or a steerable-guidewire (Magic Torque guidewire or Terumo guidewire, Tokyo, Japan) is used in combination with a multipurpose-shaped catheter and advanced across the lesion under fluoroscopic guidance. A bronchogram is then performed as the catheter is pulled back proximal to the lesion (Figures 15.4A and 15.5A). Radiographs are obtained in the presence of a sizing wire or an overlying reference guide to help determine the diameter and length of the diseased airway (Figure 15.8A). Since Dionosil (Glaxo/Wellcome,

Middlesex, England) is no longer available, a number of other agents have been used for bronchography: isosmolar, nonionic contrast (Iotrolan-300, Schering, Berlin, Germany), dilute barium, or Hytrast (Guerbet Labs, Paris, France).[39,53,54] Occasionally, balloon dilatation of the lesion will help to further define the exact location and "shoulders" of the lesion. We do not routinely balloon dilate the lesion prior to stent deployment.

Once the exact location of the lesion and the stent diameter and length to be used are determined, the stent is deployed. Although most of our experience has been with the Palmaz stent, granulation tissue formation and partial collapse of the stent have been somewhat problematic (Figures 15.6C and 15.7). Therefore, we have begun using the Wallstent. As previously described, the Wallstent is deployed by retracting the constraining membrane. The stent will foreshorten during its expansion. Therefore, subtle adjustments need to be made during the deployment process to ensure proper stent positioning. Following stent deployment, either repeat bronchoscopic or bronchographic evaluation is performed to document appropriate positioning of the stent (Figures 15.4D, 15.5B,D, and 15.6B). Although the Palmaz stent needs to be balloon expanded to its desired diameter, the Wallstent will generally continue to expand to its nominal diameter over several days to weeks (Figures 15.8B,C).

Prior to the procedure, the patient is given atropine to minimize bronchial secretions. A broad-spectrum cephalosporin is also given for 24 hours. If the patient has an ongoing pulmonary infection, appropriate antibiotics are administered until the infection resolves. Prior to advancing any devices or guidewires into the peripheral bronchi, 20 to 50 mg of lidocaine (Abbott Labs, North Chicago, IL) is administered into the airways to minimize bronchospasm.

Following a recovery period, the patient is extubated and usually discharged the next morning. A chest X-ray and baseline pulmonary function tests with flow loops are obtained prior to discharge. The patient's clinical status is followed closely, and a repeat chest X-ray and pulmonary function tests are obtained whenever clinically indicated. If there is concern about progression of disease or recurrent airway obstruction, pulmonary function tests, CT (Figure 15.10), and/or bronchoscopy are performed.[55,56] In our experience, a deterioration in the peak expiratory flow rate and flattening of the expiratory flow loop pattern on pulmonary function testing will be observed with recurrent obstruction (Figure 15.11). Bronchoscopy is the single best study to obtain if there is any question about the status of the airway.

When growth of granulation tissue into the stent leads to recurrent airways obstruction, we have used endoscopic bipolar electrocautery and balloon dilatation with good success.[57,58] Other investigators have used endoscopic laser photoresection.[39]

DISCUSSION

Obstruction of the large airways can present a significant therapeutic problem, especially when the underlying disease process is extensive. Whenever possible, benign lesions should be managed with surgical reconstruction. Unfortunately, surgery on lesions exceeding 6 cm in length is often associated with recurrent anastomotic stenoses. For such long lesions, interposition conduits to replace or support the airway have not gained wide acceptance.[59,60] Substitutions for the wall of the trachea by absorbable synthetic materials are not yet clinically applicable.[61]

Balloon dilatation has been proposed for management of benign stenoses of the airways, but this technique is of little value in the treatment of malacic segments or airway narrowing secondary to extrinsic compression. In addition, balloon angioplasty has failed to be of benefit in lung transplant anastomotic strictures.[39,62] Although silicone endobronchial stents have been successful in the treatment of benign lesions, mucociliary clearance is impaired, leading to encrustation of bronchial secretions

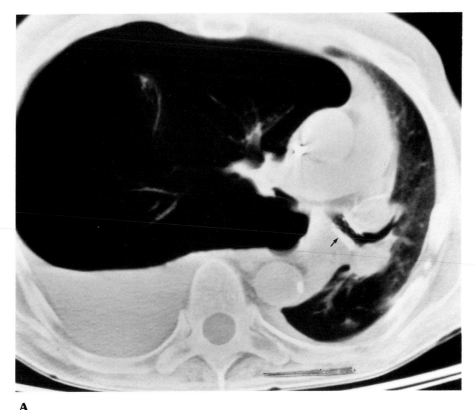

A

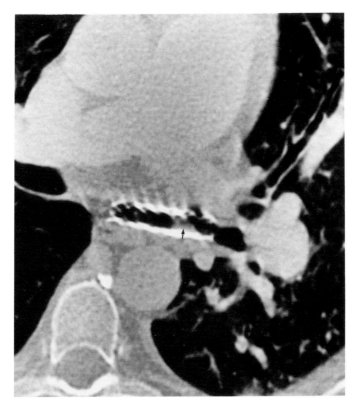

B

Figure 15.10 A. A chest CT scan in a patient with a left lung transplant demonstrates the presence of a Palmaz stent (arrow). There is no soft tissue within the lumen of the stent. B. A chest CT scan in a different patient demonstrates ingrowth of tissue through the distal aspect of the Palmaz stent (arrow).

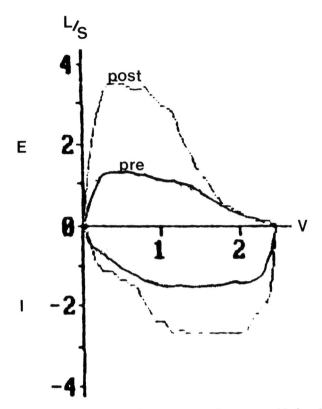

Figure 15.11 A flow loop pulmonary function test is demonstrated before (solid lines) and after (dotted lines) stent placement. There is marked improvement in the inspiratory (I) and expiratory (E) flow-volume loops following stent placement. With recurrent airway obstruction, the flow loop pattern will flatten out, similar to the pre-stent pattern. L/S = liters per second; V = volume.

within the stent. In addition, granulation tissue overgrowth at either end of the plastic stent can occur. In one series, six transplant anastomoses were treated by placement of a silicone stent. In four of the six patients, significant problems occurred: stent dislodgement in one patient, overgrowth of granulation tissue at the stent ends in two patients, and inability to clear secretions in one patient.[63] Migration has also been a problem when plastic stents were placed in malacic strictures.[45]

Malignant lesions are difficult to treat with endoscopic techniques alone. Despite initial improvement in the symptoms following cryotherapy, laser photoresection, or radiation therapy, recurrent symptoms are frequent. Although plastic stents prevent ingrowth of tumor, stent migration is a frequent occurrence when the stent is being used for the treatment of an intraluminal tumor.[46]

The theoretical advantages for using a metal stent to treat complex airway obstruction include the following: metal stents have a small profile and are fairly easy to insert; the open lattice of the stent allows maintenance of the mucociliary clearance mechanism; the open lattice design allows treatment of more peripheral bronchi with less fear of causing obstructive pneumonia and/or atelectasis; covered stents can be used to prevent ingrowth of tumor; and some of the stents are flexible. The major disadvantage of a metal stent is that it is difficult to remove after it becomes incorporated into the airway wall.

Of the metal stents currently available in the United States, the Wallstent endoprosthesis appears to be most compatible with the tracheobronchial airways. Because it is self-expanding, migrations have not been a significant problem. The stent is flexible, allowing its contour to conform to the curves of the airway. Traversing segmental bronchi with the wire mesh should be avoided whenever possible. However, covering the origins of the peripheral bronchi has not caused recurrent pneumonias or atelectasis in some series.[45,64] In cases in which traversing the ostium of a bronchus with stent filaments led to a clinically significant problem, endoscopic laser techniques have been used to remove the filaments without compromising the integrity of the stent.[39] Although formation of granulation tissue within the stent occurs in approximately 20% of patients, this appears to be self-limiting in the absence of an active inflammatory process.[24,39,45] Lastly, the covered version of the Wallstent allows its application in the presence of intraluminal tumor. Whether the silicone covering will adversely affect the mucociliary clearance mechanism is not known at this time. Crossing a bronchial orifice with the covered portion of the stent should be avoided.

The Gianturco stent seems well suited for tracheal lesions, but its rigid design and the concentration of its expanding pressure to a very small surface area have led to tracheal perforations, stent fractures, and migrations. In one series, a 30% complication rate was experienced.[39] The Palmaz stent allows precise deployment of the stent, but excessive granulation tissue formation has been demonstrated both in animals and in the clinical setting.[48,58] Stents constructed from nitinol material may prove useful in the tracheobronchial system, but further clinical experience and follow-up are needed.

In summary, whenever possible, short-segment, benign lesions of the airway should be treated with surgical reconstruction. Use of metal stents in the pediatric population should be tempered with the recognition that metal stents are not easily removed once neoepithelialization occurs. Therefore, in the pediatric population, balloon dilatation and plastic stents should be employed whenever possible to allow growth of the child until a more definitive procedure can be performed. Metal endoprostheses are most effective in the treatment of long-segment, noninflammatory stenoses, long-segment areas of tracheobronchial malacia, and compression of the airways by extrinsic pathology. Fibroinflammatory lesions appear to be associated with excessive granulation tissue formation. Therefore, these lesions are best managed with plastic stents until the inflammatory tissue matures. The use of covered metal stents for the treatment of airway obstruction secondary to intraluminal tumor appears to have theoretical merit, and the initial clinical experience is encouraging.

Acknowledgments

The authors would like to acknowledge Ms. Tammy Amos for her expert help in preparing this chapter.

REFERENCES

1. Slawson RG, Scott RM. Radiation therapy for bronchogenic carcinoma. *Radiology* 132:175–176, 1979.
2. Zajac AJ, Kohn ML, Heiser D, et al. High-dose-rate intraluminal brachytherapy in the treatment of endobronchial malignancy. *Radiology* 97:571–575, 1993.
3. Ledingham SJN, Goldstraw P. Diathermy resection and radiative gold grains for palliation of obstruction due to recurrence of bronchial carcinoma after external radiation. *Thorax* 44:48–51, 1989.
4. Beamis JF Jr, Rebeiz EE, Vergos K, et al. Endoscopic laser therapy for obstructing tracheobronchial lesions. *Ann Otol Rhinol Laryngol* 100:413–419, 1991.
5. Marasso A, Gallo E, Massaglia GN, et al. Cryosurgery in bronchoscopic treatment of tracheobronchial stenosis: Indications, limits, and personal experience. *Chest* 103:472–474, 1993.
6. Mulliken JB, Grillo HC. The limits of tracheal resection with primary anastomosis: Further anatomical studies in man. *J Cardiovasc Surg* 55:418–421, 1968.
7. Grillo HC. Primary reconstruction of the airway after resection of subglottic laryngeal and upper tracheal stenosis. *Ann Thorac Surg* 33:3–18, 1982.

8. Mathisen DJ. Surgical management of tracheobronchial disease. *Clin Chest Med* 13: 151–171, 1992.

9. Cohen RC, Filler RM, Konuma K, et al. A new model of tracheal stenosis and its repair with free periosteal grafts. *J Thorac Cardiovasc Surg* 92:296–304, 1986.

10. Grillo HC. Tracheal surgery. *Scand J Cardiovasc Surg* 17:67–77, 1983.

11. Ball JB, Delaney JC, Evans CC, et al. Endoscopic bougie and balloon dilatation of multiple bronchial stenoses: Ten year follow-up. *Thorax* 46:933–935, 1991.

12. Fowler CL, Aaland MO, Harris FL. Dilatation of bronchial stenosis with Grüentzig balloon. *J Thorac Cardiovasc Surg* 93:308–315, 1987.

13. Brown SB, Hedlund GO, Glasier CM, et al. Tracheobronchial stenosis in infants: Successful balloon dilation therapy. *Radiology* 164:475–478, 1987.

14. Carlin BW, Harrell JH, Moser KM. Treatment of endobronchial stenosis using balloon catheter dilatation. *Chest* 93:1148–1151, 1988.

15. Cohen MD, Weber TR, Rao CC. Balloon dilatation of tracheal and bronchial stenosis. *AJR* 142:477–478, 1984.

16. Colt HG, Janssen JP, Dumon JF, et al. Endoscopic management of bronchial stenosis after double lung transplantation. *Chest* 102:10–16, 1992.

17. Keller C, Frost A. Fiberoptic bronchoplasty: Description of a simple adjunct technique for the management of bronchial stenosis following lung transplantation. *Chest* 102:995–998, 1992.

18. Montgomery WW. T-tube tracheal stent. *Arch Otolaryngol* 82:820–821, 1965.

19. Westaby S, Shepherd MP. Palliation of intrathoracic tracheal compression with a silastic tracheobronchial stent. *Thorax* 38:314–315, 1982.

20. Dumon JF. A dedicated tracheobronchial stent. *Chest* 97:328–332, 1990.

21. Insall RL, Morritt GN. Palliation of malignant tracheal strictures using silicone T tubes. *Thorax* 46:168–171, 1991.

22. Cooper JD, Pearson FG, Patterson GA, et al. Use of silicone stents in the management of airway problems. *Ann Thorac Surg* 47:371–378, 1989.

23. Tsang V, Goldstraw P. Endobronchial stenting for anastomotic stenosis after sleeve resection. *Ann Thorac Surg* 48:568–571, 1989.

24. Irving JD, Goldstraw P. Tracheobronchial stents. *Semin Intervent Radiol* 8:295–304, 1991.

25. Bolliger CT, Probst PR, Tschopp K, et al. Silicone stents in the management of inoperable tracheobronchial stenoses: Indications and limitations. *Chest* 104:1653–1659, 1993.

26. Gaer JAR, Tsang V, Khaghani A, et al. Use of endotracheal silicone stents for relief of tracheobronchial obstruction. *Ann Thorac Surg* 54:512–516, 1992.

27. Becker HE, Wagner B, Liermann E, et al. Stenting of central airways. In Liermann D (ed): *Stents—State of the Art and Future Developments*. Watertown, MA, Boston Scientific, 1995, pp 249–255.

28. Grewe P, Krampe K, Muller KM, et al. Microscopic and histomorphological alterations of the bronchial wall after implantation of Nitinol stents. In Liermann D (ed): *Stents—State of the Art and Future Developments*. Watertown, MA, Boston Scientific, 1995, pp 256–259.

29. Insall R, Morritt GN. Use of a fenestrated silicone drain to stent a malignant tracheobronchial stenosis. *Thorax* 45:711–712, 1990.

30. Bucher RM, Burnett WE, Rosemond GP. Experimental reconstruction of tracheal and bronchial defects with stainless steel wire mesh. *J Thorac Surg* 21:572–583, 1951.

31. Harkins WB. An endotracheal prosthesis in the treatment of stenosis of the upper trachea. *Ann Otol Rhinol Laryngol* 61:663–675, 1952.

32. Pagliero KM, Shepherd MP. Use of stainless steel wire coil prosthesis in treatment of anastomotic dehiscence after cervical tracheal resection. *J Thorac Cardiovasc Surg* 67:932–935, 1974.

33. Wallace MJ, Charnsangavej C, Ogawa K, et al. Tracheobronchial tree: Expandable metallic stents used in experimental and clinical applications. *Radiology* 158:309–312, 1986.

34. Sawada S, Tanagawa N, Kobayashi M, et al. Malignant tracheobronchial obstructive lesions: Treatment with Gianturco expandable metallic stents. *Radiology* 188:205–208, 1993.

35. de Souza AC, Keal R, Hudson NM, et al. Use of expandable wire stents for malignant airway obstruction. *Ann Thorac Surg* 57:1573–1578, 1994.

36. Egan AM, Dennis C, Flower CDR. Expandable metal stents for tracheobronchial obstruction. *Clin Radiol* 49:162–165, 1994.

37. George PJ, Irving JD, Khaghani A, et al. Role of the Gianturco expandable metal stent in the management of tracheobronchial obstruction. *Cardiovasc Intervent Radiol* 15:375–381, 1992.

38. Higgins R, McNeil K, Dennis C, et al. Airway stenosis after lung transplantation: Management with expanding metal stents. *J Heart Lung Transplant* 13:774–778, 1994.

39. Rousseau H, Dahan M, Lauque D, et al. Self-expandable prosthesis in the tracheobronchial tree. *Radiology* 188:199–203, 1993.

40. Nashef SA, Dromer C, Velly JF, et al. Expanding wire stents in benign tracheobronchial disease: Indications and complications. *Ann Thorac Surg* 54:937–940, 1992.

41. Hind CR, Donnelly RJ. Expandable metal stents for tracheal obstruction: Permanent or temporary? A cautionary tale. *Thorax* 47:757–758, 1992.

42. Maynar M, Lopez L, Gorriz E, et al. Massive brachiocephalic artery bleeding due to a Gianturco tracheal stent. *JVIR* 4:289–291, 1993.

43. Tan BS, Watkinson AF, Dussek JE, et al. Metallic endoprosthesis for malignant tracheobronchial obstruction: Initial experience. *Cardiovasc Intervent Radiol* 19:91–96, 1996.

44. Spinelli P, Meroni E, Cerrai FG. Self-expanding tracheobronchial stent using flexible bronchoscopy: Preliminary clinical experience. *Surg Endosc* 8:411–413, 1994.

45. Brichon PY, Blanc-Jouvan F, Rousseau H, et al. Endovascular stents for bronchial stenosis after lung transplantation. *Transplant Proc* 24:2656–2659, 1992.

46. Tsang V, Williams AM, Goldstraw P. Sequential silastic and expandable metal stenting for tracheobronchial strictures. *Ann Thorac Surg* 53:856–860, 1992.

47. Santoro G, Picardo S, Testa G, et al. Balloon-expandable metallic stents in the management of tracheomalacia in neonates. *J Thorac Cardiovasc Surg* 110:1145–1148, 1995.

48. Rauber K, Syed-Ali S, Terpe HJ, et al. Endotracheal Palmaz stents and Ni-Ti stents in endotracheal use: Experimental study (abstract). *Cardiovasc Intervent Radiol* 16(Suppl 2):S39, 1993.

49. Liermann D, Rust M. First experiences with a new memory metallic endoprosthesis in the tracheobronchial system. In Liermann D (ed): *Stents—State of the Art and Future Developments.* Watertown, MA, Boston Scientific, 1995, pp 260–265.

50. Liermann D, Becker HD. Balloon-expandable and self-expandable stents in the tracheobronchial system: A study with more than 100 stent implantations (abstract). *JVIR* 4:38, 1993.

51. George PJ, Irving JD, Mantell BS, et al. Covered expandable metal stent for recurrent tracheal obstruction. *Lancet* 335:582–584, 1990.

52. Kishi K, Kobayashi H, Suruda T, et al. Treatment of malignant tracheobronchial stenosis by Dacron mesh-covered Z-stents. *Cardiovasc Intervent Radiol* 17:33–35, 1994.

53. Morcos SK, Anderson PB. Airways and lung: Bronchography through the fiberoptic bronchoscope. *Radiology* 200:612–614, 1996.

54. Nelson SW, Christoforidis AJ, Pratt PC. Further experience with barium sulfate as a bronchographic contrast medium. *Radiology* 72:829–838, 1959.

55. Maeda M, Otsuji H, Uchida H, et al. Tracheobronchial Z-stent placement: Evaluation using respiratory function tests. *Cardiovasc Intervent Radiol* 16(Suppl 2):S99, 1993.

56. Quint LE, Whyte RI, Kazerooni EA, et al: Stenosis of the central airways: Evaluation by using helical CT with multiplanar reconstructions. *Radiology* 194:871–877, 1995.

57. Cunningham L, Wendell G, Berkowitz L, et al. Treatment of tracheobronchial granular cell myoblastomas with endoscopic bipolar cautery. *Chest* 96:427–429, 1989.

58. Matsumoto AH, Tegtmeyer CJ, Rose CE, et al. Benign bronchial stenoses: Treatment with Palmaz stents (abstract). *JVIR* 4:61, 1994.

59. Toohill RJ. Autogenous graft reconstruction of the larynx and upper trachea. *Otolaryngol Clin North Am* 12:909–917, 1979.

60. Neel B. Gore-Tex implants. *Arch Otolaryngol* 109:427–433, 1983.

61. Greve H. Substitution of the wall of the trachea by absorbable synthetic material. *Thorac Cardiovasc Surg* 36:20–26, 1988.

62. Schäfer HJ, Haverich A, Wagner TOF, et al. Decreased incidence of bronchial complications following lung transplantation. *Eur J Cardiothorac Surg* 6:174–179, 1992.

63. Carre P, Rousseau H, Lombart L, et al. Balloon dilatation and self-expanding metal Wallstent insertion for management of bronchostenosis following lung transplantation. *Chest* 105:343–348, 1994.

64. Bjarnason H, Cahill B, Urness MC, et al. Tracheobronchial stents: Bridging the bronchial ostium and its effects on the lung segment (abstract). *JVIR* 8(Suppl):215, 1997.

C H A P T E R
16

Management of Esophageal Foreign Bodies, Strictures, and Leaks

Hubert A. Shaffer, Jr., Eduard E. de Lange

Esophageal foreign bodies, strictures, and leaks are clinically significant and sometimes can be life-threatening. In many cases, these conditions can be managed nonoperatively by a radiologist interested in fluoroscopically guided interventional procedures. The recommended radiologic procedures described in this chapter are relatively safe, cost-effective, and efficient methods of addressing these serious problems.

FOREIGN BODIES AND FOOD IMPACTIONS

Every year in the United States, 1,500 people die from ingestion of foreign bodies.[1] Although most swallowed objects pass through the gastrointestinal (GI) tract spontaneously, 10–20% have to be removed by a nonoperative procedure, and approximately 1% require surgery.[1-3] Most foreign body ingestions occur in infants and children, who swallow such things as coins, disk batteries, and small toys.[3-6] Adults typically have problems with impacted food and bones. Meat accounts for 70–80% of food impactions.[6-9] In most cases, a preexisting benign esophageal narrowing, such as a Schatzki ring, inflammatory stricture, or area of spasm, predisposes the patient to food impaction. In 65–83% of cases, the food lodges in the distal one-third of the esophagus.[8-11] It is unusual for food impaction to be the initial presentation of cancer. It is also uncommon for patients with foreign bodies other than food to have significant preexisting pathology in the esophagus.[6,8,10-18]

Radiologic Evaluation

Plain film radiography is generally recommended for patients with a suspected esophageal foreign body. In addition to anteroposterior and lateral radiographs of the chest and upper abdomen, a lateral radiograph of the neck should be obtained using soft tissue technique.[19,20] These radiographs are used to search for radiopaque foreign bodies and to look for any associated complication, such as a pneumonia, lung abscess, pneumothorax, pneumomediastinum, pleural effusion, pneumoperitoneum, or subcutaneous emphysema.[3,5,21]

Esophagography is employed if there is a high clinical suspicion of an esophageal foreign body and preliminary plain films are negative or equivocal. The contrast study is performed to determine whether a nonopaque foreign body is present, to define its nature and location, and to determine if there is an associated esophageal perforation or stricture.[19,20] A water-soluble contrast medium (Gastrografin; Bracco Diagnostics Inc., Princeton, NJ) is the preferred initial contrast agent because leakage of a water-soluble contrast agent into the mediastinum or pleural space is well tolerated;[3] and if endoscopy is necessary, it is easier for the endoscopist to see through water-soluble contrast than through opaque barium,[6,8] However, fatalities have occurred following aspiration of ionic water-soluble agents; therefore, if aspiration is the primary concern, a dilute suspension of barium sulfate should be used because it is inert and has minimal reactivity in the lungs.[3,8] When both leakage outside the GI tract and aspiration are potential problems, a water-soluble, nonionic contrast agent (Omnipaque; Nycomed Inc., New York, NY or Isovue; Bracco Diagnostics Inc.) is the safest choice.[3] Since 25% of perforations will be missed when esophagography is only performed with a water-soluble contrast agent,[22] if no perforation is demonstrated with use of a water-soluble contrast, the esophageal study should then be repeated with dilute barium sulfate.[19,20]

The combined use of plain films and contrast esophagography is very sensitive in detecting an esophageal foreign body.[23] In rare instances when conventional radiologic studies fail to demonstrate a foreign body, computed tomography (CT) may be useful.[3,24] Esophagoscopy should also be considered in any patient who remains symptomatic following a negative radiologic evaluation.[3,5,20]

Treatment

When a foreign body becomes lodged in the esophagus, appropriate management depends on the symptoms, the nature of the swallowed object, its location, and the length of time it has been in place. If the patient has no respiratory distress and can manage oral secretions, emergency removal of the foreign body may not be necessary. If the foreign body has smooth surfaces and is nontoxic, delaying extraction may be justified, because most blunt objects will pass spontaneously through the GI tract without incident.[1,2,13,25–27] However, sharp-edged or pointed foreign bodies and disk batteries, which may leak caustic material, should be removed promptly because of their potential for esophageal injury and perforation.[13,28,29] In any case, no foreign body should be allowed to remain in the esophagus for more than 24 hr, as the incidence of complications begins to rise.[5]

Blindly pushing impacted food or a foreign body from the esophagus into the stomach with a dilator or large tube is not recommended. This procedure risks worsening entrapment of the foreign body, extrinsic compression of the airway by the expanded esophagus, and esophageal perforation.[3,6,27]

Foreign body management has traditionally involved esophagoscopy with removal of the foreign body with forceps or a snare. Endoscopy provides the ability to visualize the foreign body during its capture and removal to protect the airway, and to evaluate the esophagus for injury and underlying pathology. It is the method most widely used for removing sharp objects. The disadvantages of endoscopic techniques include its high cost, the frequent need for general anesthesia in children, and the risk of esophageal perforation when the forceps or snare is passed around the foreign body. In experienced hands, endoscopy has a reported success rate of at least 90% and a complication rate of 1–13%.[5,6,13,15,27,30,31–34]

Our algorithm for managing foreign bodies in the esophagus depends on the location of the foreign body and its characteristics (magnetism, shape, and sharpness of its edges) (Figure 16.1).[19,20] The algorithm is organized into a logical sequence that proceeds from the least invasive and cheapest method to the more invasive and expensive ones.

Equipment required for a fluoroscopically guided extraction procedure includes the following: (1) a fluoroscope with a table that is capable of tilting at least 30° in both directions from a horizontal position; (2) radiation shielding (lead aprons, gloves, thy-

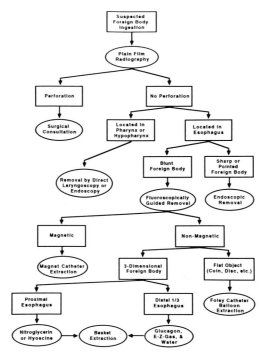

Figure 16.1 Algorithm for managing esophageal foreign bodies. (Modified from Shaffer and de Lange.[19] Reproduced by permission.)

roid shields, lead glasses, etc.); (3) universal precautions equipment (gowns, gloves, masks, and eye shields); (4) topical anesthetic spray (Xylocaine 10% Oral Spray, Astra USA Inc., Westboro, MA) for the patient's throat; and (5) viscous lidocaine (Xylocaine Viscous Solution, Astra USA Inc.) to lubricate instruments. For safe removal of foreign bodies in infants and young children, an immobilization device to firmly restrain an uncooperative child, and a bite block or a tongue depressor wrapped with adhesive tape to keep the child's teeth apart may be needed.[19,20] In all cases of an esophageal foreign body, protection of the airway is an important consideration. Emergency equipment to deal with acute airway obstruction should be immediately available. A physician capable of managing the patient's airway should also be present.[35]

Ferromagnetic Foreign Bodies

Ferromagnetic objects include disk batteries, nails, paper clips, and ball bearings. A disk battery lodged in the esophagus constitutes a true emergency because it can leak an alkaline substance that can rapidly lead to tissue necrosis, esophageal perforation, an esophagotracheal fistula, and an esophagoaortic fistula.[6,36–40] These complications can occur as soon as 4 hr after its ingestion.[37,40] Under no circumstances should a disk battery be left in the esophagus in the hope that it will pass spontaneously.[6,37]

The traditional treatment for a disk battery in the esophagus has been immediate endoscopic removal;[36,37,40] however, a failure rate of 10–62% has been reported.[36,37,39] Some authors advocate removing disk batteries and other ferromagnetic foreign bodies from the esophagus by using a fluoroscopically guided magnet attached to the end of a catheter (Magnetic Retriever Catheter; Cook Inc., Bloomington, IN or FE-EX Orogastric Tube Magnet; Effner & Spreine GmbH, Berlin, Germany).[40–42]

To extract an esophageal foreign body with a magnet catheter requires patient cooperation. Infants and young children must be securely restrained in an immobilizer. The posterior oropharynx is anesthetized with a small amount of a topical anesthetic spray. The patient is then placed in the right lateral decubitus position. The magnet catheter is lubricated with viscous lidocaine and passed through the mouth into the esophagus. A sterile bite block can be placed between the teeth to prevent the patient from biting the catheter. The magnet is coupled to the foreign body using fluoroscopic guidance. After the magnet engages the object, the patient is turned into the right anterior oblique position (semiprone). The head end of the x-ray table is lowered approximately 40° from the horizontal. With a smooth, continuous motion, the magnet with the attached foreign body is withdrawn from the esophagus into the mouth and retrieved (Figure 16.2).[19,20,40–42]

If the foreign body disengages from the magnet while in the esophagus, removal may be achieved by using a Foley catheter in combination with the magnet catheter. Using fluoroscopic visualization, the Foley catheter is passed beyond the foreign body, and its balloon is inflated. The magnet catheter is then advanced, sandwiching the foreign body between the magnet above and the balloon below. The magnet catheter, foreign body, and Foley catheter are withdrawn as a unit (Figure 16.3).[32] With the newer, stronger, rare-earth cobalt magnets, the assistance of a Foley catheter is rarely needed.[41,42]

Removal of metal foreign bodies with a magnet catheter is relatively safe, effective, and quick. It is considerably less expensive than endoscopy or surgery.[40,41] The method does not require hospitalization or general anesthesia. The success rate of the procedure is greater than 90%, and no complications have been reported.[41] Indications for this procedure include: (1) the presence of a blunt, ferromagnetic object in the esophagus; and (2) no evidence of perforation, mediastinitis, or peritonitis.[19,20]

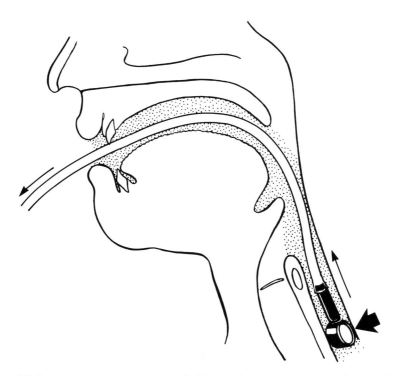

Figure 16.2 Removal of a disk battery (bold arrow) using a magnet catheter with fluoroscopic guidance. The oral route is preferred for extraction to avoid epistaxis or foreign body impaction in the nose. (Modified from Shaffer and de Lange.[19] Reproduced by permission.)

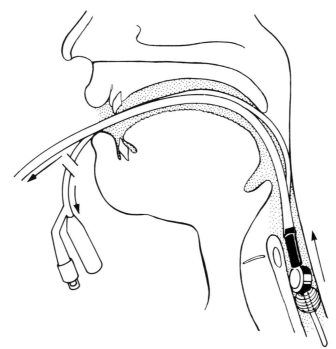

Figure 16.3 A Foley catheter balloon and a magnet catheter are used in combination to extract a metallic foreign body when the magnet alone is not strong enough to remove the object. The foreign body is sandwiched between the balloon below and the magnet above, and they are withdrawn as a unit. (From Shaffer and de Lange.[19] Reproduced by permission.)

Coins and Other Flat Objects

In 1966, Bigler first described the use of a Foley catheter to extract blunt radiopaque foreign bodies from the esophagus.[43] Campbell et al. further refined and popularized the technique.[35,44,45] The procedure involves advancing a Foley catheter distal to the foreign body. The balloon on the catheter is inflated, and the Foley catheter and the object are withdrawn using fluoroscopic guidance. The vast majority of experience has been with coins and other smooth, radiopaque objects, but nonopaque foreign bodies, including food impactions, have also been successfully removed with a Foley catheter.[3,35,44,45]

Materials needed for this procedure include: (1) several 10 to 14-Fr Foley catheters with 5-cc balloons; (2) a small syringe of contrast media to inflate the balloon; (3) nonionic contrast media to opacify the balloon, and to check the esophagus for perforation after the procedure; and (4) a Kelley surgical clamp. The Foley catheter balloon is tested to make sure that it inflates symmetrically prior to its use. If it inflates asymmetrically, it is replaced.

Before the procedure is begun, the patient must either be cooperative or restrained. If necessary, a bite block is inserted between the teeth. The patient is then placed in the right lateral decubitus position. The deflated Foley catheter is inserted by mouth to avoid the complications associated with a transnasal approach, such as epistaxis and displacement of the foreign body into the nasopharynx.[3,5,45] The catheter is advanced past the foreign body using fluoroscopic guidance, and the balloon is inflated with the water-soluble contrast agent (Figure 16.4). Overdistention of the balloon should be avoided because it may compress the adjacent airway and cause respiratory compromise.[3] The patient is turned into a semiprone position, and the table is tilted

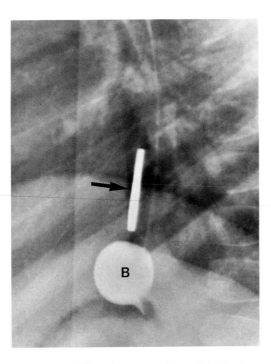

Figure 16.4 Radiograph of a child with a penny (arrow) in the lower esophagus. A Foley catheter has been passed orally, and the balloon (**B**) has been inflated with contrast medium distal to the coin in preparation for its removal. (From Shaffer and de Lange.[19]. Reproduced by permission.)

head down 30° to minimize the chance of displacing the foreign body into the larynx. The catheter is then withdrawn with moderate, steady traction to deliver the foreign body into the mouth (Figure 16.5). Once the foreign body appears in the mouth, it may be expelled or grasped with a Kelley clamp.[3,5,45,46] Moderate resistance to withdrawal of the foreign body and balloon will be encountered at the level of the cricopharyngeus muscle. Continuous, moderate traction on the balloon will usually result in relaxation of the upper esophageal sphincter and subsequent passage of the foreign body. Occasionally, asking the patient to "retch" will cause the upper sphincter to relax. If the balloon slips past the object, the deflated Foley catheter is reinserted and the procedure is repeated.

In tall adults, a Foley catheter may be too short to reach the foreign body; in smaller patients, its diameter may be too large to pass beyond a tight impaction. In these circumstances, an angiographic catheter and guidewire can be used to pass the obstruction. An angioplasty balloon catheter, appropriately sized for the patient's esophagus, can be advanced over the guidewire and beyond the foreign body. The balloon catheter is then inflated, and the catheter and foreign body are withdrawn into the mouth.[19,20]

In the presence of a stricture, Foley catheter balloon extraction should be performed with extra care. The esophageal anatomy is defined with a small amount of barium. The balloon is only partially inflated in the region of the stricture to minimize chances for perforating the esophagus. The impacted material is then withdrawn from the narrowed area. After the object has been retracted above the stricture, the balloon can be distended to its full diameter for the remainder of the extraction.[47,48]

Foley catheter balloon extraction is an easily performed, relatively effective, and safe method for removing blunt foreign bodies from the esophagus. The procedure avoids the morbidity and costs of endoscopy, general anesthesia, and hospitaliza-

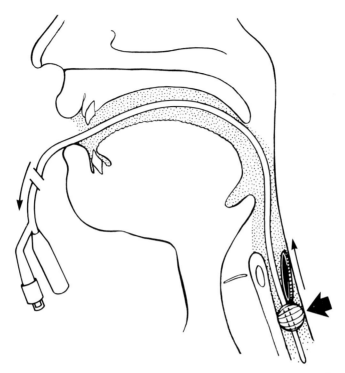

Figure 16.5 Line drawing of a Foley catheter being used to remove a coin from the esophagus. By applying steady traction on the catheter, the inflated balloon (bold arrow) is used to withdraw the coin into the patient's mouth. (From Shaffer and de Lange.[19] Reproduced by permission.)

tion.[3,5,25,44–46] The technique is most appropriate for removing flat foreign bodies, such as coins and discs, because the relatively large Foley catheter can slide easily beyond these objects. The reported success rate for this procedure in more than 2,500 patients is 95%, with a complication rate of 0.4%.[35] Only one procedure-related death has been documented in the literature, and that was due to airway occlusion by a coin that was aspirated during its withdrawal.[34]

Generally accepted contraindications to Foley catheter balloon extraction are: (1) sharp or ragged foreign bodies or those of unknown type; (2) clinical or radiographic evidence of esophageal perforation; and (3) complete esophageal obstruction, precluding passage of a guidewire or catheter.[3,46–49] Impaction for more than 72 hr is a relative contraindication.[3] In the past, a radiolucent foreign body was considered a contraindication. However, more recent experience has shown that nonopaque objects can be safely and successfully removed if the objects are first coated with a contrast agent.[35,47,48]

Food Impactions and Blunt Three-dimensional Foreign Bodies

Initial management of food impactions in the esophagus should involve methods that facilitate passage of the food into the stomach. These methods will be successful and obviate the need for a more invasive intervention.

Gas-forming Agents

Carbonated beverages have been used to dislodge impacted food from the esophagus. Mohammed and Hegedüs had patients rapidly drink 100 ml of a carbonated beverage, and impacted meat or other foreign material was propelled from the esophagus into the stomach in 16 of 20 patients (80%) without complications.[10] Karanjia and Rees successfully treated eight episodes of food impaction with no complications by administering Coca-Cola.[14] Carbonated beverages are readily available, inexpensive, and free of systemic side effects.

Gas-forming mixtures of weak acid and sodium bicarbonate have also been used to facilitate passage of impacted food from the esophagus. One package of effervescent granules (E-Z-Gas II; E-Z-EM Co. Inc., Westbury, NY), which is marketed for use in double-contrast barium studies of the stomach, produces at least 400 ml of carbon dioxide gas when added to 30 ml of water. The patient is asked to swallow this mixture in the upright position and if possible avoid belching. The acute gaseous distention of the esophagus will frequently allow the impacted food to pass.[20]

Using a gas-forming mixture of tartaric acid and sodium bicarbonate, Rice et al. reported immediate relief of meat impaction in 8 of 8 (100%) patients. Although no complications occurred, retching was observed in all of their patients.[12] Zimmers and coworkers described treating 26 esophageal food impactions with a gas-forming mixture of tartaric acid and sodium bicarbonate.[9] However, their success rate was only 65%. One patient with preprocedural chest pain sustained an esophageal mucosal tear. Of their 7 patients with impaction lasting more than 6 hrs, 6 (85%) were treatment failures. Based on their observations, these authors recommended that gas-forming agents be limited to patients without chest pain and with impactions less than 6 hr old.

Other Noninvasive Treatments

Other noninvasive interventions have been advocated for the treatment of blunt, nontoxic, esophageal foreign bodies, but most of the methods are less effective or more dangerous than using gas-forming agents.

Papain (Adolph's Meat Tenderizer; Adolph's Limited, North Hollywood, CA) is a crystalline proteolytic enzyme extracted from the papaw plant. In 1945, Richardson first described the successful use of orally administered papain to digest and dislodge meat impactions in the esophagus in 16 of 17 (94%) cases.[50] Although the method is effective,[51-53] papain can digest the injured esophageal wall or produce life-threatening acute hemorrhagic pulmonary edema if aspirated.[6,54-56]

Glucagon, a pancreatic hormone, has the ability to relax smooth muscle spasm near the gastroesophageal (GE) junction.[57,58] It has no effect on the body of the esophagus and does not relax esophageal strictures or rings.[6,57] When 1 mg of glucagon (Eli Lilly & Co., Indianapolis, IN) is given intravenously (IV), its onset of action is within 1 min.[59,60] Following its administration, the patient is given water or a barium suspension to drink in the upright position to utilize the effect of gravity and hydrostatic pressure.[3,5,8,60] Glucagon is a relatively safe drug but is successful in relieving food impactions in only 29–50% of cases.[6,8,31,52,59] Glucagon is contraindicated in patients with a pheochromocytoma, insulinoma, or history of glucagon hypersensitivity.[60]

Nifedipine (Procardia; Pfizer Inc., New York, NY) is a calcium channel blocker that reduces pressure in the lower esophageal sphincter (LES) and the amplitude of esophageal contractions adjacent to the LES.[61-63] There have been anecdotal reports of mixed success with the use of nifedipine to relieve esophageal impactions. A single 10-mg dose of nifedipine is administered sublingually by puncturing the gelatin capsule and squeezing it to express the drug beneath the patient's tongue. The effect of the drug begins within a few minutes.[64] Transient hypotension frequently occurs with sublingual nifedipine. Therefore, the patient should be treated in the supine position, and vital signs should be closely monitored during its administration. Unfortunately, the effects of gravity and hydrostatic pressure cannot be used to dislodge the impaction. Nifedipine should also be used cautiously in patients with cardiovascular disease.[64]

Nitroglycerin, unlike glucagon and nifedipine, relaxes smooth muscle spasm in the body of the esophagus as well as in the LES.[25,65] One nitroglycerin tablet containing 0.4 mg (1/150 grain) is administered sublingually. If there is a therapeutic response, it will occur within 1 min and last for several minutes.[65] Because nitroglycerin is a potential peripheral vasodilator, the patient should be treated in the supine position while vital signs are monitored. With the patient recumbent, the effects of gravity and hydrostatic pressure cannot be used to dislodge the impaction. The success rate of esophageal disimpaction with nitroglycerin approaches 50%.[19,20] The drug should be used cautiously in patients with volume depletion and in those who have a systolic blood pressure below 90 mm Hg. Nitroglycerin is contraindicated in patients who have had an idiosyncratic or hypersensitivity reaction to nitrates or nitrites.[66]

Hyoscine butylbromide (Buscopan) is an antispasmodic that produces hypotonia in the smooth muscle of the entire esophagus.[67,68] The therapeutic dose is 20 mg administered IV and may be repeated as necessary.[68] The two advantages of hyoscine over glucagon are that it produces muscle relaxation of the entire esophagus, not just the LES, and vomiting is not a side effect.[68,69] Worldwide experience with Buscopan has been extensive,[67–69] but the drug is not approved by the Food and Drug Administration (FDA) for use in the United States.

In theory, *combination therapy* with glucagon, a gas-forming agent, and water should be more effective than use of any single agent. When using this method, 1.0 mg of glucagon is given IV. After approximately 1 min, the patient is asked to drink one packet of E-Z-Gas II granules in 30 ml of water, followed by one cup (240 ml) of water.[7] The reported success rate of combined therapy in relieving food impaction is 75% to 80%.[7,70] This method seems to be less effective than simply having the patient drink a carbonated beverage.[10,14]

Fluoroscopically Guided Basket Extraction

In 1986, a method for removing impacted food and blunt foreign bodies from the esophagus using a Dormia-type wire basket with fluoroscopic guidance was introduced.[71] This method is particularly useful for extracting objects that have become impacted above an esophageal stricture. A selection of biliary stone baskets measuring 13 to 30 mm in diameter will permit extraction of most foreign bodies. A basket diameter is chosen that matches the size of the esophagus so that there will be no space outside the basket into which the foreign body can escape. In our experience, a 30-mm Dotter Retrieval Basket (Cook Inc.) is usually effective for most adults. Either a cut-off nasogastric tube or a 7- to 8-Fr angiographic catheter with a slight curve near its tip can be used to introduce and guide the basket into the esophagus. The working length of the basket must be slightly longer than the guiding catheter.[19,20,71]

A preprocedure barium swallow allows the radiologist to select a basket of proper diameter and tailor a curve at the tip of the catheter to facilitate its passage around the foreign body. After the posterior pharynx is sprayed with a topical anesthetic, the catheter is passed through the mouth into the esophagus above the impaction. If the esophageal wall and foreign body are no longer outlined by barium, coating is reestablished by injecting a small amount of medium density barium through the catheter (Figure 16.6A). This is done with the head of the x-ray table elevated about 30° to reduce the chance of barium aspiration.[19,20,71]

A 0.035–0.038-inch Teflon-coated or hydrophilic guidewire with a flexible tip is then inserted into the catheter and carefully advanced around the impacted object using fluoroscopic guidance (Figure 16.6B). The catheter is then advanced over the guidewire beyond the foreign body. This usually places the end of the catheter within or below an underlying esophageal stricture (Figure 16.6C).[19,20,71]

The guidewire is removed from the catheter, and an appropriate-size basket is advanced inside the catheter until it is located beside the foreign body (Figure 16.6D).

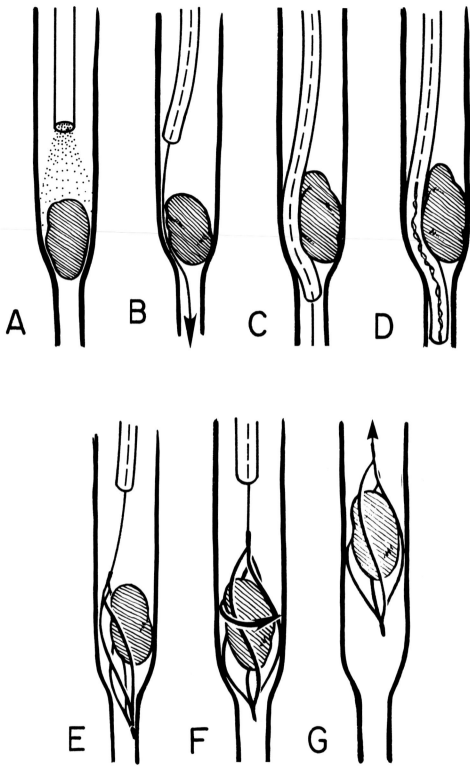

Figure 16.6 Sequential steps in the fluoroscopically guided basket extraction technique.
A. A small amount of barium is injected through an orally passed catheter to outline the
esophageal stricture and foreign body. B. A guidewire is inserted into the catheter and advanced
around the impacted foreign body. C. The catheter is advanced over the guidewire and beyond
the foreign body. D. After removal of the guidewire, a basket is advanced inside the catheter until the midpoint of the basket is positioned just below the lower edge of the foreign body. E. The
catheter is withdrawn to unsheathe the basket. F. The foreign body is engaged in the basket by
twirling the shaft of the instrument. G. After the foreign body is trapped in the basket, the
catheter and basket are withdrawn as a unit from the esophagus. (Adapted from Shaffer et al.[71]
Reproduced by permission.)

The midpoint of the basket must be positioned at or below the lower margin of the foreign body in order to capture the object when the basket is unsheathed. The catheter is withdrawn to unsheathe the basket. At first, the basket may not open fully because it is deformed by the adjacent foreign body or restricted by an underlying esophageal stricture (Figure 16.6E). If the basket is withdrawn a short distance at this time, it may dislodge the foreign body upward and away from the stricture where the basket has more room to expand. The foreign body is trapped in the basket by twirling the instrument clockwise until the object is fully enclosed within the wire cage (Figure 16.6F). Advancement of the basket should only be done within the protective cover of the catheter to avoid any risk of penetrating the esophageal wall with the stiff tip of the basket.[19,20,71]

The patient is turned onto his right side, and the x-ray table is tilted approximately 30° head-down to reduce the risk of aspiration during the extraction. With the foreign body entrapped by the basket, the catheter and basket are withdrawn as a unit in a smooth, continuous motion from the esophagus through the mouth (Figure 16.6G). Resistance may be encountered during passage of the upper esophageal sphincter (cricopharyngeus muscle), but this can be overcome by keeping steady traction on the basket or asking the patient to "retch."[19,20,71]

Occasionally, food or a foreign body will be so tightly impacted in an esophageal stricture that passage of a guidewire and catheter cannot be performed. In these circumstances, it may be necessary to use the catheter suction technique (see below) to dislodge the object a short distance upward from the esophageal stricture. Then, the guidewire and catheter can be advanced around the foreign body.

We have used the basket extraction method 47 times in 42 patients, aged 3 months to 84 yr. We have successfully removed 89% of the impactions, all located above esophageal strictures. There have been no complications. Advantages to fluoroscopically guided basket extraction of esophageal foreign bodies include: (1) it is an outpatient procedure and relatively inexpensive when compared with endoscopy of inpatient treatment; (2) general anesthesia is not required, nor is sedation needed in most cases; (3) the risk of an iatrogenic esophageal perforation is minimized because the basket is advanced within a protective sheath using fluoroscopic guidance; and (4) tracheal aspiration is unlikely because the foreign body is controlled within the basket during withdrawal.[19,20,71]

For removal of three-dimensional blunt foreign bodies, fluoroscopically guided basket extraction is the procedure of choice, especially when there is an underlying esophageal stricture (Figure 16.7). However, this method is not appropriate for removal of coins and other discoid objects from the esophagus. These flat, two-dimensional foreign bodies are difficult to secure in the basket.[19,20]

Suction Catheter Technique

In 1980, Kozarek and Sanowski reported the use of a modified 34-Fr gastric lavage tube connected to an aspirating syringe to remove meat from three patients with benign esophageal strictures.[16] The following year, McCray described the extraction of impacted food with suction using the proximal end of a standard nasogastric tube.[72] These procedures were performed without fluoroscopic or endoscopic guidance. More recently, use of a suction catheter with fluoroscopic guidance has been described for foreign body removal.[19,20]

A 12-Fr, single-lumen nasogastric tube (Argyle, St. Louis, MO) is modified by cutting off the distal end proximal to all of the side holes. This end of the tube is connected to a 60-ml syringe by using a "Christmas tree" adapter (Figure 16.8). The flared, proximal end of the tube should be made smooth with a nail file, sandpaper, or pair of scissors. The patient's throat is sprayed with a topical anesthetic. The flared proximal end of the tube is passed through the mouth and esophagus down to the level of the foreign material. Suction is applied with the 60-cc syringe, and the foreign body is sucked against the flared end of the tube. Suction is maintained as the tube and foreign body are withdrawn (Figure 16.9). If the impacted food is fragmented, the tube may have to be passed several times to extract all the pieces.[19,20] As with other esophageal extraction procedures, the patient should be placed semiprone with the fluoroscopic table tilted head-down about 30° during the actual foreign body removal.

Limited clinical experience and cadaver studies suggest that this procedure is relatively effective and safe.[16] Fluoroscopic guidance affords safer conditions for performing the procedure when compared with "blind" attempts at suction removal.

Postprocedural Considerations

After extraction of a foreign body, a radiographic contrast study of the esophagus should be done to document removal of all foreign material and to verify or exclude

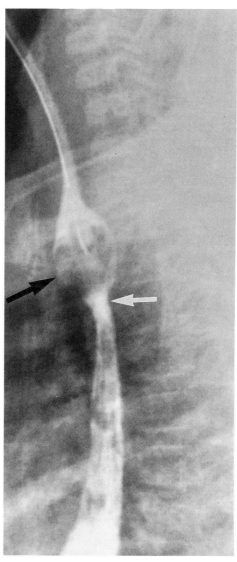

A

Figure 16.7 Basket extraction of meat from a 17-month-old boy. A. Barium esophagogram via a tube outlines a piece of meat (black arrow) impacted above a midesophageal stricture (white arrow). **B** and **C**. Following pages.

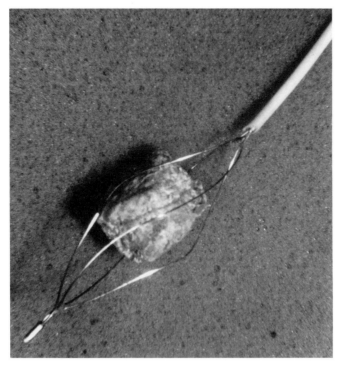

B

Figure 16.7 B. After its extraction, the piece of meat is still firmly contained inside the basket. C. Following page.

perforation.[10,12] This should be done as soon as the effects of the topical anesthetic have worn off and the patient can safely swallow. The esophagogram should first be performed with a water-soluble contrast agent. If no perforation is demonstrated, the study should be repeated immediately with a barium suspension.[19,20] Several days later, when esophageal spasm and mucosal edema have resolved, a more detailed barium esophagogram should be performed to evaluate for underlying pathology, such as a tumor, stricture, or motility disorder.[12,19,20,67]

STRICTURES

Strictures of the esophagus may be benign or malignant. Causes of benign esophageal strictures include reflux esophagitis, caustic material ingestion, inflammatory diseases (Crohn's, pemphigoid, epidermolysis bullosa, etc.), webs, muscle hypertrophy (achalasia), muscle dysfunction (spasm), and surgical anastomoses. Malignant strictures may be produced by primary neoplasms, metastases from distant primary sites, and direct invasion from a contiguous mediastinal neoplasm. A stricture manifests itself clinically when the patient develops dysphagia or symptoms of esophageal obstruction.

Fluoroscopically Guided Balloon Dilatation

Nonoperative treatment of benign esophageal strictures began in 1821, when Hildreth introduced the dilatation procedure with tapered, cylindrical instruments called bougies.[73] This bougienage technique remained the standard treatment until recently. In 1981, London et al.[74] described a new method of esophageal stricture dilatation using balloon catheters and fluoroscopic guidance. This technical advance became feasible

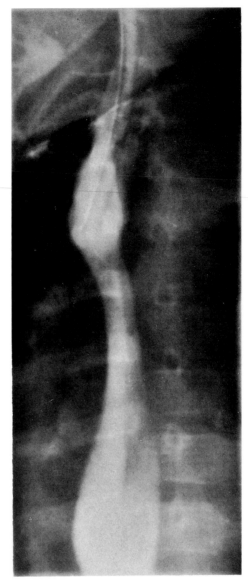

C

Figure 16.7 C. Postprocedure esophagogram shows no residual foreign body or esophageal injury. (Modified from Shaffer and de Lange.[19] Reproduced by permission.)

when a double-lumen catheter with a low-compliance balloon was introduced by Grüntzig and Hopff.[75]

Balloon dilatation offers a number of advantages over bougienage. The most important is that the inflated balloon remains in a stationary position and applies only radial forces to the esophageal wall. In contrast, the longitudinal shearing force generated by a bougie increases the risk of esophageal wall rupture, mucosal injury, and recurrence of the stenosis (Figure 16.10).[76-79] During balloon dilatation, inflation pressures can be monitored and controlled with an in-line pressure gauge. Also, balloon dilatation is more comfortable for the patient because bougienage requires multiple exchanges for progressively larger dilators. Following stricture dilatation, the symptom-free interval averages about six times longer after balloon dilatation than after bougienage.[80]

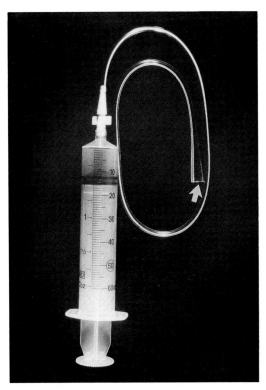

Figure 16.8 Suction catheter foreign body extractor. The distal end of a single-lumen 12-Fr nasogastric tube is cut off to remove all side holes. The cut end is attached to a 60-ml syringe with a "Christmas tree" adapter. The flared end of the tube (arrow) is used to vacuum foreign material from the esophagus. (From Shaffer and de Lange.[19] Reproduced by permission.)

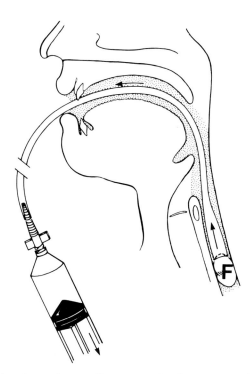

Figure 16.9 Drawing shows the use of a nasogastric tube to remove impacted food from the esophagus. The flared end of the tube is advanced through the mouth and esophagus to the level of the foreign body (F). The foreign body is sucked against the flared end of the tube by aspiration with the syringe. As continuous suction is maintained with the syringe, the flared end of the catheter is used to withdraw foreign body from the esophagus. (From Shaffer and de Lange.[19] Reproduced by permission.)

379

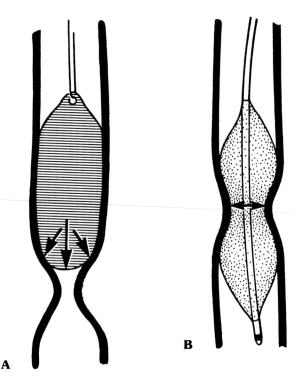

Figure 16.10 Dilatation of an esophageal stricture with a bougie or balloon. **A.** The bougie is forced longitudinally into the stricture. The dilating forces are both longitudinal and radial (arrows). **B.** The deflated balloon is positioned across the stricture. During inflation, the dilating forces (arrows) are directed radially, resulting in more effective stretching of the stricture and less injury to the normal esophageal muscles and mucosa. (From Shaffer and de Lange.[20] Reproduced by permission.)

The use of fluoroscopically guided dilatation has advantages over "blind" or endoscopically controlled procedures. When endoscopy is used to guide a dilating bougie or balloon, only the esophagus proximal to the stricture is visualized (Figure 16.11). Once the dilator enters the stricture, the instrument is advanced without visual control, and perforation by the tip of the dilator can occur.[81] Fluoroscopy allows visualization of the catheter tip, balloon status, and esophagus proximal and distal to the stricture during the entire procedure.

Prior to the balloon dilatation procedure, a barium esophagogram is obtained to define the location and character (length, diameter, mucosal surface) of the lesion, and the presence or absence of an associated ulcer or fistula (Figure 16.12A). This information is needed for planning the dilatation procedure and choosing balloon catheters of appropriate diameter and length.[20,82]

Stricture dilatation is performed using angioplasty catheters with noncompliant balloons. The diameter of the balloon to be used depends upon the diameters of both the stricture and the adjacent normal esophagus. In relatively mild strictures, a single balloon sized to the adjacent normal esophagus can be used. The largest balloon that we routinely use for an esophageal stricture is 20 mm in diameter. In patients with tight strictures, the procedure is initially performed with a small diameter balloon. If complete balloon inflation can be done without causing significant discomfort to the patient, the procedure is continued with balloons of progressively larger diameter until the desired result is achieved. If the length of the stricture extends over several centimeters, a relatively long balloon (8 cm) is more likely to remain in position and not slide away from the stricture during balloon inflation. In patients with a hiatal hernia who have strictures at the gastroesophageal junction, the position of the gastro-

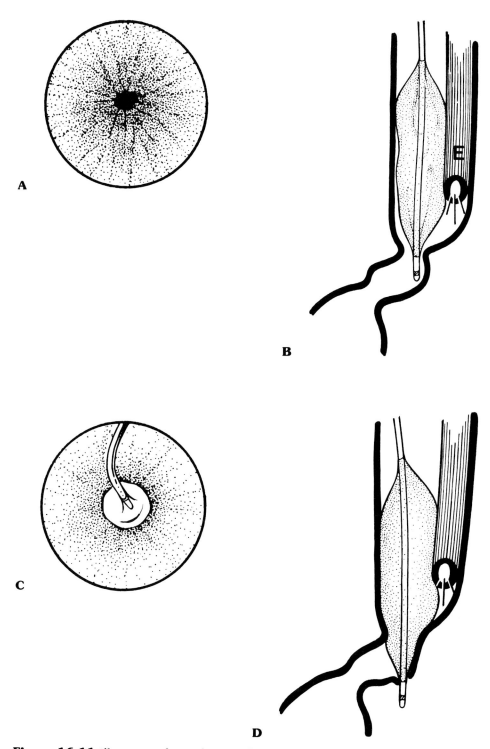

Figure 16.11 Illustration of an endoscopically guided balloon dilatation of a tight, tortuous stricture of esophagus. **A.** View through the endoscope positioned above the stricture shows only the proximal end of the narrowing. **B.** As the balloon catheter is advanced into the stricture, the view through the endoscope (**E**) becomes partially obscured. Neither the lumen inside the stricture nor the catheter tip can be seen. **C.** View through the endoscope with the balloon in the stricture. Only the proximal part of the balloon is visible to the endoscopist. **D.** When the balloon catheter is advanced, a perforation can easily occur because the tip of the catheter and the course of the tortuous esophageal lumen are not visible to the endoscopist. (From Shaffer and de Lange.[20] Reproduced by permission.)

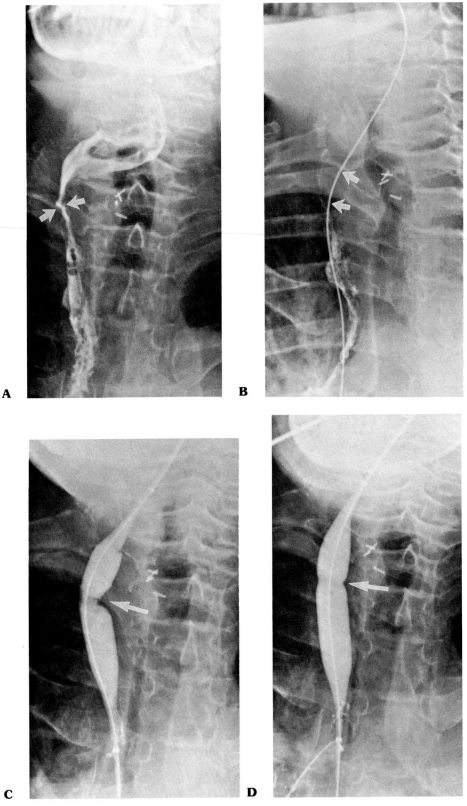

Figure 16.12 Fluoroscopically guided balloon dilatation in a patient with an anastomotic stricture after esophagectomy and colonic interposition. A. Barium esophagogram is used to define the location and characteristics of the 2-mm-diameter stricture (arrows). B. Under fluoroscopic visualization, a guidewire (arrows) is passed through an orally inserted feeding tube and carefully advanced across the stricture. C. After removal of the initial catheter, a 10-mm balloon is advanced over the guidewire and positioned so that the midportion of the balloon straddles the stricture. As it is slowly inflated, the balloon develops a waist-like deformity (arrow) that corresponds to the site of stricture. D. After several balloon inflations with increasing pressures, the "waist" (arrow) almost disappears. E, F, and G. Following page.

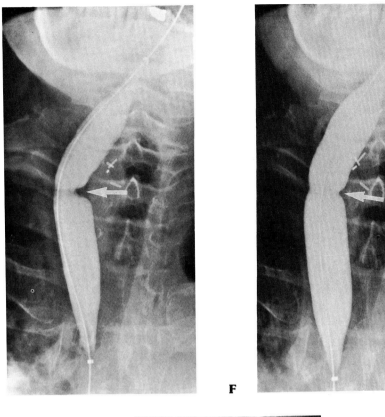

E   F

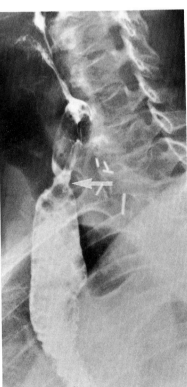

G

Figure 16.12 E. Following complete deflation, the 10-mm balloon is exchanged for a 20-mm balloon. As the 20-mm balloon is inflated, the "waist" (arrow) localizes the site of the stricture. F. The balloon is inflated to its rated pressure tolerance, but there is still a residual deformity (arrow). G. After deflation of the balloon and removal of the guidewire, the catheter is withdrawn so that its tip is above the stricture. Barium is injected through the main lumen of the catheter to opacify the esophageal stricture (arrow) and exclude perforation. Due to spasm and edema, the stricture typically appears narrower than was achieved during maximal balloon dilatation. (Modified from Shaffer and de Lange.[20] Reproduced by permission.)

esophageal junction may change when the balloon is introduced. In these patients, use of a long balloon will also increase the likelihood that the balloon will completely straddle the stricture.[20]

During the procedure, the patient is given neuroleptic analgesia with a combination of IV meperidine (Demerol; Sanofi Winthrop, New York, NY) or fentanyl (Sublimaze; Janssen Pharmaceutica, Titusville, NJ) and midazolam (Versed; Roche Laboratories, Nutley, NJ). The patient's throat is sprayed with a topical anesthetic (Xylocaine 10% Oral Spray; Astra USA, Inc.) because the instruments are passed orally. The instruments are lubricated with viscous lidocaine prior to their introduction. Oral secretions can be reduced with atropine sulfate (0.4 mg intramuscularly) or removed by means of intermittent suctioning. The patient's vital signs and oxygen saturation are continuously monitored.

A shortened 8- or 10-Fr nasogastric tube is passed through the mouth and advanced until it reaches the upper margin of the esophageal stricture. A 0.035–0.038-inch Teflon-coated guidewire is then inserted through the nasogastric tube and carefully advanced across the stricture during fluoroscopic observation (Figure 16.12B). A J-tipped guidewire is preferred for its safety in avoiding esophageal wall penetration; however, a straight wire may be required to cross a tight stricture. In some cases, it may be necessary to turn the nasogastric tube or use a curved angiographic catheter to direct the wire across the stricture. A steerable wire (Glidewire; Terumo Corp., Tokyo, Japan) will also facilitate traversal of the lesion. Once the stricture is crossed, the guidewire needs to be advanced well beyond the stricture to provide stable purchase for catheter exchange. Following this, a balloon catheter is advanced over the guidewire.

The radiopaque markers on the balloon catheter are positioned so that the midportion of the balloon will straddle the stricture. The balloon is inflated with a dilute (20–30%), water-soluble contrast medium so that it can be visualized fluoroscopically. The stricture causes a waist-like deformity on the middle of the balloon as it begins to inflate (Figure 16.12C). This "waist" corresponds to the stricture. The balloon is slowly inflated until the "waist" disappears (Figure 16.12D). In many cases, it may not be possible to stretch the stricture completely with the first balloon inflation. In these cases, the balloon is inflated until moderate resistance is felt or the patient begins to experience some discomfort, usually at about 1 atmosphere (atm) of pressure. This inflation pressure is maintained for a variable period, ranging from 30 to 180 secs, and is monitored by an in-line pressure gauge. After the initial dilatation, the balloon is deflated for approximately 1 min and subsequently reinflated as many times as necessary to obtain full distention of the stricture. With each balloon inflation, the pressure is increased by a small increment (usually 1 atm) until maximum distention of the balloon (no "waist") is achieved or the burst pressure rating is reached. Multiple balloon inflations with small incremental increases in pressure are preferred for dilating strictures. A single rapid inflation of the balloon to maximum pressure increases the risk of a mucosal tear and/or perforation. Balloon inflation is monitored fluoroscopically to ascertain that the balloon does not migrate and that no complications are occurring. The total number of inflations during each procedure may vary, but usually ranges from 3 to 5. In addition to using incremental increases in balloon inflation pressure, some cases require the use of progressively larger balloons to adequately dilate a stricture (Figure 16.12C–F).[20]

When the stricture is maximally dilated, the balloon is deflated and the guidewire withdrawn. The balloon catheter is then withdrawn so that its tip is proximal to the stricture. A dilute barium suspension or nonionic contrast material is injected through the catheter during fluoroscopic observation to check for the presence of esophageal perforation.[20,83] The stricture frequently appears little changed from the preprocedural barium examination (Figure 16.12G); however, the clinical response of the patient's dysphagia is the most important factor in judging the ultimate success or failure of the procedure.[82–86]

There are several reports with encouraging short-term results from balloon dilatation of esophageal strictures. In a series of 19 patients with anastomotic strictures, 9 (47%) patients had permanent relief of clinical symptoms after only one dilatation; the other 10 patients required 1–7 additional dilatations to obtain lasting relief.[82] Mean follow-up was 13 months. In a second series of 9 patients with esophageal webs, 100% had complete relief of dysphagia after only one dilatation session.[83] Mean follow-up was 2.6 yr. Another group of 35 patients with esophageal strictures from various causes obtained relief of dysphagia in 77% of cases during an unspecified period of follow-up. These patients each received an average of 5 balloon dilatations. In general, patients with achalasia or anastomotic strictures responded better than those caused by reflux esophagitis, caustic substance ingestion, or malignancy.[86] Another group of 50 patients with strictures of various types had an average of 2.2 dilatation procedures per patient. Dysphagia was initially relieved in 98% of the patients. The number of symptom-free patients decreased to 81% at 6 months and leveled off at 71% between 9 and 27 months after the last dilatation procedure.[84,85]

Large series and long-term follow-up of patients who have received balloon dilatation for treatment of esophageal strictures have not been reported. We are in the process of reviewing our first 700 procedures, spanning a period of more than a decade. Judging by the initial review of our data and the increasing number of patient referrals, fluoroscopically guided balloon dilatation seems to be safer, less painful, and more effective in the short term than endoscopic dilatation or bougienage. The long-term response seems to vary from patient to patient and is not entirely predictable. The most important factor determining the long-term outcome appears to be the underlying condition that caused the stricture, and whether or not the process is still active. For instance, patients with inappropriately treated gastroesophageal reflux and a stricture due to peptic esophagitis often experience a rapid recurrence of the stricture following balloon dilatation. On the other hand, patients with anastomotic strictures, mucosal rings, or webs usually receive long-term relief of dysphagia following balloon dilatation.

When fluoroscopically controlled balloon dilatation is carefully performed, the risk of a complication is very low. Potential complications include bleeding, esophageal perforation, and infection (aspiration pneumonia, abscess formation, or bacteremia). An esophageal wall perforation is suggested if there is abrupt disappearance of the "waist" on the balloon and a sudden drop in the inflation pressure. The patient may experience pain that is not relieved with balloon deflation. When such a complication is suspected, the balloon should be immediately deflated and the guidewire removed from the catheter. The balloon catheter is then slightly withdrawn so that its tip is just above the stricture and suspected leak. Water-soluble contrast medium is injected through the central lumen of the balloon catheter to search for a possible leak. If no leak is demonstrated, the esophagogram is immediately repeated with a dilute barium suspension. If a laceration or leak is demonstrated, the dilatation procedure is terminated; if not, the treatment is resumed and completed.[20]

In our experience with more than 700 dilatation procedures, significant complications have occurred in fewer than 2% of cases. Perforations occurred in 11 patients and were confirmed immediately on postprocedure contrast studies. All patients were hospitalized and treated with parenteral antibiotics and parenteral feedings, receiving nothing by mouth. Healing occurred without additional sequelae or the need for surgery. One case of aspiration pneumonia developed, and this responded to outpatient antibiotic treatment. No cases of abscess formation or significant bleeding have occurred.

Self-expanding Metal Stents

The idea of an endoprosthesis to treat esophageal strictures and fistulas is not new. Sir Charles Symonds reported the first successful insertion of an esophageal tube in 1887.[87] However, further progress in endoprosthetic devices had to await the advent of plastic materials. In 1959, Celestin described a new plastic tube that became the prototype for most of the rigid esophageal stents used in the palliation of malignant strictures.[87] In

1983, Frimberger reported the endoscopic placement of a self-expanding metallic stent for the palliation of esophageal cancer.[88] Since 1990, self-expanding metallic stents have been developed, and a number of prototypes are being evaluated by both endoscopists and radiologists.[89-99] At this writing, several stent types are being commercially manufactured and used in Asia and Europe. However, only two are currently approved by the FDA for sale in the United States: the Ultraflex Esophageal Stent (Boston Scientific Corp., Natick, MA) and the Wallstent Esophageal Prosthesis (Schneider USA Inc., Minneapolis, MN). The use of these stents is restricted to treatment of malignant esophageal strictures. The use of stents for benign lesions is currently not recommended.

The *Ultraflex™ Esophageal Stent* is also known as the nitinol, Strecker, or Elastalloy stent. This self-expanding, metal-mesh stent is made of knitted 0.15 mm nitinol (nickel–titanium alloy) wire (Figure 16.13) The ends of the stent have smooth, looped wires with a special coating to reduce trauma to the esophageal wall. The stent is flexible in its long axis and has exceptional cross-sectional elasticity. The fully expanded stent measures 18 mm in diameter. Its proximal end is flared into a 5-mm-long collar with a 21-mm diameter to provide fixation to the esophageal wall. It is manufactured in lengths of 7, 10, and 15 cm. The stent comes from the manufacturer in a sterile package and is compressed inside a delivery system. It is wrapped around the distal end of a 95-cm-long catheter that accepts an 0.038-inch guidewire. The catheter has an olive-shaped widening distal to the stent and a 4-cm-long soft tip to reduce trauma during placement. To minimize the diameter of the stent at insertion, it is longitudinally stretched, circumferentially compressed, and embedded in gelatin. The catheter and compressed stent are then encased within an 8-mm (24-Fr) Teflon outer sheath (Figure 16.14).[90,95,97]

A covered version of the Ultraflex Stent has recently received FDA approval. The central part of this stent is wrapped with a three-layer polymer to provide a barrier that resists tumor ingrowth and occludes esophageal fistulae. At both ends of the stent, a 1.5-cm segment remains uncovered to aid attachment of the stent to the esophageal wall above and below the stricture and retard stent migration. It is manufactured in lengths of 10 and 15 cm, and the delivery system is only 5 mm (15-Fr) in outside diameter. This stent is otherwise identical to the uncovered version described above.

The *Wallstent Esophageal Prosthesis* I is a self-expanding, flexible, compliant stent composed of a superalloy monofilament wire braided into a tubular mesh configuration. A proprietary silicone membrane is sandwiched between inner and outer layers

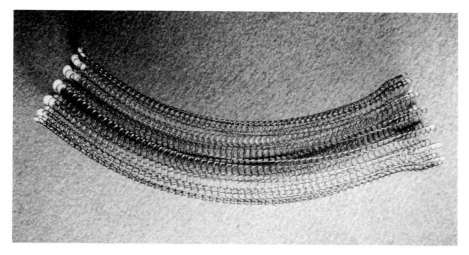

Figure 16.13 An Ultraflex Esophageal Stent is made with knitted nitinol wire. The wires at the ends of the stent are looped and coated to reduce esophageal trauma. The stent is very flexible, both longitudinally and in cross section.

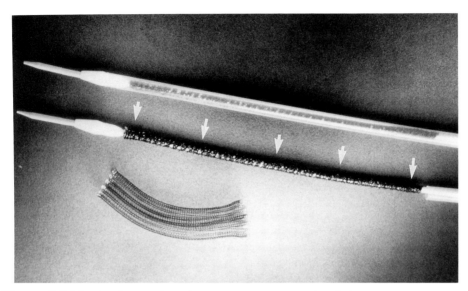

Figure 16.14 Ultraflex Esophageal Stent System. *Top:* Distal end of the 24-Fr delivery system containing the stent is shown. This catheter-based system is introduced over a 0.038-inch guidewire. *Middle:* The distal end of delivery system with outer sheath withdrawn reveals the longitudinally stretched and circumferentially compressed stent (arrows) embedded in gelatin around the inner catheter. *Bottom:* The fully expanded stent demonstrates the considerable amount of shortening that occurs during circumferential expansion of the stent.

of the mesh to inhibit tumor ingrowth or occlude an esophageal fistula (Figure 16.15). The body of the stent has an 18-mm lumen and a 20-mm outer diameter. The stent ends are flared to a diameter of 28 mm and are left uncovered to better anchor the device to the esophageal wall and retard stent migration. This stent is currently available in 4, 6, and 9-cm lengths. The stent delivery system is a system of coaxial tubes and has an outer diameter of 38-Fr. It also accommodates an 0.038-inch guidewire.

A newer version, Esophageal Prosthesis II, has recently become available. It is made from a single metal stent with an inner silicone covering. The stent delivery system has been reduced to 18-Fr. Once deployed the device has a 19-mm inner lumen. It is available in 10 cm and 15 cm lengths. The Wallstent II does not have as much hoop stength as the Wallstent I. Both esophageal Wallstents can be recaptured, if they have been less than 50% deployed.

Telestep (Schneider AG, Bülach, Switzerland) is a polyurethane-covered, self-expanding Wallstent endoprosthesis. This esophageal stent is commercially available in Europe, but not in the United States. It is manufactured in two sizes: 20 mm in diameter and 110 mm in length, or 25 mm in diameter and 105 mm in length. The middle section of the stent is covered with polyurethane. The outer diameter of the delivery system is either 18 or 22 Fr, and consists of three coaxially arranged shafts. It will slide over an 0.038-inch guidewire.[96]

Silicone-covered Song modification of the Gianturco Z-stent (Sooho Medi-Tech, Seoul, Korea). This self-expanding stent is constructed of eight 0.3–0.5 mm stainless steel wires in a cylindrical zigzag configuration and is available in diameters ranging from 14 to 20 mm and a length of 2 cm. Two to five stent segments are connected to form a stent of the desired length. Larger (22-mm) diameter segments, constructed of 10 wires each, are attached with metal struts to the proximal and distal ends to keep the stent from sliding upward or downward in the esophagus following deployment. A nylon mesh is wrapped around the outside of the stent and covered with silicone rubber to inhibit tumor ingrowth or occlude an esophageal fistula. The stent tube can be compressed and inserted into a 12-mm (36-Fr) introducer tube with an 8-mm pusher rod.[89,92]

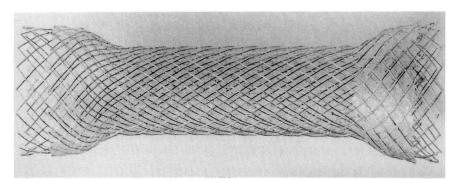

Figure 16.15 The Wallstent Esophageal Prosthesis is a self-expanding tubular stent made of two layers of braided superalloy wire. A proprietary silicone membrane is sandwiched between the inner and outer layers of the mesh to inhibit tumor ingrowth or occlude an esophageal fistula. The stent ends are flared to retard stent migration.

Silicone-covered Rösch modification of the Gianturco Z-stent. This stent is currently handmade at the Dotter Interventional Institute, Oregon Health Sciences University, Portland, Oregon, using 0.5-mm stainless steel wire bent into a zigzag configuration. Individual stent bodies are 18 mm in diameter and 2 cm in length. Multiple stents are interconnected with nonabsorbable suture material to make stent tubes ranging from 8 to 14 cm in length. The proximal end segment is flared to a diameter of 22 mm to produce a funnel for swallowed material and to retard migration of the stent. The distal end is covered with several layers of silicone material to produce a soft "bumper" to reduce esophageal wall injury. The stent has six 3-mm-long wire hooks at its midportion to facilitate anchoring within the tumor. The entire stent tube is covered with a thin silicone membrane to inhibit tumor ingrowth or occlude an esophageal fistula. Prior to its introduction into a patient, the stent tube is compressed into a 10-mm (30-Fr)-diameter delivery apparatus.[93,98]

Prior to placement of any stent, the patient should undergo barium contrast esophagography to determine the location and extent of the tumor and identify any fistula. There are several considerations that affect the choice of stent. If a fistula is demonstrated, a covered stent should be used. The stent should be 4 to 6 cm longer than any malignant stenosis to reduce the possibility of tumor overgrowth at the ends of the stent. When multiple stents are required to cover a long stricture, the most distal stent should be deployed first. The stents should be overlapped by at least 3 cm to ensure adequate stent anchoring.

The procedure is performed with neuroleptic analgesia and topical lidocaine spray for the oropharynx. A cut-off, small-caliber nasogastric tube or angiographic catheter is used in conjunction with a guidewire to traverse the stricture and enter the stomach (Figure 16.16A). Using the technique described previously under Fluoroscopically Guided Balloon Dilatation, the stricture is dilated with an 8-cm-long balloon, 12 to 15 mm in diameter, to facilitate placement of the stent (Figure 16.16B). If the stricture cannot be dilated to at least 12 mm, stent placement is generally contraindicated.

Based on the information obtained from the esophagogram and the length of the waist deformity on the balloon during its inflation in the stricture, anatomic landmarks are fluoroscopically identified inside the patient or radiopaque markers are taped to the patient's skin to demarcate the ends of the tumor. The prepackaged stent delivery system is used with fluoroscopic guidance to deploy the esophageal stent in accordance with the manufacturer's instructions.

The methods of delivery are similar for all of the self-expanding metal stents. Deployment of the Ultraflex Esophageal Stent will be described in detail. After removal of

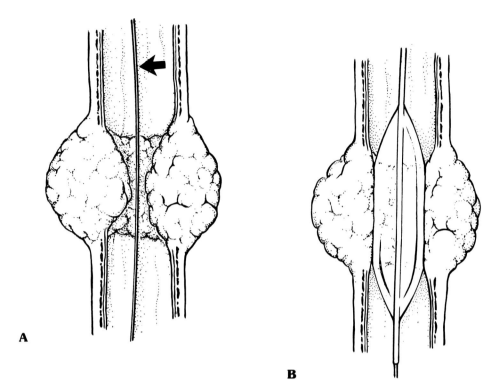

Figure 16.16 Technique of Ultraflex Stent placement. **A.** A guidewire (arrow) is passed through an orally inserted feeding tube or catheter and is carefully advanced across the stricture using fluoroscopic guidance. **B.** After removing the introducing catheter, an angioplasty catheter with a 12- to 15-mm-diameter balloon is advanced over the guidewire. After positioning the balloon astride the malignant stricture, the balloon dilatation procedure is performed as previously described. **C, D, E,** and **F.** Following pages.

the deflated balloon catheter from the esophagus, the delivery system containing the stent is advanced over the guidewire into the stricture (Figure 16.16C). The delivery system is relatively rigid, and extension of the patient's neck makes advancement easier. The position of the delivery system is adjusted until its thicker, innermost pair of radiopaque markers are symmetrically placed at least 2–3 cm beyond the proximal and distal margins of the mass. These markers indicate the final position of the ends of the stent when it is fully expanded. The safety sleeve should not be removed from the proximal shaft of the delivery catheter until the stent system is in proper position. The safety sleeve prevents inadvertent retraction of the outer sheath, which would allow moisture to enter the delivery system and initiate premature gelatin dissolution and stent expansion prior to proper positioning of the stent.

When the radiopaque markers on the shaft of the delivery catheter are properly aligned with the esophageal tumor, the outer sheath is withdrawn in one continuous motion. Upon exposure to the moisture in the esophagus, the gelatin around the stent should completely dissolve and permit the stent to expand within 5 to 10 mins (Figure 16.16D). If the stent does not expand within 10 min, a small amount of water may be instilled into the esophagus through a second catheter to accelerate stent expansion. To prevent aspiration, the procedure table should be tilted with the head up 30° to 45°.

After release and expansion of the stent are confirmed fluoroscopically, the delivery system is carefully removed, leaving the guidewire and stent in place (Figure 16.16E). The stent must be completely released from the inner catheter, otherwise removal of the delivery system may dislodge the stent.

A 12-mm balloon catheter is then passed over the guidewire and inflated to distend

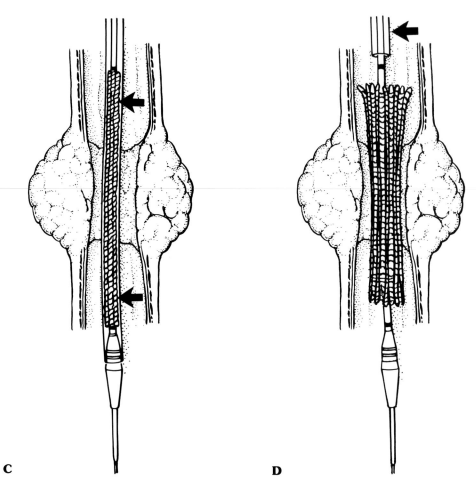

C   **D**

Figure 16.16 C. After removing the deflated balloon catheter from the esophagus, the delivery system containing the compressed stent (arrows) is advanced over the guidewire into the stricture. The delivery system is adjusted until its radiopaque markers are symmetrically placed 2–3 cm beyond each end of the stricture. **D.** When the delivery system is properly positioned, its outer sheath (arrow) is withdrawn, exposing the gelatin covered stent to esophageal moisture. The gelatin gradually dissolves, and the stent expands spontaneously over a 5- to 10-min interval. E and F. Following page.

and attach the stent more firmly to the esophageal wall (Figure 16.16F). Careful insertion and removal of the deflated balloon with fluoroscopic guidance is mandatory to avoid inadvertent stent displacement.

The guidewire is removed, and the patient is monitored until the effects of the topical anesthetic and IV conscious sedation have disappeared. Barium esophagography is then performed to evaluate stent patency and position and to rule out any significant iatrogenic injury to the esophagus (Figures 16.17A and B). If the procedure is done in an outpatient setting, the patient may be discharged after an uneventful 4-hr period of close observation.

For the 48 hr following the procedure, the patient should be restricted to a liquid diet even if the stent seems to be fully expanded. If the stent is not fully expanded by 48 hr, the patient's diet should be advanced to include only liquids and soft foods. Follow-up esophagograms should be performed at 5- to 7-day intervals until the stent is adequately expanded. As soon as the stent is fully expanded, the patient may have a regular diet with the admonition to avoid swallowing large pieces of solid food. If the patient drinks carbonated beverages with meals, the possibility of food impactions will

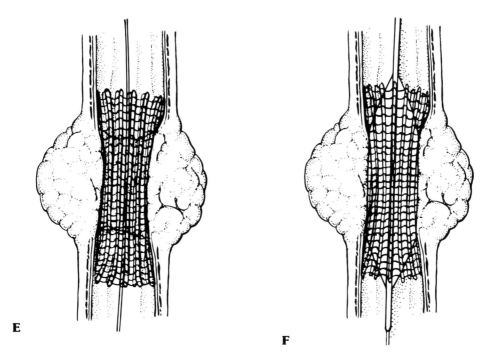

Figure 16.16 E. After release from the delivery catheter and expansion of the stent are confirmed fluoroscopically, the delivery system is carefully removed, leaving the guidewire and stent in place. F. A 12-mm balloon catheter is carefully advanced over the guidewire, and the balloon is inflated inside the stent to further expand it and more firmly attach it to the esophageal wall.

be reduced. If the esophageal stent protrudes across the lower esophageal sphincter, antireflux instructions should be given to the patient, and a daily 20-mg dose of omeprazole (Prilosec Delayed Release Capsules; Merck & Co. Inc., West Point, PA) should be prescribed to minimize the anticipated symptoms and complications of gastroesophageal reflux.[93,96] Endoscopic or fluoroscopic follow-up examinations should be performed every 4 months or sooner, if dictated by the patient's symptoms. Close follow-up will allow evaluation of stent function and early diagnosis of tumor ingrowth or overgrowth.

Initial technical failures and procedure-related complications are extremely rare. Reports in the literature describe successful stent placement in nearly 100% of patients.[90,91,93,95–97,99] Only 1–2% of stents fail to expand enough for the patient to maintain adequate nutrition.[97] The decrease in dysphagia is described as good or very good by most reports. Following stent placement, 78–80% of patients can eat a normal diet, 13–20% can eat soft foods, and 0–7% are restricted to liquids only.[90,97] Most patients die without recurrence of debilitating dysphagia.

Late complications of self-expanding metal stents include stent migration (0–25%), esophageal perforation (0–2%), esophagorespiratory fistula (0–5%), food impaction (0–14%), tumor ingrowth (0–14%), tumor overgrowth (3–10%), severe hemorrhage (0–6%), benign stricture at stent end (0–6%), gastroesophageal reflux (0–7%), and intractable chest pain requiring narcotic analgesia (0–7%).[91–93,96,97] Migration occurs more frequently with covered stents, especially those that sit astride the gastroesophageal junction with the distal end free in the gastric lumen, and with stents used for benign strictures.[92,93,95–97] Tumor ingrowth occurs primarily through noncovered metal stents; however, most patients usually die of their cancer before the stent can become occluded.[91,92,95,96] When tumor ingrowth does occur, it can be man-

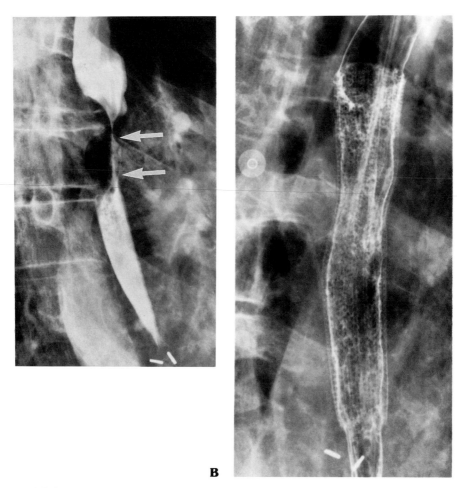

Figure 16.17 Squamous cell carcinoma of the esophagus in a 66-yr-old man with 2–3 months of dysphagia and 30 lb weight loss. **A.** Preprocedure barium esophagogram demonstrates a tight stricture (arrows) of 5 cm length in the midthoracic esophagus. **B.** Postprocedure air-contrast esophagogram shows nearly complete expansion of the Ultraflex Stent. The patient was able to resume a normal diet.

aged successfully with endoscopic laser coagulation.[90,91] Severe bleeding is more frequent with the larger-sized Gianturco-type stents, especially in patients who receive radiation therapy after stent placement.[92,98] Severe chest discomfort requiring narcotics for pain control is seen almost exclusively after placement of Gianturco-type stents.[92,95,96,98] Stent-related mortality is reported to be 0% to 6%.[96–98] By comparison, nonexpandable plastic tube stents have an insertion failure rate of 10% and a complication rate of 36–40%.[90]

LEAKS

Esophageal Perforations

Treatment for esophageal perforation has traditionally been surgery, but the development of more effective antibiotics and parenteral nutrition has led to a cautious trend toward nonoperative management. At present, surgery remains the preferred treatment in the following situations: (1) Boerhaave's syndrome; (2) unstable patients with systemic sepsis, respiratory failure, or shock; (3) large perforations with widespread contamination; (4) intraperitoneal perforations; (5) perforations with an associated pneumothorax; (6) perforations with retained foreign bodies; and (7) perforations associated with an underlying esophageal lesion (such as achalasia, nondilatable stricture, or carcinoma) for which surgery would be chosen even in the absence of a perforation. We believe that nonoperative (medical) treatment should be considered only in the following circumstances: (1) clinically stable patients; (2) iatrogenic perforations in which the patient was taking nothing by mouth (NPO) and the leak is detected promptly before major mediastinal contamination has occurred; (3) perforations with such a long delay in diagnosis that the patient has already demonstrated tolerance for the perforation without surgery; and (4) esophageal disruptions that are well contained within the mediastinum or a pleural loculus.[100] Basic medical treatment consists of in-hospital observation, triple antibiotic coverage, nothing by mouth, and parenteral nutrition until closure of the perforation is documented by esophagography.

Covered self-expanding metal stents have been used successfully in a few patients to treat esophageal perforations caused by endoscopic balloon dilatation of esophageal malignancies. The technique used for stent placement is identical to that described previously for the management of malignant strictures. In a small series of seven patients with iatrogenic perforation, prompt covered-stent placement is reported to have sealed the leakage in all cases with no evidence of mediastinitis or other related complications.[96]

Esophagoenteric Anastomotic Leaks

Disruption of an esophagogastrostomy or esophagocolonic interposition surgical anastomosis occurs in 6% to 35% of cases.[101,102] The leak usually develops within 2 wk after surgery and may lead to a chronic enterocutaneous fistula. Spontaneous healing may require several weeks or months and result in an extended and expensive hospital stay.[103]

It is reported that the healing can be accelerated by dilating the leaking esophagoenteric anastomosis with a bougie or balloon.[103–105] Balloon dilatation is performed in a fashion similar to the previously described technique. The procedure is performed with a 15 or 20 mm balloon, regardless of whether or not the anastomosis is visibly narrowed (Figure 16.18)[20,104,105]

We recently evaluated our experience with fluoroscopically guided balloon dilatation for the treatment of esophagoenteric anastomotic leaks. In a group of 16 consecutive patients with this complication, 14 (88%) responded successfully to balloon dilatation. The anastomotic leakage ceased immediately in 10 patients and within 5 days in the remaining 4. The procedure was performed 7–32 days (mean, 13 days) after surgery. Earlier intervention seemed to increase the effectiveness of the procedure. In no case was there further disruption of the anastomosis or another associated complication.[105]

The probable explanation as to why the dilatation procedure is effective in controlling an anastomotic leak is that it relieves the stenosis that develops at the site of the disrupted anastomosis. This luminal narrowing is probably caused by postoperative edema and granulation tissue. The narrowing obstructs flow of swallowed saliva through the esophageal lumen and diverts some of it through the leak (Figure 16.19). The leakage continues as long as the anastomotic narrowing persists. Balloon dilatation increases the diameter of the anastomosis and reduces the resistance to flow of saliva through its lumen. Consequently, the secretions are no longer directed through the leak, and the fistula can begin to heal.[20,103–105]

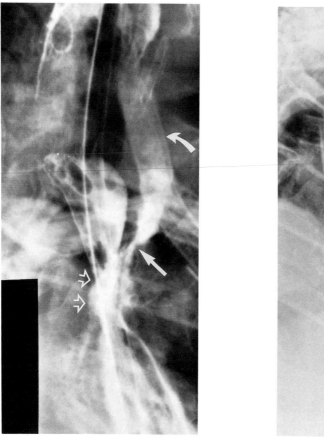
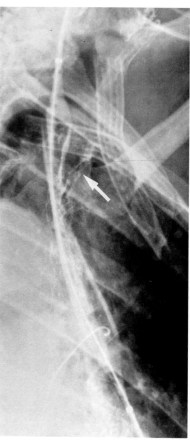

A   **B**

Figure 16.18 Balloon dilatation of a leaking esophagoenteric anastomosis. **A.** Esophagogram through an orally placed nasogastric tube shows a narrowed anastomosis (open arrows). Barium leaking from anastomosis (straight arrow) is tracking toward a surgical drain (curved arrow) in the patient's neck. **B.** After crossing the anastomosis with a J-tipped guidewire, a deflated 15-mm balloon is advanced across the narrowing and positioned so that its midportion straddles the leaking anastomosis. The leak is faintly visible (arrow). **C** and **D.** Following page.

Esophagorespiratory Fistulas

A debilitating complication of an esophageal malignancy is an esophagorespiratory fistula (ERF). This complication develops in 5% to 15% of esophageal cancer patients.[93] Untreated ERF invariably leads to paroxysmal coughing, profound malnutrition, recurrent pneumonias, and ultimately, early death. Until recently, the treatment of choice in these patients has been to place a rigid plastic tube in the esophagus. However, these devices have been associated with significant complications, such as esophageal perforation, hemorrhage, obstruction, and stent migration.[93,96] Preliminary experience with use of covered, self-expanding metal stents in the treatment of an ERF suggests that these endoprostheses produce a more favorable result.[93,96,98,99]

In patients with an ERF due to a malignancy, an associated esophageal stricture is almost always present. The procedure for placement of a covered, self-expanding metal stent to occlude the fistula is identical to that for treatment of a malignant stricture alone (Figure 16.20). However, after stent placement, patients with ERF should be instructed to begin eating a soft food diet, initially avoiding liquids. If no symptoms

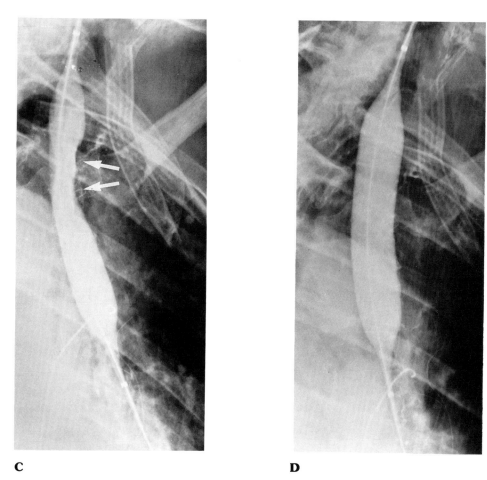

C   **D**

Figure 16.18 C. After partial inflation of the balloon, a waist-like deformity in the middle of the balloon (arrows) confirms the presence of an anastomotic stricture. D. After applying additional inflation pressure, the balloon is fully distended, indicating that the anastomosis has been dilated to 15 mm. (From de Lange et al.[104] Reproduced by permission.)

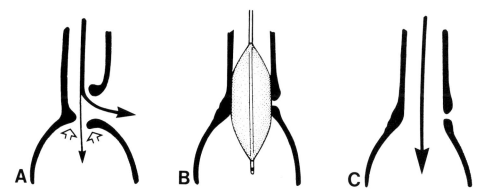

Figure 16.19 Effect of dilatation on a leaking anastomosis. A. When there is a breakdown of the suture line, most swallowed saliva is diverted through the leak (curved arrows) because the anastomosis is narrowed (open arrow) by postoperative edema and granulation tissue. Continued flow of saliva keeps the disruption open. B. Balloon dilatation increases the luminal diameter of the anastomosis. C. After dilatation, flow in the esophageal lumen is unrestricted, and swallowed saliva is no longer diverted through the leak. This promotes more rapid healing. (From de Lange et al.[105] Reproduced by permission.)

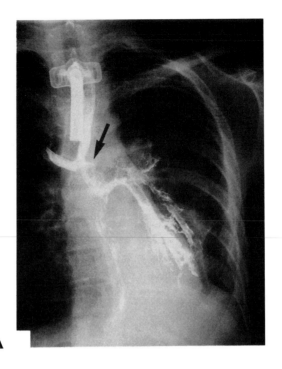

A

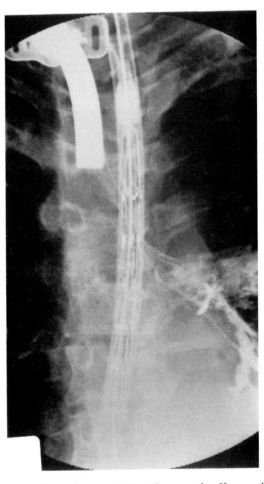

B

Figure 16.20 Treatment of a malignant ERF with covered self-expanding metallic stent.
A. Barium esophagogram demonstrates a fistula (arrow) between the midthoracic esophagus and
the left mainstem bronchus due to a squamous cell carcinoma. B. Immediately after insertion, the
Gianturco-Rösch silicone-covered Z-stent appears to be in excellent position. C. Following page.

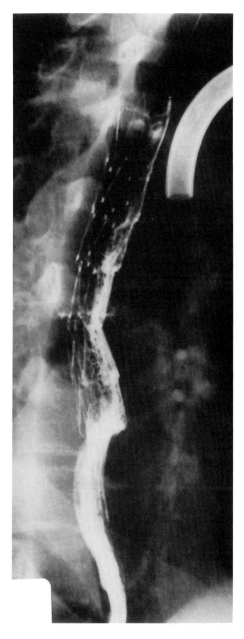

C

Figure 16.20 C. A follow-up barium esophagogram shows unimpeded flow through the stent with complete sealing of the ERF. (From Wu et al.[93] Reproduced by permission.)

of aspiration occur with soft food, then liquid intake can be introduced.[93] Other than the diet modification, postprocedure monitoring is identical to that described previously.

Covered stent placement in patients with an ERF has been reported to achieve sustained relief of aspiration symptoms in 70–75% of patients, with lesser degrees of improvement in the remainder.[89,98] Fluoroscopic guidance permits precise localization of the fistula and strictured segment and allows more accurate stent placement than endoscopic guidance.[89]

REFERENCES

1. Schwartz GF, Polsky HS: Ingested foreign bodies of the gastrointestinal tract. *Am Surg* 42:236–238, 1976.

2. Perelman H: Toothpick perforation of the gastrointestinal tract. *J Abdom Surg* 4:51–53, 1962.

3. Taylor RB: Esophageal foreign bodies. *Emerg Med Clin North Am* 5(2):301–310, 1987.

4. Erbes J, Babbitt DP: Foreign bodies in the alimentary tract of infants and children. *Appl Ther* 7:1103–1109, 1965.

5. Chaikhouni A, Kratz JM, Crawford FA: Foreign bodies of the esophagus. *Am Surg* 51:173–179, 1985.

6. Webb WA: Management of foreign bodies of the upper gastrointestinal tract. *Gastroenterology* 94:204–216, 1988.

7. Kaszar-Seibert DJ, Korn WT, Bindman DJ, et al.: Treatment of acute esophageal food impaction with a combination of glucagon, effervescent agent, and water. *Am J Roentgenol* 154:533–534, 1990.

8. Trenkner SW, Maglinte DDT, Lehman GA, et al: Esophageal food impaction: treatment with glucagon. *Radiology* 149:401–403, 1983.

9. Zimmers TE, Chan SB, Kouchoukos PL, et al: Use of gas-forming agents in esophageal food impactions. *Ann Emerg Med* 17:693–695, 1988.

10. Mohammed SH, Hegedüs V: Dislodgement of impacted oesophageal foreign bodies with carbonated beverages. *Clin Radiol* 37:589–592, 1986.

11. Friedland GW: Opinion. The treatment of acute esophageal food impaction. *Radiology* 149:601–602, 1983.

12. Rice BT, Spiegel PK, Dombrowski PJ: Acute esophageal food impaction treated by gas-forming agents. *Radiology* 146:299–301, 1983.

13. Vizcarrondo FJ, Brady PG, Nord HJ: Foreign bodies of the upper gastrointestinal tract. *Gastrointest Endosc* 29:208–210, 1983.

14. Karanjia ND, Rees M: The use of Coca-Cola in the management of bolus obstruction in benign oesophageal stricture. *Ann Royal Coll Surg Eng* 75:94–95, 1993.

15. Nandi P, Ong GB: Foreign body in the esophagus: review of 2,394 cases. *Br J Surg* 65:5–9, 1978.

16. Kozarek RA, Sanowski RA: Esophageal food impaction. Description of a new method for bolus removal. *Dig Dis Sci* 25:100–103, 1980.

17. Norton RA, King GD: "Steakhouse syndrome". The symptomatic lower esophageal ring. *Lahey Clin Bull* 13:55–59, 1963.

18. Saeed ZA, Michaletz PA, Feiner SD, et al: A new endoscopic method for managing food impaction in the esophagus. *Endoscopy* 22:226–228, 1990.

19. Shaffer HA Jr, de Lange EE: Diagnosis and treatment of food impactions and foreign bodies in the esophagus. In Taveras JM, Ferrucci JT (eds): *Radiology: Diagnosis/Imaging/Intervention*. Philadelphia, Lippincott, 1994, Volume 4, Chapter 15B, pp 1–11.

20. Shaffer HA Jr, de Lange EE: Gastrointestinal foreign bodies and strictures: radiologic interventions. *Curr Probl Diagn Radiol* 23(6):205–252, 1994.

21. Hüpsher DN: *Radiology of the Esophagus*. New York, Thieme Medical Publishers, 1988.

22. Foley MJ, Ghahremani GG, Rogers LF: Reappraisal of constant media used to detect upper gastrointestinal perforations. *Radiology* 144:231–237, 1982.

23. Haglund S, Haverling M, Kuylenstierna R, et al: Radiographic diagnosis of foreign bodies in the esophagus. *J Laryngol Otol* 92:1117–1125, 1978.

24. Douglas M, Sistrom CL: Chicken bone lodged in the upper esophagus: CT findings. *Gastrointest Radiol* 16:11–12, 1991.

25. Spiro HM: *Clinical Gastroenterology*, ed 3. New York, Macmillan, 1983.

26. Selivanov V, Sheldon GF, Cello JP, et al: Management of foreign body ingestion. *Ann Surg* 199:187–191, 1984.

27. Shaffer RD, Klug T: A comparative study of techniques for esophageal foreign body removal with special emphasis on meat bolus obstruction. *Wis Med J* 80:33–36, 1981.

28. Borden S IV: Removal of esophageal foreign bodies by balloon catheter. In Athanasoulis CA, Pfister RC, Greene RE, et al (eds): *Interventional Radiology*. Philadelphia, WB Saunders, 1982.

29. Jaffe RB, Corneli HM: Fluoroscopic removal of ingested alkaline batteries. *Radiology.* 150:585–586, 1984.

30. Ricote GC, Torre LR, Perez De Ayala VP, et al: Fiberendoscopic removal of foreign bodies of the upper part of the gastrointestinal tract. *Surg Gynecol Obstet* 160:499–504, 1985.

31. Giordano A, Adams G, Boies L Jr, et al: Current management of esophageal foreign bodies. *Arch Otolaryngol* 107:249–251, 1981.

32. Classen M, Farthmann EF, Seifert E, et al: Operative and therapeutic techniques in endoscopy. *Clin Gastroenterol* 7:741–763, 1978.

33. Crysdale WS, Sendi KS, Yoo J: Esophageal foreign bodies in children. 15-year review of 484 cases. *Ann Otol Rhinol Laryngol* 100:320–324, 1991.

34. Hawkins DB: Removal of blunt foreign bodies from the esophagus. *Ann Otol Rhinol Laryngol* 99:935–940, 1990.

35. Campbell JB, Condon VR: Catheter removal of blunt esophageal foreign bodies in children. Survey of the Society for Pediatric Radiology. *Pediatr Radiol* 19:361–365, 1989.

36. Litovitz TL: Button battery ingestions. A review of 56 cases. *JAMA* 249:2495–2500, 1983.

37. Litovitz T, Schmitz BF: Ingestion of cylindrical and button batteries: an analysis of 2382 cases. *Pediatrics* 89:747–757, 1992.

38. Votteler TP, Nash JC, Rutledge JC: The hazard of ingested alkaline disk batteries in children. *JAMA* 249:2504–2506, 1983.

39. Blatnik BS, Toohill RJ, Lehman RH: Fatal complications from an alkaline battery foreign body in the esophagus. *Ann Otol* 86:611–615, 1977.

40. Volle E, Beyer P, Kaufmann HJ: Therapeutic approach to ingested button-type batteries. Magnetic removal of ingested button-type batteries. *Pediatr Radiol* 19:114–118, 1989.

41. Paulson EK, Jaffee RB: Metallic foreign bodies in the stomach: fluoroscopic removal with a magnetic orogastric tube. *Radiology* 174:191–194, 1990.

42. Towbin RB, Dunbar JS, Rice S: Magnet catheter for removal of magnetic foreign bodies. *Am J Roentgenol* 154:149–150, 1990.

43. Bigler FC: The use of a Foley catheter for removal of blunt foreign bodies from the esophagus. *J Thorac Cardiovasc Surg* 51:759–760, 1966.

44. Campbell JB, Foley LC: A safe alternative to endoscopic removal of blunt esophageal foreign bodies. *Arch Otolaryngol* 109:323–325, 1983.

45. Campbell JB, Quattromani FL, Foley LC: Foley catheter removal of blunt esophageal foreign bodies. Experience with 100 consecutive children. *Pediatr Radiol* 13:116–119, 1983.

46. Kirks DR: Fluoroscopic catheter removal of blunt esophageal foreign bodies. A pediatric radiologist's perspective. *Pediatr Radiol* 22:64–65, 1992.

47. Nixon GW: Foley catheter method of esophageal foreign body removal: extension of applications. *Am J Roentgen* 132:441–442, 1979.

48. Kushner DC, Cleveland RH: Removal of esophageal foreign bodies in childhood. In Ferrucci JT Jr, Wittenberg J, Mueller PR, et al (ed): *Interventional Radiology of the Abdomen.* Baltimore, Williams & Wilkins, 1984.

49. McGuirt WF: Use of Foley catheter for removal of esophageal foreign bodies. A survey. *Ann Otol Rhinol Laryngol* 91:599–601, 1982.

50. Richardson JR: A new treatment for esophageal obstruction due to meat impaction. *Ann Otol Rhinol Laryngol* 54:328–348, 1945.

51. Robinson AS: Meat impaction in the esophagus treated by enzymatic digestion. *JAMA* 181:1142–1143, 1962.

52. Hargrove MD Jr, Boyce HW Jr: Meat impaction of the esophagus. *Arch Intern Med* 125:277–281, 1970.

53. Nighbert E, Dorton H, Griffen WO Jr: Enzymatic relief of the "steakhouse syndrome." *Am J Surg* 116:467–469, 1968.

54. Hall ML, Huseby JS: Hemorrhagic pulmonary edema associated with meat tenderizer treatment for esophageal meat impaction. *Chest* 94:640–642, 1988.

55. Andersen HA, Bernatz PE, Grindlay JH: Perforation of the esophagus after use of a digestant agent. Report of a case and experimental study. *Ann Otol Rhinol Laryngol* 68:890–896, 1959.

56. Holsinger JW Jr, Fuson RL, Sealy WC: Esophageal perforation following meat impaction and papain ingestion. *JAMA* 204:734–735, 1968.

57. Hogan WJ, Dodds WJ, Hode SE, et al.: Effect of glucagon on esophageal motor function. *Gastroenterology* 69:160–165, 1975.

58. Jaffer SS, Makhlouf GM, Schorr BA, et al: Nature and kinetics of inhibition of lower esophageal sphincter pressure by glucagon. *Gastroenterology* 67:42–46, 1974.

59. Ferrucci JT Jr, Long JA Jr: Radiologic treatment of esophageal food impaction using intravenous glucagon. *Radiology* 125:25–28, 1977.

60. Marks HW, Lousteau RJ: Glucagon and esophageal meat impaction. *Arch Otolaryngol* 105:367–368, 1979.

61. Berger K, McCallum RW: Nifedipine in the treatment of achalasia. *Ann Intern Med* 96:61–62, 1982.

62. Nasrallah SM: Nifedipine in the treatment of diffuse oesophageal spasm. *Lancet* 2:1285, 1982.

63. Nasrallah SM, Tommaso CL, Singleton RT, et al: Primary esophageal motor disorders: clinical response to nifedipine, *South Med J* 78:312–315, 1985.

64. Bell AF, Eibling DE: Letter. Nifedipine in the treatment of distal esophageal food impaction. *Arch Otolaryngol Head Neck Surg* 114:682–683, 1988.

65. Swamy N: Esophageal spasm: clinical and manometric response to nitroglycerin and long acting nitrites. *Gastroenterology* 72:23–27, 1977.

66. Nickerson M: Vasodilator drugs. In Goodman LS, Giman A (eds): *Pharmacological Basis of Therapeutics*, ed 4. New York, Macmillan, 1971.

67. Ignotus PI, Grundy A: Disimpaction of swallowed bolus. *Br Med J* 298:1359, 1989.

68. Zalev AH: Radiologic treatment of a patient with the "steakhouse syndrome": case report. *J Can Assoc Radiol* 39:59–61, 1988.

69. Caravati EM, Bennett DL, McElwee NE: Pediatric coin ingestion: a prospective study on the utility of routine roentgenograms. *Am J Dis Child* 143:549–551, 1989.

70. Smith JC, Janower ML, Geiger AH: Use of glucagon and gas-forming agents in acute esophageal food impaction. *Radiology* 159:567–568, 1986.

71. Shaffer HA Jr, Alford BA, de Lange EE, et al: Basket extraction of esophageal foreign bodies. *Am J Roentgenol* 147:1010–1013, 1986.

72. McCray RS: Foreign body endoscopy. *Gastrointest Endosc* 27:236–237, 1981.

73. Hildreth CT: Stricture of the esophagus. *N Engl J Med Surg* 10:235–240, 1821.

74. London RL, Trotman BW, Di Marino AJ, et al: Dilatation of severe esophageal strictures by an inflatable balloon catheter. *Gastroenterology* 80:173–175, 1981.

75. Grüntzig A, Hofff H: Perkutane Rekanalisation chronischer arterieller Verschlüsse mit einem neuen Dilatationskatheter: Modification der DotterTechnik. *Dtsch Med Wochenschr* 99:2502–2505, 1974.

76. Starck E, Paolucci V, Herzer M, et al: Esophageal stenosis: treatment with balloon catheters. *Radiology* 153:637–640, 1984.

77. Dawson SL, Mueller PR, Ferrucci JT, et al: Severe esophageal strictures: indications for balloon catheter dilatation. *Radiology* 153:631–635, 1984.

78. Götberg S, Afzelius LE, Hambraeus G, et al: Balloon-catheter dilatation of strictures in the upper digestive tract. *Radiology* 22:479–483, 1984.

79. Kollath J, Starck E, Paolucci V: Dilation of esophageal stenosis by balloon catheter. *Cardiovasc Intervent Radiol* 7:35–39, 1984.

80. Starck E, Paolucci V, Onneken M, et al: Konservativen Behandlung von Oesophagusstenosen mit Ballon Katheter. *Dtsch Med Wochenschr* 110:1025–1030, 1985.

81. Kozarek RA: Hydrostatic balloon dilation of gastrointestinal stenosis: a national survey. *Gastrointest Endosc* 32:15–19, 1986.

82. de Lange EE, Shaffer HA: Anastomotic strictures of the upper gastrointestinal tract: results of balloon dilation. *Radiology* 167:45–50, 1988.

83. Huynh PT, de Lange EE, Shaffer HA Jr: Symptomatic webs of the upper esophagus: treatment with fluoroscopically guided balloon dilation. *Radiology* 196:789–792, 1995.

84. McLean GK, Cooper GS, Hartz WH, et al: Radiologically guided balloon dilation of gastrointestinal strictures. Part I. Technique and factors influencing procedural success. *Radiology* 165:35–40, 1987.

85. McLean GK, Cooper GS, Hartz WH, et al: Radiologically guided balloon dilation of gastrointestinal strictures. Part II. Results of long-term follow-up. *Radiology* 165:41–43, 1987.

86. Maynar M, Guerra C, Reyes R, et al: Esophageal strictures: balloon dilatation. *Radiology* 167:703–706, 1988.

87. Celestin LR: Permanent intubation in inoperative cancer of the esophagus and cardia. *Ann R Coll Surg Engl* 25:165–170, 1959.

88. Frimberger E: Expanding spiral—a new type of prosthesis for the palliative treatment of malignant esophageal stenoses. *Endoscopy* 15:213–214, 1983.

89. Do YS, Song H-Y, Lee BH, et al: Esophagorespiratory fistula associated with esophageal cancer: treatment with a Gianturco stent tube. *Radiology* 187:673–677, 1993.

90. Cwikiel W, Stridbeck H, Tranberg K-G, et al: Malignant esophageal strictures: treatment with a self-expanding nitinol stent. *Radiology* 187:661–665, 1993.

91. Knyrim K, Wagner H-J, Bethge N, et al: A controlled trial of an expansile metal stent for palliation of esophageal obstruction due to inoperable cancer. *N Engl J Med* 329:1302–1307, 1993.

92. Song H-Y, Do Y-S, Han Y-M, et al: Covered, expandable esophageal metallic stent tubes: experiences in 119 patients. *Radiology* 193:689–695, 1994.

93. Wu WC, Katon RM, Saxon RR, et al: Silicone-covered self-expanding metallic stents for the palliation of malignant esophageal obstruction and esophagorespiratory fistulas: experience in 32 patients and a review of the literature. *Gastrointest Endosc* 40:22–33, 1994.

94. Goldin E, Beyar M, Safra T, et al: A new self-expandable, nickel-titanium coil stent for esophageal obstruction: a preliminary report. *Gastrointest Endosc* 40:64–68, 1994.

95. Cwikiel W: Esophageal stenting. In Cope C: *Current Techniques in Interventional Radiology.* Philadelphia, Current Medicine, 1995, pp 134–142.

96. Watkinson AF, Ellul J, Entwisle K, et al: Esophageal carcinoma: initial results of palliative treatment with covered self-expanding endoprosthesis. *Radiology* 195:821–827, 1995.

97. Cwikiel W: Esophageal nitinol stents: long-term results. In Liermann DD: *Stents—State of the Art and Future Developments.* Watertown, MA, Boston Scientific Corp, 1995, pp 218–221.

98. Rösch J, Saxon RR, Barton RE, et al: Silicone-covered self-expandable Z-stents in the treatment of malignant esophageal obstructions and esophagorespiratory fistulas. In Liermann DD: *Stents—State of the Art and Future Developments.* Watertown, MA, Boston Scientific Corp, 1995, pp 222–228.

99. Yang R-J, Wang X-D, Song S-W, et al: Digestive duct stenting: report of primary cases. In Liermann DD: *Stents—State of the Art and Future Developments.* Watertown, MA, Boston Scientific Corp, 1995, pp 239–245.

100. Shaffer HA, Valenzuela G, Mittal RK: Esophageal perforation: a reassessment of the criteria for choosing medical or surgical therapy. *Arch Int Med* 152:757–761, 1992.

101. Orringer MB, Orringer JS: Esophagectomy without thoracotomy: a dangerous operation? *J Thorac Cardiovasc Surg* 85:72–80, 1983.

102. Orringer MB: Transhiatal esophagectomy for benign disease. *J Thorac Cardiovasc Surg* 90:649–655, 1985.

103. Orringer MB, Lemmer JH: Early dilatation in the treatment of esophageal disruption. *Ann Thorac Surg* 42:536–539, 1986.

104. de Lange EE, Shaffer HA, Daniel TM, et al: Esophageal anastomotic leaks: preliminary results of treatment with balloon dilation. *Radiology* 165:45–47, 1987.

105. de Lange EE, Shaffer HA Jr, Holt PD: Esophagoenteric anastomotic leaks: treatment with fluoroscopically guided balloon dilatation. *Am J Roentgenol* 162:51–54, 1994.

C H A P T E R
17

Interventional Breast Procedures

Ellen Shaw de Paredes, Phan T. Huynh, Melinda M. Dunn

INTERVENTIONAL BREAST PROCEDURES

The role of the breast imager has expanded to encompass the performance of several interventional procedures, such as galactography, percutaneous breast biopsy, cyst aspiration, and lesion localization techniques. In this chapter, we will discuss patient selection, indications, contraindications, techniques, diagnostic considerations, and outcome for each of these procedures.

NEEDLE LOCALIZATION OF NONPALPABLE BREAST LESIONS

For mammographic abnormalities that are suspicious but nonpalpable, needle localization (NL) is performed prior to excisional biopsy or lumpectomy. The purpose of NL is to facilitate precise excision of the lesion and minimize the amount of surrounding normal tissue that is removed. If there is a large volume of normal tissue resected, the risk of missing the lesion in the pathologic specimen increases, particularly if the lesion is small. The accuracy of excisional biopsy in determining the diagnosis can be improved when less normal tissue is excised. Removing a minimum amount of surrounding normal tissue is also important for cosmesis.

The localization of a nonpalpable breast lesion has been affected most by the development of two instruments—the localization grid or plate and a needle loaded with a hookwire.[1] Before the advent of localizer plates, the radiologist triangulated from the mammographic images to determine the location of the lesion. This approach often required multiple needle passes to accurately place the needle tip in the region of interest. Although the patient was sent to the operating room with the needle taped in position, the needle tip could be easily displaced from its position in the breast.

The development of flexible hookwire systems permits much more patient mobility with decreased likelihood of displacement of the localization device. Kopans and Deluca[2] described the development of a commonly used spring-loaded hookwire and localizer needle (Cook, Inc., Bloomington, IN). Homer[3] later described the development of a J wire with a Mammalok system (Namic, Great Falls, NY) that allowed retraction and replacement of an already released wire without the need for placement of a second wire. This wire is thicker and less flexible than many varieties of spring-loaded hookwires.

Typical needles used for localization are 20-gauge in caliber and 3.0–15.0 cm in length. The choice of needle length depends upon the depth of the lesion in the breast and the compressibility of the intervening tissue. It is best to choose a needle and wire longer than necessary, because a wire that is too short can completely retract into the breast and out of sight when breast compression is released. The most commonly used wire configurations are nonretractable V shapes or retractable J hooks. Total wire lengths are at least 10.0 cm greater than the needle length.

Prior to the procedure, the mammograms must be reviewed to determine the appropriate mode of imaging guidance for NL (mammographic, sonographic, or stereotactic), the direction of needle placement, and the needle length to be used. If a 90° lateral (mediolateral) mammogram is not available, it should be performed to define the exact location of the lesion. The skin surface closest to the lesion is determined (medial, lateral, superior, or inferior) on the basis of two orthogonal views of the lesion (craniocaudal and mediolateral). If mammographic guidance is to be used, a localization plate with either multiple round perforations or a rectangular aperture is placed on the surface of the breast, and a film is made. Compression is not released until the localization procedure is complete. By reading the alphanumeric coordinates of the aperture on the compression plate over the lesion, the correct location for needle insertion is determined.

The skin is cleansed with an antiseptic solution. Local anesthesia is not necessary for most patients undergoing NL unless multiple needle passes are anticipated.[4] If a needle and hookwire are used without any injection of dye, the wire is kept inside the needle but is withdrawn slightly from the needle tip to avoid premature deployment. The needle is placed through the appropriate aperture (X and Y dimension) and is advanced parallel to the chest wall. The required depth of needle advancement (Z dimension) is estimated from the relative location of the lesion, with allowances being made for the compressed thickness of the breast. A film is made to confirm accurate placement of the needle in the X and Y dimensions (Figure 17.1A). The localizer plate is then carefully removed while the needle is held in position. The orthogonal view is obtained to determine the depth of the needle (Z dimension) relative to the lesion (Figure 17.1B). It is better to place the needle too deep than too shallow to avoid having to advance the needle without the localizer plate for guidance (Figure 17.1C). If the needle has been advanced beyond the lesion, it can be withdrawn so that its tip is in the lesion. When the needle is in satisfactory position, the wire can be deployed by inserting it until its tip is just beyond the tip of the needle. The needle is then removed as the wire is held in position (Figure 17.1D). For the J system, the wire is advanced into the breast to form the J configuration, and then the needle is removed.

Dye (methylene or isosalfan blue) can be injected through the localization needle after radiographic confirmation of accurate needle placement to mark the tissue containing the lesion.[5] The needle may be withdrawn as dye is also injected into the tract, marking the path to the lesion for the surgeon. A needle or hookwire can also be deployed in the lesion. Because the dye quickly diffuses into the adjacent tissues, the excisional biopsy must immediately follow the dye localization procedure. Diffusion of the dye over time produces a less accurate localization. However, if a localizing wire has been inadvertently displaced, previous dye instillation can still direct the surgeon to the correct area.

Final films in the mediolateral and craniocaudal projections are made to demonstrate the tip of the wire relative to the lesion. The hook of the wire should be within 1 cm of the lesion. It is helpful if the radiologist marks the lesion on the final films and sends the films to the operating room with the patient (Figure 17.2). In addition, the approach used, the length of wire inside the breast (total wire length minus length outside the skin), and the relationship of the lesion to the hook should be described for the surgeon. The wire is taped to the breast and covered with a gauze bandage. The patient then goes to the operating room for surgical excision of the lesion.

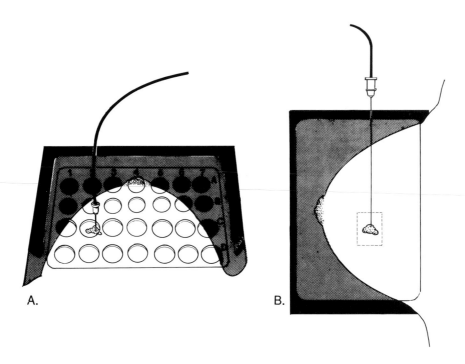

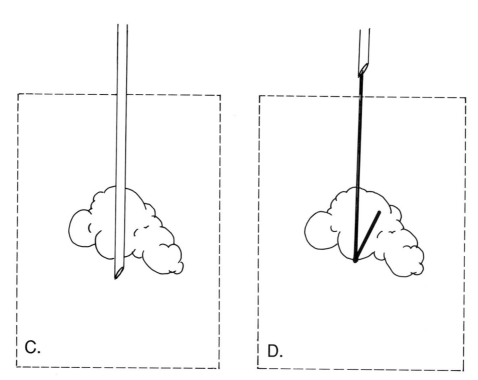

Figure 17.1 **A.** An alphanumeric grid is placed over the skin surface closest to the lesion, and the X Y coordinates are determined. **B.** The orthogonal view is performed to determine the depth (Z coordinate) of the needle relative to the lesion. **C.** The needle is placed in the lesion and is withdrawn as the hookwire is inserted. **D.** Once deployed, the hookwire is pulled back slightly to engage the hook in tissue.

The surgical approach for needle-localized lesions varies. Some surgeons cut down along the path of the wire. Others triangulate and make the incision cephalad or caudad to the entry point of the wire, dissecting back toward the hook. Knowledge of the length of wire within breast tissue is particularly important for surgeons who use the triangulation technique for resection.

A specimen radiograph should always be performed. The surgeon must be immediately informed whether the tissue specimen contains the lesion and the relationship of the lesion to the margins of the specimen.[6–9] Once the biopsy sample is considered satisfactory, the specimen is placed in a holder with an alphanumeric grid system for radiography to facilitate localization of the lesion for the pathologist (Figure 17.3). The specimen is transported in the grid system to the pathologist, and the region of interest is indicated. If microcalcifications are present, the pathologist must search for the calcium deposits in the specimen to ensure complete specimen analysis.

Specimen radiography is performed with compression and magnification using 22–23 kVp and low mAs.[9] Although microcalcifications are readily visible on mammography, they may not be visualized on routine hematoxylin and eosin stained histologic specimens. Therefore, for specimens containing microcalcifications, the paraffin-fixed tissue slices prepared by the pathology laboratory can be radiographed to determine in which section the microcalcifications are located.[10] Polarized light may be required to demonstrate these birefringent calcium-containing particles.[11]

Potential complications of an NL procedure include: hematoma, infection, migration of the wire (including into the pleural space), and pneumothorax.[12–15] Rappaport et al. found an infection rate of about 8% in patients who underwent NL prior to exci-

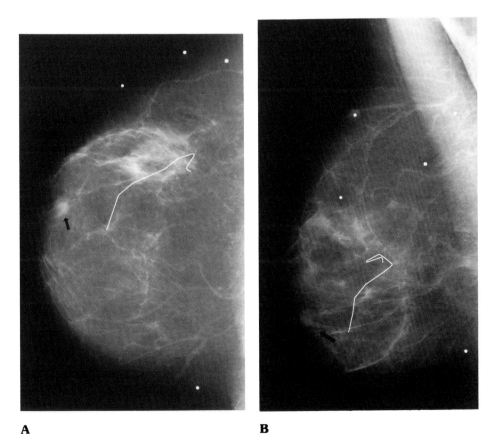

A　　　　　　　　**B**

Figure 17.2 A. Left craniocaudal (CC) and B. mediolateral oblique (MLO) views show a 9-mm indistinct mass in the subareolar area at the 4 o'clock position (arrows). C, D, E, F, and G. Following pages.

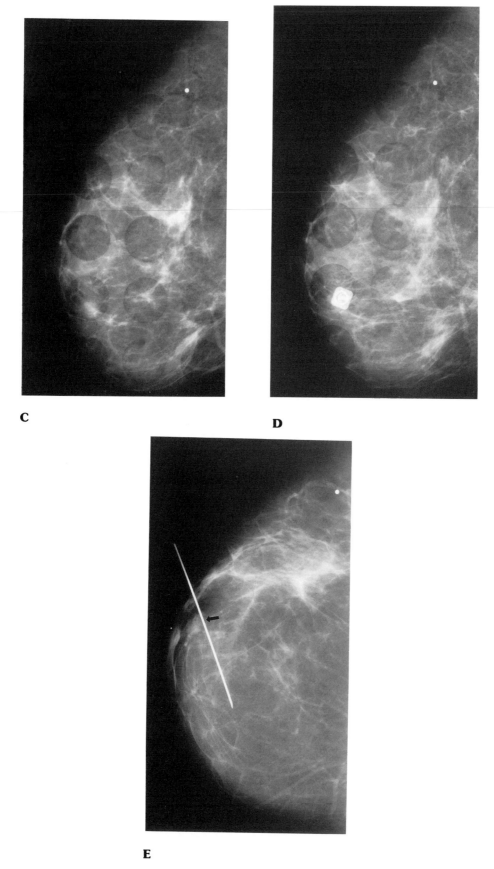

C

D

E

Figure 17.2 C. The localizer plate is placed over lateral aspect of breast on lateromedial (LM) view. D. The needle is placed into breast through the aperture and a confirmatory film is made. E. Craniocaudal film demonstrates the needle tip to be 3 cm deep to lesion. F and G. Following page.

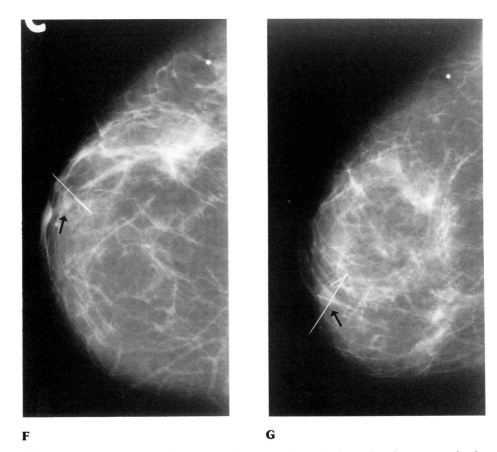

F   **G**

Figure 17.2 The needle has been withdrawn and the hookwire has been inserted. The hookwire passes directly through the mass (arrow) and the hook of the wire is located just deep to it. F. Final CC and G. LM films are made and sent with the patient. Pathology: mucinous carcinoma.

sional biopsy.[13] The infection rate in this series may be high because of factors not related to the NL procedure, such as use of surgical drains. Pneumothoraces and wire migrations can be prevented by inserting the needle parallel to the chest wall and using a wire of sufficient length, respectively.

Complete absence of the targeted lesion on an NL excisional biopsy has been reported in 0–17% of procedures.[16–19] If the lesion is not documented to be within the biopsy sample on specimen radiography, the surgeon should remove additional tissue. If the abnormality cannot be found within the removed specimen(s), repeat mammography in 2 to 3 months is required. Occasional difficulties encountered in the interpretation of the specimen radiograph may make an immediate postoperative mammogram useful.[20]

Ultrasound-guided Localization

Ultrasound is an excellent guidance modality for localizing masses not detectable on mammographic films, for lesions difficult to approach through a mammographic localizer grid, or in women who are unable to sit up for a mammographic localization.[21] It is especially helpful for cyst aspiration procedures and is being used with increasing frequency for NL, fine needle aspiration biopsy (FNAB), and large-gauge core biopsy (LGCB) of breast lesions. The development of high-resolution and high-frequency

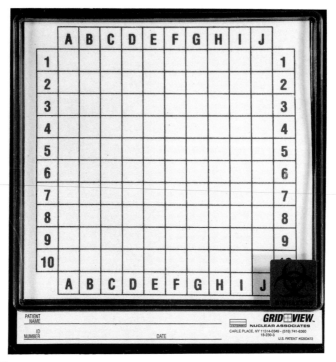

Figure 17.3 Specimen transport device incorporates an alphanumeric grid system to indicate the region of interest on specimen radiography to the pathologist.

transducers (7.5% MHz or greater) has significantly facilitated the ability to directly visualize the needle as it is advanced into the abnormality. Videotape documentation can be used to demonstrate accurate needle placement, the path of sampling for FNAB, and the area sampled by the LGCB needle[22] (Figure 17.4).

In preparation for the ultrasound-guided procedure, the transducer is covered with a sterile sleeve and the skin overlying the abnormality is sterilely prepared. Sterile coupling gel is used on the patient. A biopsy guide can be used but is usually not necessary. The needle can be inserted along the long or short axis of the transducer[21] (Figure 17.5). With the long-axis approach, the ultrasound transducer is positioned along the axis of needle insertion. It is usually safer than the short-axis approach because the needle is inserted almost parallel to the chest wall. This approach may also be easier because the needle tip is observed as it is advanced toward and into the lesion. This technique is preferred for LGCB to minimize the chance of advancing the needle into the chest wall and pleural space. The disadvantages of the long-axis approach are that the needle path is longer than with a short-axis approach and the lesion may be displaced as the needle is advanced toward it.

The short-axis approach is preferred for superficial lesions or big breasts. It is more difficult for the operator because the needle shaft is not seen until its tip is in the plane of the lesion. Therefore, the operator must be able to triangulate the location of the lesion based upon the predetermined estimate of the depth of the lesion and the angle of needle insertion. To approach a superficial lesion, a flat or shallow angle is used, whereas a deep lesion requires a more vertical angle of needle insertion (Figure 17.6).[22]

Specimen radiography is unlikely to be useful for NLs performed with sonographic guidance since most of the lesions are not well-delineated with radiography. Instead, sonography of the surgical specimen with a high-frequency linear-array transducer (i.e., at least 7.5 MHz) and a water path (step-off pad) is performed for documentation of lesion removal.

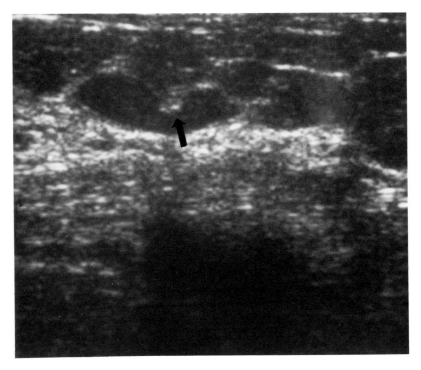

Figure 17.4 Sonographic guidance for needle placement in a solid mass demonstrates needle tip in the lesion (arrow).

Stereotactic Needle Localizations

Guidance using stereotactic breast imaging has significantly improved the ability to accurately place a needle into small, nonpalpable lesions. Stereotactic guidance can also be used for needle aspiration of a cyst, NL for surgical biopsy, FNAB, and LGCB. This technology has had a large impact on the diagnostic algorithm for breast abnormalities, with more and more biopsies being obtained by percutaneous techniques rather than open or surgical methods. The two basic components of a stereotactic unit are the imaging components (compression device, x-ray tube, receptor, and biopsy apparatus) and the equipment used for determining the location of the lesion (a computer with a digital workstation or a light box for viewing the film screen images).[23] Stereo-

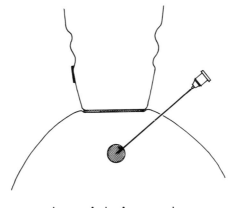

Long Axis Approach

Figure 17.5 Long-axis approach shows needle shaft and the needle tip in the lesion.

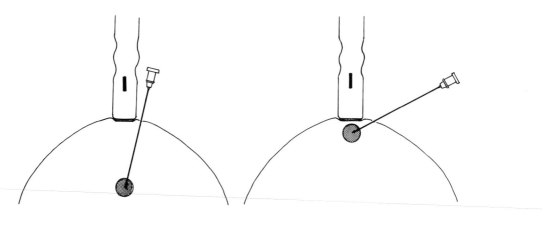

A. Deep Lesion   B. Superficial Lesion

Short Axis Approach

Figure 17.6 Short-axis approach for needle placement into a deep lesion **A.** and superficial lesion **B.** demonstrates the needle tip in the target lesion and the angle of obliquity used.

tactic guidance can also be performed using upright attachments to mammographic units or with dedicated prone table units.

In preparation for a stereotactic-guided biopsy, two 15° oblique films are made over the area of interest while the breast is compressed by a fenestrated compression device. This is accomplished by shifting the tube 15° from midline while the breast and receptor remain in a stationary position. These spot views of the breast should demonstrate the lesion relative to a reference point that is located in the film holder. The exact three-dimensional (X, Y, and Z) coordinates of the lesion relative to the reference point are determined by the computer. Depending on the type of system being used, reference points are initially indicated as the zero position. The lesion is then identified on the images obtained and the point or points for needle placement are targeted. For NL, the center of the lesion is targeted; for FNAB and LGCB, multiple areas within the abnormality are targeted. The computer then reads the X, Y, and Z coordinates of the lesion and transmits this information to the needle holder component on the machine. The shortest needle length that will reach the lesion is indicated by the computer. The length of the needle used for the biopsy must either be determined by the computer program or measured on the images. The calculation of needle length is crucial, because the change in the Z (ΔZ) position of the needle guide is determined relative to the needle length. The needle guide is then moved into a position where the ΔX, ΔY, and ΔZ or the change in distance between the targeted lesion and the guide position for each dimension (X, Y, and Z) s turned to 0.00 mm. Once the guide is positioned directly over the lesion, a needle of appropriate length is inserted until its hub is in contact with the top of the needle guide. At this point, the needle tip should be in the center of the lesion.

Repeat stereotactic images are performed to document accurate needle placement. For NLs, the needle is advanced 5 mm beyond the lesion in the Z coordinate.[24,25] The hookwire is advanced to the end of the needle. The shaft of the wire is then held firmly as the needle is withdrawn. The stereotactic guides are carefully pulled back over the shaft of the hookwire extending outside the breast and compression is released. Final craniocaudal and mediolateral films are obtained to confirm accurate wire placement.

Occasionally, a small, irregular density or mass may not be evident on one of the two orthogonal mammographic views because of superimposed dense parenchyma. In this situation, stereotactic guidance is much more reliable than standard mammographic guidance techniques. The lesion can be localized by placing the stereotactic guidance aperture over the surface of the breast in the projection in which the lesion is seen. With stereotactic guidance, an NL procedure can also be performed rapidly and with a minimum number of x-ray exposures.

The primary drawback to stereotactic NL is that the guidance aperture is small and the technologist may have a difficult time centering the lesion directly under the aperture.[24] The center of the lesion must be accurately targeted to avoid creating a significant disparity in the actual and measured depth (Z coordinate) of the lesion. Early experience with stereotactic NL was disappointing because the hookwire was often too shallow or too deep.[24,25] When the needle tip is placed 5 mm beyond the lesion in the Z coordinate and the hookwire is carefully deployed, localization will be accurate. When breasts are large or fatty, or when the lesion is in a deep, central position, compensation for the effect of breast reexpansion after release of compression is necessary. In this setting, the Z coordinate of the guiding needle may need to be as much as 10 mm deep to the lesion.[26]

In most NL series from the United States, the presence of malignancy is demonstrated in about 10–40% of biopsies.[27–31] This positive biopsy rate is similar to the rate found with surgical excision of palpable lesions. The majority of lesions biopsied are some form of fibrocystic change.[32] In a series of 220 patients who underwent NL and biopsy, Herman et al.[33] classified mammographic abnormalities as "probably benign" or "probably malignant" and were correct in only 68% of the cases. Therefore, an aggressive approach to sampling indeterminate lesions is needed to avoid missing a significant number of nonpalpable breast cancers.

PERCUTANEOUS BREAST BIOPSY

Because the majority of breast lesions are benign, it is imperative that less costly and less invasive methods be developed to evaluate breast abnormalities. Percutaneous biopsies are less expensive and less morbid than surgical biopsies and can be used to confirm a benign diagnosis for indeterminate lesions and to confirm the presence of malignancy in highly suspicious lesions. Those lesions that are probably benign (likelihood of malignancy less than 2%) should not be sampled percutaneously; instead, follow-up mammography should be performed in 3–6 months.

Palpable Breast Lesions

Initial experience with palpable breast lesions began with excisional or incisional biopsy techniques. Refinements in FNAB and cytologic analysis have led to a significant trend toward using percutaneous biopsy techniques to sample breast abnormalities.[34] The initial recommended intervention for a palpable breast mass is FNAB. This technique is less costly and less invasive than surgical biopsy, and the results can be used to plan the best therapeutic regimen for the patient. Fine needle aspiration biopsy has a sensitivity of 70–95%[35–37] and a specificity of 98–100%. It is a quick, easy, and cost-effective method of obtaining tissue from a breast lesion.[38] The combination of mammography, clinical examination, and FNAB for the evaluation of a palpable mass is a reliable method of managing most breast lesions.[35,39] If the FNAB is negative, but the lesion is clinically suspicious, excision of the mass is performed for a more definitive diagnosis. Patients with palpable, nonsuspicious lesions and a negative FNAB should still receive close clinical and mammographic follow-up.[36,37] With the addition of an unremarkable breast ultrasound to a negative mammogram and FNAB and a nonsuspicious clinical examination, Bucchi et al. found a negative predictive value for malignancy of 100%.[40]

When performing FNAB, a 22-g or smaller needle is used for solid masses and an 18- to 21-g needle is used for cyst aspiration. The skin over the mass is cleansed, and the mass is grasped between two fingers. Local anesthesia (1% lidocaine; Astra Corp., Westboro, MA) can be used, particularly if multiple passes or the use of a larger gauge needle are anticipated. The needle is advanced into the mass and suction is applied to the biopsy needle with a 20-cc syringe. The use of short plastic tubing to connect the needle to the syringe provides better control of the needle by the operator while an assistant applies suction to the syringe. The needle is moved rapidly in and out in multiple areas of the mass.[41] When material is observed in the hub of the needle, suction is released and the needle is removed from the breast. The aspirate should not be allowed to enter the tubing or syringe, because it may be difficult to empty the contents completely. The material is expelled in droplets onto glass slides and smeared. The method for fixation of the specimen depends upon the cytology laboratory. The specimen slides can be air dried or the smears may be immediately fixed with such substances as 95% alcohol. Slide fixation must be coordinated with the cytopathologist.

If fluid is obtained on needle insertion, the mass is drained completely. Manual pressure can be applied to the mass to effect more complete drainage. Clear straw-colored fluid aspirated from a presumed cyst is not generally sent for analysis.[42] If fluid from a benign cyst is sent for cytologic analysis, the typical findings consist of apocrine metaplasia, which reflects the cells that line the cyst cavity. However, if the fluid is turbid or sanguinous, it is sent for pathologic review.

For noncystic masses or for masses that are still palpable or unresolved even after all the fluid is aspirated, FNAB is performed.[40] For palpable lesions, three needle samples are commonly obtained. For nonpalpable lesions, even more passes may be needed to acquire sufficient cytologic material.[41,43] For FNAB to be successful, it is necessary for the cytology laboratory to be highly reliable and positive breast aspirates be definitive for carcinoma.

Nonpalpable Cyst Aspiration

Most breast cysts do not need to be aspirated. The indications for aspiration of a cystic mass are (1) drainage to provide symptomatic relief of a painful mass, and (2) the cystic nature of the mass is equivocal on ultrasound because of internal echoes, wall thickening, or a filling defect. Nonpalpable cysts that are 1 cm or greater in diameter and are visualized on both ultrasound and mammography can be aspirated under the guidance of either modality.

For mammographic-guided aspiration, the localizing plate is placed on the skin surface closest to the cyst and a film is made. A 20-g needle of appropriate length is advanced parallel to the chest wall into the breast through the aperture overlying the lesion. A repeat film is made to confirm the accuracy of needle placement. A syringe is connected to the needle and suction applied as the needle is slowly withdrawn. When fluid begins to fill the syringe, the needle is maintained in position as the aspiration is completed. When no more fluid can be withdrawn, the needle is kept in position with its tip in the cyst. The syringe containing fluid is disconnected and replaced with a syringe filled with room air equal to the amount of fluid removed from the cyst. The air is injected into the cyst and the needle and localizing plate are removed from the breast. Final craniocaudal and mediolateral views are obtained to evaluate the cyst cavity. Pneumocystography will demonstrate the internal characteristics of the cyst cavity and define the presence of any filling defects that might suggest a papilloma or papillary carcinoma. A cyst with a smooth inner wall contour is benign. Injecting air into the cyst cavity may also have some therapeutic value in decreasing the likelihood of fluid reaccumulation.[44]

If no fluid is obtained during mammographically guided cyst aspiration, the localizer plate can be removed and the orthogonal view can be obtained to show the relationship of the needle tip to the mass.[45,46] Once the appropriate placement of the needle tip in the lesion is confirmed, either cyst aspiration or FNAB of a noncystic mass can then be performed.

Sonography is an excellent guidance modality for cyst aspiration because it is relatively easy, requires no radiation, and offers real-time documentation of the outcome of the procedure. Once the needle tip is visualized within the mass (see Figures 17.5 and 17.6), suction is applied and fluid is removed. Aspiration is continued until the cyst disappears.

Stereotactic guidance affords a highly accurate method of needle placement in small circumscribed nodules that are poorly visualized with ultrasound. Postaspiration radiographs are obtained to verify successful drainage of a cyst. If fluid is not obtained, FNAB is performed.

Fine Needle Aspiration Biopsy of Nonpalpable Lesions

Fine needle aspiration biopsy of nonpalpable breast lesions was performed in Sweden in the late 1970s and in the U.S. in the 1980s using standard mammographic guidance.[45-48] This procedure has become more accurate with stereotactic and sonographic guidance and has provided an excellent alternative to surgical biopsy for the evaluation of many breast lesions. For well-circumscribed masses that are likely to be cysts, for some fibroadenomas and for many carcinomas, FNAB is generally diagnostic.[49] Even for malignant microcalcifications without an associated mass, FNAB has been found to be successful in the diagnosis of carcinoma.[49,50] However, many lesions that mimic carcinoma mammographically actually are various forms of benign fibrocystic change, a difficult diagnosis to establish by FNAB. Therefore, indeterminate groups of microcalcifications and some indistinct masses are not suitable for this technique. In addition, since cytopathologic analysis of a breast biopsy relies on the identification of duct cells, lesions such as fibrosis and sclerotic fibroadenomas that are primarily fibrotic and lack epithelium may present a problem.[49,51,52] In such instances, it is important that the cytologic and mammographic features of the lesion be correlated in order to determine the most appropriate course of action.[49,52-54]

Reported sensitivities with stereotactic FNAB of nonpalpable lesions range from 73% to 97%, with specificities of 72% to 100%.[50,55] The rate of insufficient samples has ranged from 0% to 26%.[56] A distinct advantage of FNAB with a cytopathologist on-site is that slides can be reviewed immediately, and the sufficiency of the sampling as well as the diagnosis can be determined before the patient leaves the department.

Supplies that are used for FNAB with stereotactic guidance include the following: sterile needle guides of appropriate caliber to fit the biopsy needle, antiseptic solution, sterile gauze, 1% lidocaine in a syringe equipped with a 25-g needle, 20-cc syringe for aspiration, short plastic tubing, 20-g outer cannula (for a coaxial biopsy technique), 22-g aspirating needle (usually 7.5 to 10.5 cm long), sterile glass slides, and fixative (if needed by the laboratory). Specifically designed needle sets for use with a coaxial biopsy technique include the Precision Guide (II) (Becton and Dickinson, Franklin Lakes, NJ) and the Jackson aspirating set (MD Tech, Gainesville, FL). A coaxial technique provides increased stability of the biopsy needle, less deflection of the needle on entering a firm lesion, and the ability to obtain multiple samples rapidly.

For stereotactic FNAB, the lesion is placed in the field of the aperture and 15° stereotactic images are obtained. The center of the lesion and peripheral points at the 12, 3, 6, and 9 o'clock positions are targeted. The coordinates for these points are transmitted from the computer to the stereotactic device. The minimum needle length that will reach the lesion is determined by the computer. The length of needle to be used is programmed into the machine. The needle guides are then moved to the ΔX, ΔY, and ΔZ positions at 0.00 mm. The ΔZ coordinate of the needle guide is set at 5 to 10 mm deep to the lesion. The needle is placed into the breast until its hub is in contact with the top of the needle guide. Stereotactic images are performed to verify needle position in the lesion. The aspiration biopsy is then performed by traversing the lesion with a back and forth motion.

With the coaxial technique, a 20-g outer cannula or guiding needle is placed 5 mm above or proximal to the center of the lesion. A 22-gauge Chiba needle (Cook, Inc.) or a 22-gauge Wescott-type needle (Cook, Inc.) with a sharp open point as well as a cutting trough at its edge is advanced through the lumen of the outer, guiding needle into the lesion. Once the biopsy sample is obtained, the biopsy needle is removed. Additional samples can be rapidly acquired if the guiding needle has not been displaced.

Sampling for FNAB can be optimized by following several steps: performing multiple needle passes in the lesion at different ΔX and ΔY positions; aspirating for at least 5 sec with each pass; avoiding the loss of cells by minimizing material being withdrawn out of the needle hub into the tubing or syringe; and using a larger bore needle for lesions that do not yield many cells.

Large-gauge Core Biopsy

The difficulty in obtaining a definitive diagnosis of benign lesions by FNAB prompted the development of large-gauge core biopsy (LGCB) techniques. Early experience with breast biopsy by automated core biopsy sampling involved use of 18-g needles.[57] Because of tissue fragmentation and poor sampling, larger gauge needles were used. Good samples have been routinely achieved with 14-g needles.[58,59] Lesions that are amenable to LGCB are the following: well-defined solid masses, indistinct or spiculated masses, and clustered microcalcifications.[58,60,61] Percutaneous LGCB is particularly advantageous in the evaluation of multiple clusters of suspicious microcalcifications or multiple malignant-appearing masses in the same breast because biopsies can be performed at multiple sites without causing much cosmetic deformity.

Problematic lesions for LGCB are those that are difficult to target, very small lesions, and lesions in small breasts. Posterior lesions near the chest wall and superficial and periareolar lesions, indistinct masses, and fine microcalcifications may present problems in targeting.[62] Not only are lesions smaller than 5 mm difficult to target, but also a good portion of the lesion may be removed with LGCB. Since the volume of the lesion is reduced, it may not be visualized on follow-up mammography. If the biopsy is positive for malignancy, a therapeutic problem arises because complete surgical resection of the tumor is needed, yet the residual portion of the lesion cannot be localized.[63] It is also very difficult to obtain an LGCB in breasts that compress to 25 mm or less because of the length required for needle excursion during the biopsy procedure. For extremely suspicious lesions in which one may not be satisfied with a benign result, NL and excisional biopsy may be preferred.[63] Another particularly problematic lesion to diagnose by LGCB is a radial scar. Because the pathologic architecture of the entire lesion needs to be studied, biopsy of a segment of a radial scar can produce a suspicious histologic appearance. Therefore, architectural distortion that might represent a radial scar should be completely excised.[60,62]

Prior to an LGCB, a brief clinical assessment of the patient should be made to determine the presence of any factors that might increase the risk of bleeding or infection. Assessment of the prebiopsy studies allows one to plan the approach, the needle to use, and the potential management decisions based on the likely histologic findings.

The most commonly used needles are 14-g cutting needles that fit into a spring-loaded biopsy gun. The biopsy needle consists of an inner needle with a trough for tissue sampling and an outer needle sleeve that cuts the sample free from the breast tissue. The inner needle typically has a 4–5 mm beveled tip and a trough or slot 8–19 mm in length for the core of tissue. The total forward distance that the needle moves is termed the "throw". The "throw" of most needles ranges from 12 to 25 mm and typically equals the length of the beveled tip plus the trough. Needles having a throw of 20 to 25 mm are best because a larger tissue sample is acquired. Some biopsy systems, such as the BIP High Speed-Multi (Turkenfeld, Germany) or BD Precision Cut (Becton-Dickinson, Franklin Lakes, NJ) have an adjustable needle throw that allows use of the same needle for various throw distances and sample lengths desired. Other guns such as the Pro-mag (Manan Medical Products, Northbrook, IL) have a fixed throw, necessitating the use of a specific needle and trough size for each biopsy.

The needle is always placed into the breast in the pre-fire or cocked position. When the gun is fired, a split-second mechanism causes the inner slotted needle to move forward engaging the targeted breast tissue, and the outer needle sleeve moves over it, cutting the tissue. Before firing the biopsy gun, the radiologist must verify that the distance from the lesion to the opposite breast surface is greater than the "throw" of the needle. The distance between the lesion and the opposite breast surface minus the throw of the needle is called the stroke margin. The stroke margin should be greater than 5 mm to avoid puncturing the opposite skin surface and bending the needle tip against the film holder.

Stereotactic guidance aids in the performance of an LGCB. The lesion is usually approached from the closest skin surface. An exception to this rule is a very superficial lesion, because the needle position is not stable unless it is advanced past the abnormality. Superficial lesions should be approached from a direction that ensures needle stability and a safe stroke margin. The patient may be seated or placed prone on a dedicated table unit or in a lateral decubitus position for a stereotactic device with an upright attachment. With an upright unit, if the lesion is in the upper, outer quadrant of the breast, it may be approached via the lateral skin surface of the breast with the patient in a left-side down decubitus position.

A scout image is obtained by the technologist to verify that the localizing aperture has been positioned over the region of interest. Two stereotactic images are obtained 15° to the left and right of midline. The lesion is targeted and the skin is cleansed and locally anesthetized. A small skin nick is made with a #11 scalpel blade to allow easy insertion of the needle.

With the guides moved to a ΔX, ΔY, and ΔZ position of 0.00 mm, the needle is inserted into the breast and images are obtained to verify that the needle tip is in the center of the lesion (Figure 17.7A). The stroke margin should be greater than 5 mm. The needle is then withdrawn approximately 5 mm to allow optimum sampling of the lesion with the needle trough. The biopsy device is fired and a set of stereotactic images is made to assess the accuracy of sampling. On the post-fire images, the needle tip should project over the upper outer aspect of the lesion on both views (Figure 17.7B). The biopsy needle is removed from the breast, and the specimen is retrieved. Additional biopsies are targeted at the 12, 3, 6, and 9 o'clock positions for masses or at another collection of calcifications for a cluster of microcalcifications (Figure 17.8). Liberman et al. found that five LGCB samples achieved a 99% diagnostic yield for breast masses.[64] For microcalcifications, additional core samples may be needed.[64]

Manual pressure is applied to the breast for 5 min or until bleeding has ceased after each sample is obtained. Steristrips (3M Medical Division, St. Paul, MN) are used to cover the biopsy site on the skin and an ice pack is applied for 10–15 min. Written postprocedure instructions are given to the patient, including information about pain control (acetaminophen), level of activity (nonvigorous for 12–24 hr), signs to observe, (i.e., infection, bleeding, or pneumothorax) and the manner in which the patient will receive the results of the biopsy.[62]

Prefire

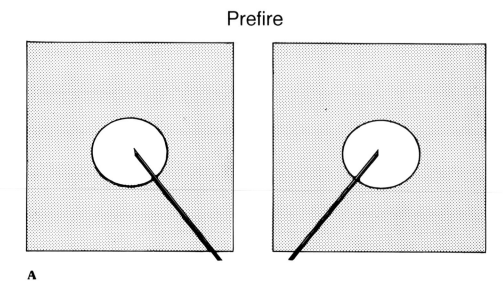

A

Postfire

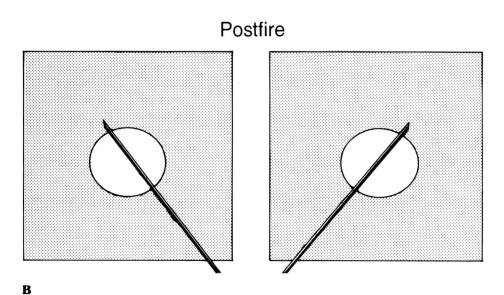

B

Figure 17.7 A. Pre-fire stereotactic images demonstrate needle tip in the center of lesion on both views. B. On post-fire images, the needle tip projects into upper outer aspect of lesion, confirming successful path of needle excursion.

For clusters of microcalcifications, the LGCB specimens are radiographed to verify the excision of calcium deposits (Figure 17.9).[65,66] The biopsy samples are placed on a glass slide or a piece of lens paper and are moistened with a few drops of lactated Ringer's solution. Magnification mammography without compression is performed using a technique of approximately 23 kVp at 20 mAs.[66] After radiography, the specimens are placed in formalin for fixation and transportation to the pathology laboratory.

For ultrasound-guided LGCB, the lesion is visualized with a 7.5-MHz (or greater frequency) linear-array transducer. A biopsy guide or a free-hand technique may be used. The needle is inserted lateral to the edge of the transducer and its tip and shaft are visualized as it is inserted along the long axis of the transducer. This approach per-

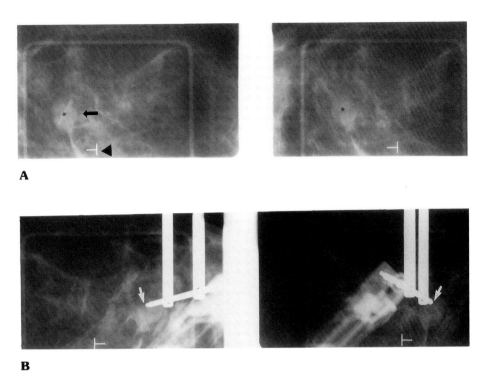

A

B

Figure 17.8 A. Stereotactic 15° images show the lesion to be targeted (arrow) and the reference cursor (arrowhead) in the cassette. **B.** Stereotactic images demonstrate the needle tip at the 12 o'clock position in the lesion on both views (arrow).

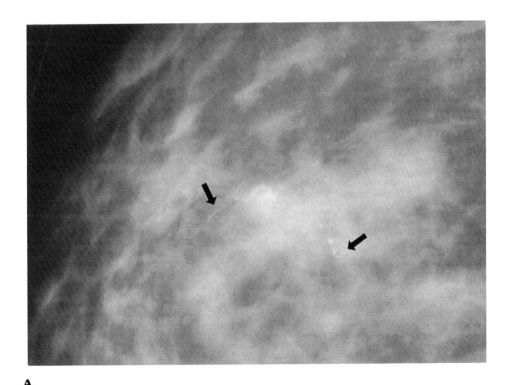

A

Figure 17.9 A. Preliminary magnification view shows malignant, linear microcalcifications (arrows). **B.** Following page.

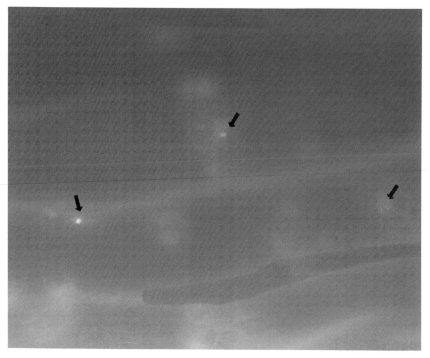

B

Figure 17.9 B. The specimen radiograph from the core biopsy shows multiple areas of calcifications (arrows). Pathology: Intraductal carcinoma.

mits a needle angle that is almost parallel to the chest wall, and is particularly important for deep lesions to avoid penetration of the chest wall with the throw of the needle.

For LGCB, the needle tip is positioned just proximal to the lesion and the gun is fired (Figure 17.10). Demonstration of the needle tip transversing the lesion is a distinct advantage of ultrasound guidance. Because of the ease of the needle placement and the rapidity of the procedure, ultrasound has replaced stereotaxis as the guidance modality for many LGCBs.[58,67,68]

Experienced operators using either stereotactic or sonographic guidance achieve a sensitivity with LGCB of at least 85%; many report a sensitivity of 95% or more.[58,59,64,67] Insufficient sampling by LGCB occurs in only 1% to 2% of cases.

The most frequent complications associated with LGCB include hematoma formation and infection. To avoid more serious complications such as needle penetration of the chest wall and pneumothorax, the needle should be inserted parallel to the chest wall. Seeding of the needle tract with tumor during LGCB of a mucinous carcinoma has been reported.[69] No other cases of tumor seeding along the biopsy track have been reported with use of automated LGCB devices. However, following LGCB of a carcinoma, excision of the biopsy tract during a lumpectomy should be considered. Although breast biopsies are rarely performed on lactating women, a milk fistula can develop from either a surgical biopsy or LGCB.[70]

After a negative result from a percutaneous breast biopsy, surgical excision is undertaken to remove lesions considered highly suspicious at mammography or to further evaluate lesions not adequately assessed by percutaneous techniques. Lesions that are diagnosed as atypical duct hyperplasia by LGCB may reflect adjacent, undetected carcinoma. Therefore, an LGCB that demonstrate histologic findings of atypical hyperplasia should prompt excision of the entire lesion.[71]

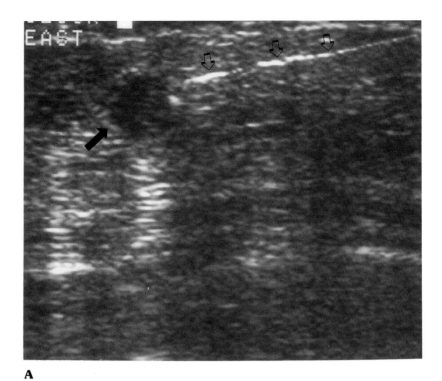

A

B

Figure 17.10 A. Large core needle (open arrow) is at the proximal edge of a solid mass (arrow) on ultrasound. B. The needle (open arrow) traverses the lesion after the gun has been fired.

For all percutaneous biopsies, the level of mammographic suspicion of the lesion, the accuracy of needle targeting, and the histologic findings must be considered. Appropriate lesion and patient selection, close follow-up, and good communication with the pathologist and surgical team are critical for establishing a successful percutaneous breast biopsy program.

GALACTOGRAPHY

The evaluation of a patient with a nipple discharge includes physical examination of both breasts and mammography. If the discharge is bilateral and galactorrhea is suspected, a serum prolactin level should be obtained. Galactorrhea, or production of a milky discharge, can occur when serum prolactin levels become elevated secondary to lactation or a pituitary abnormality, or by the ingestion of a variety of medications. Galactorrhea is not caused by an abnormality within the lactiferous ducts and therefore does not warrant galactographic examination.

A nipple discharge that is spontaneous and unilateral, whether serous, serosanguinous, or bloody, may be associated with an intraductal tumor.[72] Galactography or ductography is indicated to determine whether there is an intraductal lesion and to map its location for the surgeon.[73] Galactography facilitates preoperative mapping of abnormal ducts and allows accurate excision of the involved area without removing excessive amounts of surrounding normal tissue.

Prior to the galactogram, the patient should not express discharge from the breast for 2 to 3 days, so that there will be sufficient discharge present for the study. If the duct orifice to be cannulated cannot be identified based upon visualization of the site of discharge, the galactogram cannot be performed.

In preparation for the study, the patient is positioned on a table, preferably near the mammographic unit. The breast is thoroughly cleansed with an antiseptic solution. The cannulas used for galactography are the same blunt, straight, or right-angled metallic cannulas used for sialography. Occasionally, small-gauge plastic intravenous catheters have been used. The typical cannula used is 27-gauge. A 10-cc plastic syringe is filled with contrast material and the cannula is flushed to clear out any air bubbles.

The radiologist then expresses very small amounts of the discharge from the patient's nipple while attempting to visualize the orifice of the abnormal duct. It is absolutely necessary to identify the correct orifice. Once the duct is identified, the cannula is very gently advanced into it. If the cannula is in the proper position and the duct is distended because of the discharge, it should be possible to position the cannula without using any pressure, because the abnormal duct is usually distended by the residual discharge.[2] If the duct is not distended, its caliber may be too small to allow insertion of the cannula. Once the proper duct is cannulated, contrast is injected into the duct until the patient feels pressure in the breast. Care should be taken to avoid injection of air which can stimulate a filling defect. The amount of contrast typically used ranges from 0.1 to 3.0 cc, varying with the degree of ductal dilation and the extent of the system drained by the cannulated duct. The cannula is taped into position and the patient is moved to the mammographic unit for imaging.

Compression, to a slightly lesser degree than used for screening mammography, is applied to the breast. Craniocaudal and mediolateral views of the breast are obtained. Magnification views may also be helpful, particularly to evaluate for the presence of any filling defect. One may need to inject additional contrast and obtain additional films to visualize the entire duct system. After the procedure, a final film is made immediately after withdrawal of the cannula to allow visualization of the most distal segment of the duct.

Should the patient feel pain during contrast injection, the injection should be stopped. A film should be obtained to verify that the cannula is within the duct and that contrast has not extravasated from the duct system. Extravasated contrast appears as a dense area of contrast and is often associated with lymphatic filling. The lymphatics appear as fine, linear contrast-filled vessels that are oriented toward the axilla.

Normal ductal anatomy includes the collecting ducts, segmental and subsegmental ducts, and the terminal ducts. The collecting ducts open onto the nipple and are cannulated during galactography. There are 5 to 8 collecting ducts, normally 2–3 mm in diameter. A normal widening in the collecting duct, known as the lactiferous sinus, is located in the subareolar region; several segmental ducts drain into each lactiferous sinus. As the ducts arborize in the breast, they gradually decrease in caliber. In the normal breast, the duct walls are smooth and there are no filling defects, areas of beading, abrupt narrowing, or obstruction.

Duct ectasia is a condition that is part of the spectrum of plasma cell mastitis or secretory disease; nipple discharge may be present, but if so, it is often bilateral, white to yellow, and expressible. If galactography is performed on a patient with duct ectasia, the ducts appear dilated, particularly in the subareolar area. The degree of dilatation may be so great as to cause cystic spaces to form in the major lactiferous ducts (Figure 17.11).[74] Although duct hyperplasia tends to occur in the smaller terminal ducts, it may also be present in larger ducts.

Findings on galactography that suggest an intraductal lesion include the following: solitary or multiple filling defects, beading, abrupt angulation, or obstruction of the duct. The most likely etiology of a solitary filling defect is a papilloma.[75] Papillomas are benign pedunculated lesions of the major lactiferous ducts. They appear as smooth or irregular solitary intraductal filling defects and are most often located in the subareolar region. When papillomas cause major duct obstruction, they appear as a convex edge defect in an obstructed lactiferous duct. Papillomas are also the most common cause of a bloody nipple discharge.

Multiple filling defects on galactography can be caused by multiple papillomas, but more commonly, they are associated with more diffuse processes such as papillomatosis, duct adenoma, duct hyperplasia, and intraductal carcinoma.[76] Papillomatosis is a papillary form of hyperplasia. Nonpathologic entities causing multiple defects on galactography are air bubbles injected with the contrast, inspissated secretions, or blood clots associated with a sanguinous discharge. These can usually be recognized because they are not fixed and vary in position with the injection of the contrast.

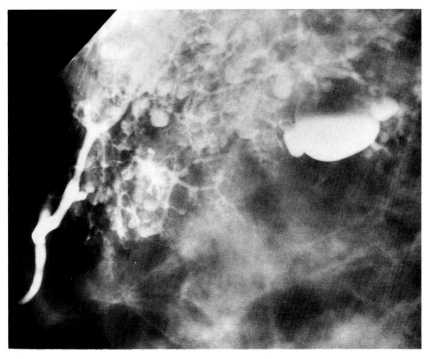

Figure 17.11 Mediolateral (ML) galactographic view in a patient with duct ectasia demonstrates dilated ducts with contrast-filled cystic spaces.

When one identifies multiple irregular fixed defects, multiple areas of beading, duct encasement, or areas of obstruction, the possibility of an intraductal carcinoma must be strongly considered. Intraductal carcinoma can be a solitary lesion on galactography, but the more common appearance is that of multiple lesions.

The identification of a filling defect that appears pathologic should prompt surgical examination. Sometimes, the abnormal area found on galactography can be identified as a dilated duct or an area of increased density on mammography, and needle localization can be performed. However, if the area of the lesion identified with galactography is not seen on mammography, repeat galactography can be performed to map out the exact location of the lesion for the surgeon.

ACKNOWLEDGMENT

The authors gratefully acknowledge the assistance of Karren O'Connell in the skillful preparation of the manuscript.

REFERENCES

1. Muhlow A: A device for precision needle biopsy of the breast at mammography. *Am J Roentgenol* 121:843–845, 1974.
2. Kopans DB, Deluca SA: A Modified needle hookwire technique to simplify preoperative localization of occult breast lesions. *Radiology* 134:781, 1980.
3. Homer MJ: Nonpalpable breast lesion localization using a curved-end retractable wire. *Radiology* 157:259–260, 1985.
4. Reynolds HE, Jackson VP, Musick BS: Preoperative needle localization in the breast: utility of local anesthesia. *Radiology* 187:503–505, 1993.
5. Edeiken S, Suer WE, Vitale SF, et al: Needle localization of nonpalpable breast lesions using methylene blue. *Breast Dis* 3:75–80, 1990.
6. Snyder RE: Specimen radiography and preoperative localization of nonpalpable breast cancer. *Cancer* 46:950–956, 1980.
7. Stomper PC, Davis SP, Sonnenfeld MR, et al: Efficacy of specimen radiographically of clinically occult noncalcified breast lesions. *Am J Roentgenol* 151:43–47, 1988.
8. Rebner M, Pennes DR, Baker DE, et al: Two view specimen in radiography in surgical biopsy of nonpalpable breast masses. *Am J Roentgenol* 149:283–285, 1987.
9. D'Orsi CJ: Management of the breast specimen. *Radiology* 194:297–302, 1995.
10. Cardenosa G, Eklund GW: Paraffin block radiography following breast biopsies: use of orthogonal views. *Radiology* 180:873–874, 1991.
11. Surratt JT, Monsees BS, Mazoujian G: Calcium oxalate microcalcifications in the breast. *Radiology* 181:141–142, 1991.
12. Sistrom C, Abbitt PL, Paredes ES: Hematoma of the breast: a complication of needle localization. *Virginia Med Monthly* 115(2):78–79, 1988.
13. Rappaport W, Thompson S, Wong R, et al: Complications associated with needle localization biopsy of the breast. *Surg Gynecol Obstet* 172:303–306, 1991.
14. Davis PS, Wechsler RJ, Reig SA, et al: Migration of breast biopsy localization wire. *Am J Roentgenol* 150:787–788, 1988.
15. Bristol JB, Jones PA: Transgression of localization wire to the pleural cavity prior to mammography. *Br J Radiol* 54:139–140, 1981.
16. Pitzen RH, Urdaneta LF, Al-Jurf AS, et al: Specimen xeroradiography after needle localization and biopsy of non-calcified, non-palpable breast lesions. *Am Surg* 51:50–57, 1985.
17. Proudfoot RW, Mattingly SS, Stelling CB, et al: Non-palpable breast lesions. Wire localization and excisional biopsy. *Am Surg* 52:117–122, 1986.
18. Powell RW, McSweeney MB, Wilson CE: X-ray calcifications as the only basis for breast biopsy. *Ann Surg* 197:555–559, 1983.
19. Norton LW, Zeligman BE, Pearlman NW: Accuracy and cost of needle localization breast biopsy. *Arch Surg* 123:947–950, 1988.

20. Hasselgren P, Hummel RP, Georgian-Smith D, et al: Breast biopsy with needle localization: accuracy of specimen x-ray and management of missed lesions. *Surgery* 114:836–842, 1993.

21. D'Orsi CJ, Mendelson EB: Interventional breast ultrasonography. *Semin Ultrasound CT MR* 10:132–138, 1989.

22. Fornage BD: Percutaneous biopsies of the breast: state of the art. Cardiovasc Intervent *Radiol* 14:29–39, 1991.

23. Dershaw DD, Fleischman RC, Liberman L, et al: Use of digital mammography in needle localization procedures. *Am J Roentgenol* 161:559–562, 1993.

24. Kopans DB: Review of stereotaxic large-core needle biopsy and surgical biopsy results in nonpalpable breast lesions. *Radiology* 189:665–666, 1993.

25. Elvecrog EL, Lechner MC, Nelson MT: Nonpalpable breast lesions: correlation of stereotaxic large-core needle biopsy and surgical biopsy results. *Radiology* 188:453–455, 1993.

26. Kopans DB: Preoperative imaging guided needle placement and localization of non-palpable breast lesions. In syllabus of 26th National Conference on Breast Cancer, American College of Radiology 1994, pp 27–41.

27. Shaw de Paredes E: Interventional procedures. In: Shaw de Paredes E. *Atlas of Film-Screen Mammography*, ed 2. Baltimore, Williams and Wilkins, 1992, pp 513–548.

28. McCreery BR, Frankl G, Frost DB: An analysis of the results of mammographically guided biopsies of the breast. *Surg Gynecol Obstet* 172:223–226, 1991.

29. Rosenberg AL, Schwartz GF, Feig SA, et al: Clinically occult breast lesions: localization and significance. *Radiology* 162:167–170, 1987.

30. Sailors DM, Crabtree DJ, Land RL, et al: Needle localization for nonpalpable breast lesions. *Am Surg* 60:186–189, 1994.

31. Alexander RH, Candela FC, Dershaw DD, et al: Needle-localized mammographic lesions. *Arch Surg* 125:1441–1444, 1990.

32. Rubin E, Visscher DW, Alexander RW, et al: Proliferative disease and atypia in biopsies performed for nonpalpable lesions detected mammographically. *Cancer* 161:2077–2082, 1988.

33. Hermann G, Janus C, Schwartz IS, et al: Nonpalpable breast lesions: accuracy of prebiopsy mammographic diagnosis. *Radiology* 165:323–326, 1987.

34. Shabot MM, Goldberg IM, Schick P, et al: Aspiration cytology is superior to Tru-Cut needle biopsy in establishing the diagnosis of clinically suspicious breast masses. *Ann Surg* 196:122–126, 1982.

35. Martelli G, Pilotti S, Coopmans de Yoldi G, et al: Diagnostic efficacy of physical examination, mammography, fine needle aspiration cytology (triple-test) in solid breast lumps: an analysis of 1708 consecutive cases. *Tumori* 76:476–479, 1990.

36. Costa MJ, Tadros T, Hilton G, et al: Breast fine needle aspiration cytology: utility as a screening tool for clinically palpable lesions. *Acta Cytol* 37:461–471, 1993.

37. Atamdede FI, Isaacs JH: The role of fine-needle aspiration in the diagnosis of breast lesions. *Gynecol Oncol* 50:159–163, 1993.

38. Layfield LJ, Chrischilles EA, Cohen MB, et al: The palpable breast nodule. *Cancer* 72:1642–1651, 1993.

39. Kaufman Z, Shpitz B, Shapiro M: Triple approach in the diagnosis of dominant breast masses: combined physical examination, mammography, and fine-needle aspiration. *J Surg Oncol* 56:254–257, 1994.

40. Bucchi L, Schincaglia P, Melandri G, et al: Performance of fine needle aspiration cytology of the breast. Clincial experience in Ravenna (Italy). *Tumori* 79:413–417, 1993.

41. Wilkinson EJ, Bland KI: Techniques and results of aspiration cytology for diagnosis of benign and malignant diseases of the breast. *Surg Clin North Am* 70:801–812, 1990.

42. Donegan WL: Evaluation of a palpable breast mass. *N Engl J Med* 327:937–942, 1992.

43. Pennes DR, Naylor B, Rebner M: Fine needle aspiration biopsy of the breast: influence of sample size on breast FNA. *Acta Cytol* 34:673–676, 1990.

44. Tabar L, Pentek A, Dean PB: The diagnostic and therapeutic value of breast cyst puncture and pneumocystography. *Radiology* 141:659–663, 1981.

45. Layfield LJ, Parkinson B, Wong J, et al: Mammographically guided fine-needle aspiration biopsy of nonpalpable breast lesions. Can it replace open biopsy? *Cancer* 68:2007–2011, 1991.

46. Masood S, Frykberg ER, McLellan GL: Prospective evaluation of radiologically directed fine-needle aspiration biopsy of nonpalpable breast lesions. *Cancer* 66:1480–1487, 1990.

47. Helvie MA, Baker DE, Adler DD, et al: Radiographically guided fine-needle aspiration of nonpalpable breast lesions. *Radiology* 174:657–661, 1990.

48. Arishita GI, Cruz BK, Harding CT, et al: Mammogram-directed fine-needle aspiration of nonpalpable breast lesions. *J Surg Oncol* 48:153–157, 1991.

49. Shaw de Paredes E: Stereotactic needle biopsies: FNA. In syllabus of 26th National Conference on Breast Cancer, American College of Radiology 1994, pp 14–16.

50. Dowlatshahi K, Yaremko LM, Kluskens LF, et al: Nonpalpable breast lesions: findings of stereotaxic needle-core biopsy and fine-needle aspiration cytology. *Radiology* 181:745–750, 1991.

51. Lofgren M, Andersson I, Lindholm K: Stereotactic fine-needle aspiration for cytologic diagnosis of nonpalpable breast lesions. *Am J Roentgenol* 154:1191–1194, 1990.

52. Azavedo E, Auer G, Svane G: Stereotactic fine-needle biopsy in 2594 mammographically detected non-palpable lesions. *Lancet* 1(8646):1033–1035, 1989.

53. Fajardo LL, Davis JR, Wiens JL, et al: Mammography-guided stereotactic fine-needle aspiration cytology of nonpalpable breast lesions. *Am J Roentgenol* 155:977–981, 1990.

54. Oliver DJ, Frayne JR, Sterrett G: Stereotactic fine needle biopsy of the breast. *Surgery* 62:463–467, 1992.

55. Mitnick JS, Vazquez MF, Roses DF, et al: Stereotaxic localization for fine-needle aspiration breast biopsy. *Arch Surg* 126:1137–1140, 1991.

56. Jackson VP: The status of mammographically guided fine needle aspiration biopsy of nonpalpable breast lesions. Radiol Clin North Am 30:155–166, 1992.

57. Parker SH, Lovin JD, Jobe WE, et al: Stereotactic breast biopsy with a biopsy gun. *Radiology* 176:741–747, 1990.

58. Parker SH, Lovin JD, Jobe WE, et al: Nonpalpable breast lesions; stereotactic automated large-core biopsies. *Radiology* 180:403–407, 1991.

59. Gisvold JJ, Goellner JR, Grant CS, et al: Breast biopsy: a comparative study of stereotaxically guided core and excisional techniques. *Am J Roentgenol* 162:815–820, 1994.

60. Evans P, Oberman H: Stereotactic needle biopsies: core and FNA. In syllabus of 26th National Conference on Breast Cancer. American College of Radiology 1994, pp 9–10.

61. Sullivan DC: Needle core biopsy of mammographic lesions. *Am J Roentgenol* 162:815–820, 1994.

62. Shaw de Paredes E: Patient selection and care for percutaneous breast biopsy. In Dershaw D (ed): Interventional Breast Procedures. New York, Churchill Livingstone (*in press*).

63. Dronkers DJ: Stereotaxic core biopsy of breast lesions. *Radiology* 183:631–634, 1992.

64. Liberman L, Dershaw DD, Rosen PP, et al: Stereotaxic 14-gauge breast biopsy: how many core biopsy specimens are needed? *Radiology* 192:793–795, 1994.

65. Liberman L, Evans WP, Dershaw DD, et al: Radiography of microcalcifications in stereotaxic mammary core biopsy specimens. *Radiology* 190:223–225, 1994.

66. Meyer JE, Lester SC, Frenna TH, et al: Occult breast calcifications sampled with large-core biopsy: confirmation with radiography of the specimen. *Radiology* 188:581–582, 1993.

67. Gordon PB, Goldenberg LS, Chan NHL: Solid breast lesions: diagnosis with US-guided fine-needle aspiration biopsy. *Radiology* 189:573–580, 1993.

68. Fornage BD, Coan JD, David CL: Ultrasound-guided needle biopsy of the breast and other interventional procedures. *Radiol Clin North Am* 30:167–185, 1992.

69. Harter LP, Curtis JS, Ponto G, et al: Malignant seeding of the needle track during stereotaxic core needle breast biopsy. *Radiology* 185:713–714, 1992.

70. Schackmuth EM, Harlow CL, Norton LW: Milk fistula: a complication after core breast biopsy. *Am J Roentgenol* 161:961–962, 1993.

71. Jackman RJ, Nowels KW, Shepard MJ, et al: Stereotaxic large-core needle biopsy of 450 nonpalpable breast lesions with surgical correlation in lesions with cancer or atypical hyperplasia. Radiology 193:91–95, 1994.

72. Leis HP, Greene FL, Cammarata A, et al: Nipple discharge: surgical significance. *South Med J* 81(1):20–26, 1988.

73. Cardenosa G, Doudna C, Eklund GW: Ductography of the breast: technique and findings. *Am J Roentgenol* 162:1081–1087, 1994.

74. Diner WC: Galactography: mammary duct contrast examination. *Am J Roentgenol* 137:853–856, 1981.

75. Haagenson CD: *Diseases of the Breast.* Philadelphia, WB Saunders, 1971.

76. Threatt B: Ductography. In Bassett LW, Gold RH (eds): *Mammography, Thermography and Ultrasound in Breast Cancer Detection.* New York, Grune and Stratton, 1982.

Index